theclinics.com

CARDIOLOGY CLINICS

Three-Dimensional Echocardiography

GUEST EDITORS
Edward A. Gill, MD
Navin C. Nanda, MD, and
Roberto M. Lang, MD

CONSULTING EDITOR
Michael H. Crawford, MD

May 2007 • Volume 25 • Number 2

SAUNDERS
An Imprint of Elsevier, Inc.
PHILADELPHIA LONDON TORONTO MONTREAL SYDNEY TOKYO

W.B. SAUNDERS COMPANY
A Division of Elsevier Inc.

Elsevier Inc. • 1600 John F. Kennedy Blvd., Suite 1800 • Philadelphia, Pennsylvania 19103-2899

http://www.theclinics.com

CARDIOLOGY CLINICS
May 2007
Editor: Barbara Cohen-Kligerman

Volume 25, Number 2
ISSN 0733-8651
ISBN-13: 978-1-4160-4282-2
ISBN-10: 1-4160-4282-2

Cardiology Clinics (ISSN 0733-8651) is published quarterly by Elsevier Inc., 360 Park Avenue South, New York, NY 10010-1710. Months of issue are February, May, August, and November. Business and editorial Offices: 1600 John F. Kennedy Blvd., Suite 1800, Philadelphia, PA 19103-2899. Customer Service Office: 6277 Sea Harbor Drive, Orlando, FL 32887-4800. Periodicals postage paid at New York, NY, and additional mailing offices. Subscription prices are $198.00 per year for US individuals, $302.00 per year for US institutions, $99.00 per year for US students and residents, $242.00 per year for Canadian individuals, $367.00 per year for Canadian institutions, $264.00 per year for international individuals, $367.00 per year for international institutions and $132.00 per year for Canadian and foreign students/residents. To receive student/resident rate, orders must be accompanied by name of affiliated institution, data of term, and the *signature* of program/residency coordinator on institution letterhead. Orders will be billed at individual rate until proof of status is received. Foreign air speed delivery is included in all *Clinics* subscription prices. All prices are subject to change without notice. POSTMASTER: Send address changes to *Cardiology Clinics*, Elsevier Periodicals Customer Service, 6277 Sea Harbor Drive, Orlando, FL 32887-4800. **Customer Service: 1-800-654-2452 (US). From outside of the US, call 1-407-345-1000.**

Cardiology Clinics is also published in Spanish by McGraw-Hill Interamericana Editores S. A., P.O. Box 5-237, 06500, Mexico D. F., Mexico; in Portuguese by Reichmann and Alfonso Editores Rio de Janeiro, Brazil; and in Greek by Dimitrios P. Lagos, 8 Pondon Street, GR115-28 Ilissia, Greece.

Cardiology Clinics is covered in *Index Medicus, Excerpta Medica, The Cumulative Index to Nursing and Allied Health Literature* (INAHL).

Printed in the United States of America.

CONSULTING EDITOR

MICHAEL H. CRAWFORD, MD, Professor of Medicine, University of California San Francisco; Lucie Stern Chair in Cardiology, and Interim Chief of Cardiology, University of California San Francisco Medical Center, San Francisco, California

GUEST EDITORS

EDWARD A. GILL, MD, FACC, FASE, FACP, Associate Professor of Medicine, University of Washington School of Medicine; Department of Medicine, Division of Cardiology, Director of Echocardiography, Harborview Medical Center, Seattle, Washington

NAVIN C. NANDA, MD, FACC, FAHA, FSOC, FISCU, Professor of Medicine and Director, Heart Station/ Echocardiography Laboratories, University of Alabama at Birmingham, Birmingham, Alabama

ROBERTO M. LANG, MD, FACC, FASE, FAHA, Professor of Medicine and Radiology; Director, The Cardiac Imaging Center, Departments of Medicine and Radiology, University of Chicago Hospitals, Chicago, Illinois

CONTRIBUTORS

ALICIA A. AHLGRIM, BS, RDCS, RDMS, Harborview Medical Center, Seattle, Washington

ROLF BAUMANN, MS, TomTec Imaging Systems, Unterschleissheim, Germany

ELENISE BERTHER, RDCS, Harborview Medical Center, Seattle, Washington

JOSE A. DE AGUSTIN, MD, CV Imaging Unit, University Clinic San Carlos, Madrid, Spain

LEOPOLDO PÉREZ DE ISLA, MD, PhD, CV Imaging Unit, University Clinic San Carlos, Madrid, Spain

ANDREAS FRANKE, MD, Professor of Internal Medicine, FESC, Medical Clinic I, RWTH University Hospital, Aachen, Germany

EDWARD A. GILL, MD, FACC, FASE, FACP, Associate Professor of Medicine, University of Washington School of Medicine; Department of Medicine, Division of Cardiology, Director of Echocardiography, Harborview Medical Center, Seattle, Washington

JOSEPH A. HORSTMAN, MD, University of Washington School of Medicine, Seattle, Washington

MARTIN HYCA, MD, MS, TomTec Imaging Systems, Unterschleissheim, Germany

BERTHOLD KLAS, BS, TomTec Corporation, Unterschleissheim, Germany

ROBERTO M. LANG, MD, FACC, FASE, FAHA, Professor of Medicine and Radiology; Director, The Cardiac Imaging Center, Departments of Medicine and Radiology, University of Chicago Hospitals, Chicago, Illinois

DAVID H. LIANG, MD, PhD, Division of Cardiovascular Medicine, Stanford University School of Medicine, Stanford, California

RAVI K. MALLAVARAPU, MD, Division of Cardiovascular Diseases, University of Alabama at Birmingham, Birmingham, Alabama

ANDREW P. MILLER, MD, Assistant Professor of Medicine, Division of Cardiovascular Diseases, University of Alabama at Birmingham, Birmingham, Alabama

MARK J. MONAGHAN, MD, PhD, King's College Hospital, London, United Kingdom

VICTOR MOR-AVI, PhD, Research Associate, Professor, Director of Cardiac Imaging Research, The Cardiac Imaging Center, Departments of Medicine and Radiology, University of Chicago, Chicago, Illinois

BERNHARD MUMM, MS, President & CTO, TomTec Imaging Systems, Unterschleissheim, Germany

NAVIN C. NANDA, MD, FACC, FAHA, FSOC, FISCU, Professor of Medicine and Director, Heart Station/Echocardiography Laboratories, Division of Cardiovascular Diseases, University of Alabama at Birmingham, Birmingham, Alabama

GERALD R. MARX, MD, Senior Associate of Cardiology, Department of Cardiology, Children's Hospital Boston, Boston; Associate Professor, Harvard Medical School, Boston, Massachusetts

DAVID J. SAHN, MD, Oregon Health & Science University, Pediatric Cardiology Department, Portland, Oregon

IVAN S. SALGO, MD, MS, Chief, Cardiovascular Investigations, Ultrasound Research & Development, Philips Medical Systems, Andover, Massachusetts

LISSA SUGENG, MD, Assistant Professor of Medicine, Section of Cardiology, Department of Medicine, University of Chicago Medical Center, Chicago, Illinois

XIAOHONG SU, MD, Department of Cardiology, Children's Hospital Boston, Boston, Massachusetts

MASAAKI TAKEUCHI, MD, Department of Cardiology, Tane General Hospital, Osaka, Japan

BORIS TUTSCHEK, MD, PhD, Prenatal Medicine Munich, Munich; and Heinrich Heine University, Düsseldorf, Germany

JOSE L. ZAMORANO, MD, CV Imaging Unit, University Clinic San Carlos, Madrid, Spain

CONTENTS

FORTHCOMING ISSUES

August 2007

The Athletes Heart 2007: On the Border Between Physiology and Pathology
Antonio Pelliccia, MD, *Guest Editor*

November 2007

Heart Failure, Part I
James B. Young, MD, and Jagat Narula, MD, *Guest Editors*

February 2008

Heart Failure, Part II
James B. Young, MD, and Jagat Narula, MD, *Guest Editors*

RECENT ISSUES

February 2007

Cardiovascular Magnetic Resonance Imaging
Raymond J. Kim, MD, *Guest Editor*

November 2006

Adult Congenital Heart Disease
Gary D. Webb, MD, *Guest Editor*

August 2006

Advanced 12-Lead Electrocardiography
S. Serge Barold, MD, *Guest Editor*

ELSEVIER
SAUNDERS

Cardiol Clin 25 (2007) xi

CARDIOLOGY
CLINICS

Foreword

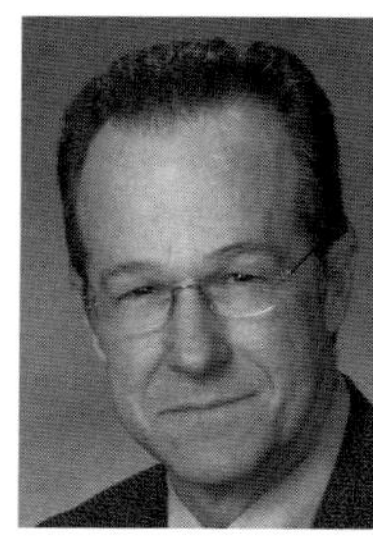

Michael H. Crawford, MD
Consulting Editor

Cardiology Clinics has a long tradition of keeping its readers up-to-date on technological advances in cardiology diagnostics. Recently we have done issues on CT angiography, contrast echocardiography and MRI. This issue focuses on 3D echocardiography. It is guest edited by three of the leaders in the field, Drs. Edward Gill, Roberto Lang and Navin Nanda. Each editor is from a different academic medical center, so this issue is well balanced. The issue starts with articles on the development and technology behind 3D echo, then launches into 14 articles on specific uses. Most of the articles deal with the three major uses of 3D echocardiography, imaging the left ventricle, cardiac valves and congenital heart disease. Finally, there is an article on using 3D echocardiography to guide intracardiac therapy.

3D echocardiography is used in most large academic medical centers now, and its use is spreading as commercially available machines are being bought to replace older models. The articles in this issue focus on the well-established uses of 3D echo, but there is much more to learn. Other uses that were not discussed because there are little data about them include the assessment of cardiac masses, aneurysms and pseudoaneurysms. Also, we have much more to learn about the utility of three-dimensional color flow imaging. I expect this to be a growing field that competes with 3D reconstruction of MR and CT images of the heart. This issue of *Cardiology Clinics* will get you up to speed in this important area.

Michael H. Crawford, MD
Division of Cardiology
Department of Medicine
University of California
San Francisco Medical Center
505 Parnassus Avenue, Box 0124
San Francisco, CA 94143-0124, USA

E-mail address: crawfordm@medicine.ucsf.edu

doi:10.1016/j.ccl.2007.07.002

ELSEVIER
SAUNDERS

Cardiol Clin 25 (2007) xiii–xiv

CARDIOLOGY
CLINICS

Preface

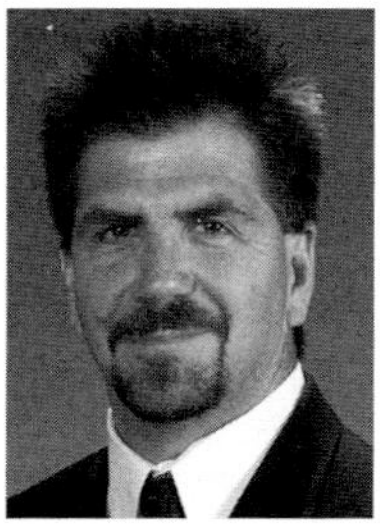
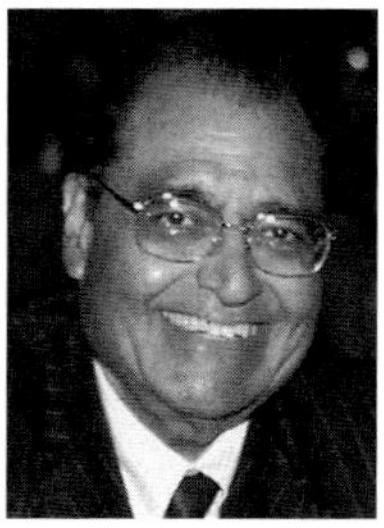
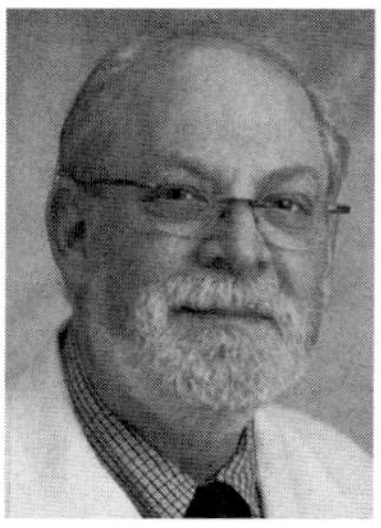

Edward A. Gill, MD, FACC, FASE, FACP

Navin C. Nanda, MD, FACC, FAHA, FSOC, FISCU

Roberto M. Lang, MD, FACC, FASE, FAHA

Guest Editors

Three-dimensional echocardiography (3DE) has transitioned from a research tool to a methodology useful in everyday clinical practice. This transition began, in earnest, in 2002 with the release of a reasonably user-friendly version of a matrix array transducer capable of real-time 3D imaging together with software that allows rapid slicing and quantification of structures. Prior to this time, 3DE had been acquired by using a two-dimensional echocardiography (2DE) transducer, wherein the movement of the transducer was followed in space, or by moving it in a prespecified pattern, acquiring multiple 2DE images with the aid of cardiac and (in some renditions) respiratory gating, and finally assembling the 2D images into a 3D image using advanced computer software and coupled with the spatial tracking information. This approach was formidable and only undertaken by those with a major interest in the research and development of the technology. Previous ultrasound imaging systems had 256 to 512 elements. The current 3D matrix transducer has approximately 3000 imaging elements, coupled with significantly enhanced computer processing power. The major breakthrough in transducer technology was the development of a microbeam former that allowed not only the acquisition of a large volume of information but also electronic steering of the transducer.

Hence the combination of the microbeam former, improved image quality, more efficient management of the images (in terms of digital storage and transfer), improved analysis packages, and reimbursement of the service combine to make 3DE a possibility for routine use in the clinical echocardiography laboratory. Most importantly, critical research has been performed that defines the current use of the technology.

The timing of this issue of the *Cardiology Clinics* is primed by the recent release of a position paper by the American Society of Echocardiography (ASE) and a message from Dr. Michael Picard, the current ASE president. The ASE position paper summarizes the data documenting the usefulness of 3D technology. Dr. Picard encourages the use of 3DE for the following reasons:

1. *Keeping up with the competition.* Currently, CT and MRI already use 3D imaging to their advantage. We as echocardiographers need to increase awareness that this approach is feasible with echocardiography.
2. *Improved assessment of the left ventricle.* There are now many publications showing the superiority of left ventricular volume, mass, and ejection fraction measurement with 3DE compared with 2DE. Volume

0733-8651/07/$ - see front matter
doi:10.1016/j.ccl.2007.06.011

and mass are important markers of prognosis in both heart failure and hypertension.

3. *Improved understanding of valve function.* As depicted in the ASE position paper, 3DE allows an "en face" view of the valve for measuring the valve area in mitral stenosis and aortic stenosis. Furthermore, in mitral regurgitation—more specifically, mitral valve prolapse—3DE can precisely define which individual scallop is involved and further delineate other mechanisms of mitral regurgitation. In addition, using 3D color Doppler, the shape and exact size of the vena contracta can be assessed, obviating assumptions made regarding its shape when using 2DE/Doppler. Thus, it provides more accurate quantitative assessment of valva regurgitation severity, unlike the proximal isovelocity surface area (PISA) method, which assumes (mostly incorrectly) the flow acceleration to be hemispherical.
4. *Improved display of congenital heart lesions.* A mainstay of 3DE is its ability to display complex spatial relationships between structures in patients with more advanced forms of congenital heart disease.
5. *Preparing for the future.* It is likely that 3DE will become a common part of all echocardiographic examinations. This will be challenging, because the technology is changing rapidly—on the positive side, it is improving rapidly as well. It is important for us as cardiologists, not just as echocardiographers, to keep up with this technology.
6. *Helping drive the technology forward.* It is our job within this issue of the *Cardiology Clinics* to challenge all cardiologists and sonographers to explore this technology and ask critical questions regarding its use and development. The more people engage from the sidelines and become part of the process, the quicker the technology will advance and be understood. Clearly improvements are needed, particularly with regard to more advanced transducers with higher frequencies and frame rates and complete Doppler capabilities.

The reader is encouraged to explore Dr. Picard's entire document, as well as the position paper [1,2].

Edward A. Gill, MD, FACC, FASE, FACP
Division of Cardiology
University of Washington
Harborview Medical Center 2EH69.2
Seattle, WA 98195-9748, USA

E-mail address: eagill@u.washington.edu

Navin C. Nanda, MD, FACC, FAHA, FSOC, FISCU
University of Alabama at Birmingham
Heart Station SW/S102
619 South 19th Street
Birmingham, AL 35249, USA

E-mail address: nanda@uab.edu

Roberto M. Lang, MD, FACC, FASE, FAHA
University of Chicago Hospitals
5841 S. Maryland Avenue, MC 5084
Chicago, IL 60637, USA

E-mail address: rlang@medicine.bsd.uchicago.edu

References

[1] Picard M. President's message: the time for 3D. J Am Soc Echocardiogr 2007;20:19A–20A.
[2] Hung J, Lang R, Flachskampf F, et al. 3D echocardiography: a review of the current status and future directions. J Am Soc Echocardiogr 2007;20:213–33.

ELSEVIER
SAUNDERS

Cardiol Clin 25 (2007) 221–229

CARDIOLOGY CLINICS

Three-Dimensional Echocardiography: An Historical Perspective

Edward A. Gill, MD, FACC, FASE, FACP[a,*], Berthold Klas, BS[b]

[a]Department of Medicine, Division of Cardiology, University of Washington School of Medicine, Harborview Medical Center, 325 Ninth Avenue, Box 359748, Seattle, WA 98104, USA
[b]TomTec Imaging Systems GmbH, Edisonstrasse 6, Unterschleissheim, 85716, Germany

Three-dimensional echocardiography (3DE) has made a dramatic transition from predominantly a research tool to a technology useful in everyday clinical practice. Clearly this transition began in earnest in 2002 with the release of a reasonably user-friendly version of real-time 3DE (RT3DE). Before this time, 3DE had relied on using a two-dimensional echo (2DE) transducer, either tracking that transducer in space, or moving it in a prespecified pattern, acquiring multiple 2DE images with the aid of cardiac, and in some renditions, respiratory gating, and finally assembling the 2D images into a 3D image using advanced computer software and the spatial information obtained from the transducer tracking device. This type of approach was formidable and was undertaken only by those with a major interest in either the commercial or research development of the technology (ie, academic centers and industry). All of that changed with the introduction of a dense array, matrix transducer that is equipped with 3000 elements compared to the conventional 256 or 512 along with enhanced computer processing speed and memory.

Early history

3DE has its roots in the early 1980s in terms of when it actually came to market as a real commercially available product. Therefore, it is interesting to note that work with 3DE actually began in the early 1970s. All early work in 3DE focused on methods of locating a standard 2D transducer in space, acquiring multiple 2D images, and melding the multiple 2D images into a 3D image. In fact, Dekker and colleagues [1] are credited as the original pioneers of 3DE, performing their first 3DE in approximately 1974. They used a long mechanical arm to locate the position of the transducer in space and allow alignment of multiple 2D images and ultimately generated a 3D image (Fig. 1). Unfortunately, the equipment was impractical for general clinical applicability, and the images were archaic (see Fig. 1). This was followed by the development of the spark-gap technique by Moritz and Shreve [2] in 1976 that located the 2D transducer by sending constant pulsed acoustic signals from a device holding the transducer, called a spark gap to a Cartesian locator grid (Fig. 2). Several other authors published early attempts at 3DE during this time period [3–7]. Other techniques were developed that operated under the assumption that both the patient and the housing of the ultrasound probe remained in a relatively fixed position. The ultrasound probe was held by a device that moved the probe in a specified, preprogrammed fashion within the housing of the mechanical device. Examples were linear, fan-like, and rotational acquisition methods. The rotational method became by far the most popular (Figs. 3–6). In 1977, Raab and colleagues [8] developed an electromagnetic locator that ultimately led to free-hand scanning. Although this technique was quite advanced for 1977, paradoxically, it would not see more than patchy use until the mid 1990s (Fig. 7).

* Corresponding author.
E-mail address: eagill@u.washington.edu (E.A. Gill).

doi:10.1016/j.ccl.2007.05.001

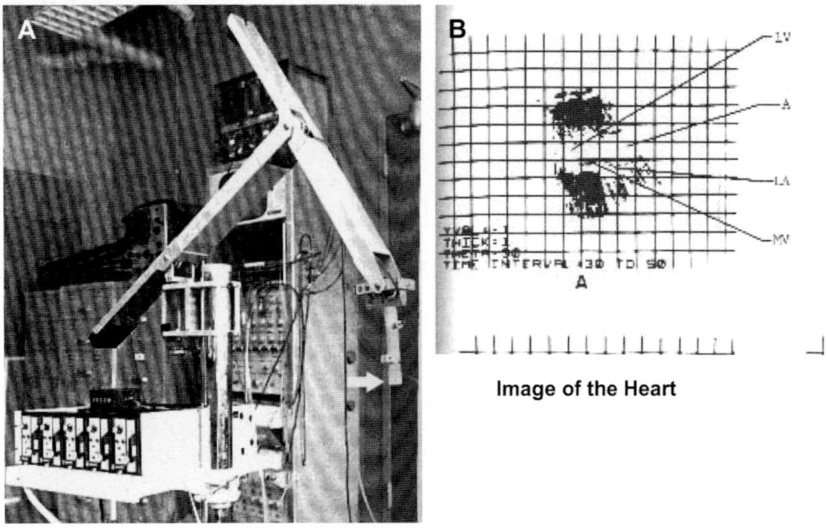

Fig. 1. (*A*) The mechanical arm. A large external beam device gives spatial data regarding an ultrasound probe to enable 3D reconstruction. The ultrasound probe is depicted by the arrow. (*B*) The image that resulted from the mechanical arm 3D reconstruction. Note that the image is barely discernable as a cardiac structure.

Rotational scanning and other transducer-prescribed methods

The development of commercially available 3DE equipment began in the early 1990s with the introduction of transesophageal 3DE. TomTec Imaging Systems (Munich, Germany) introduced a special transesophageal transducer that allowed moving a phased-array transducer element parallel within the esophagus. This movement of the transducer was controlled by a stepper motor that was in sync with the patient's ECG and respiratory cycle (Fig. 8).

The first realistic attempts at clinical 3DE began in the mid-1990s, when TomTec Incorporated developed and began marketing a product called Echo Scan that applied transthoracic 3DE acquisition methods. Mechanical devices were used to advance a standard 2DE transducer over a region of interest. A separate computer workstation monitored the patient's ECG and respiratory signals, and, accordingly, a stepper motor advanced the position of the device and inherently the transducer. Researchers evaluated several different acquisition devices like parallel scan device, fan-like scan motion, and rotational acquisition devices (see Figs. 3–6). After a rather short period of time, mostly rotational type devices achieved the greatest popularity, with others rarely used.

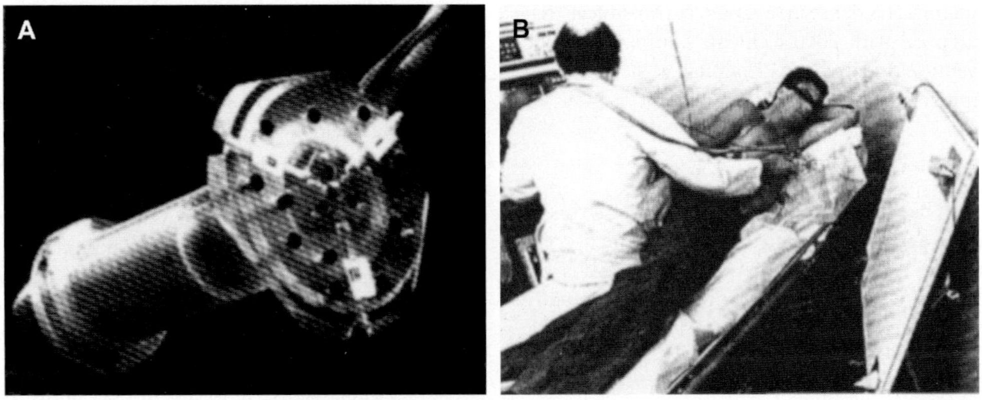

Fig. 2. (*A*, *B*) The acoustic locator or spark gap. Ultrasound probe location is tracked by a means similar to radar technology.

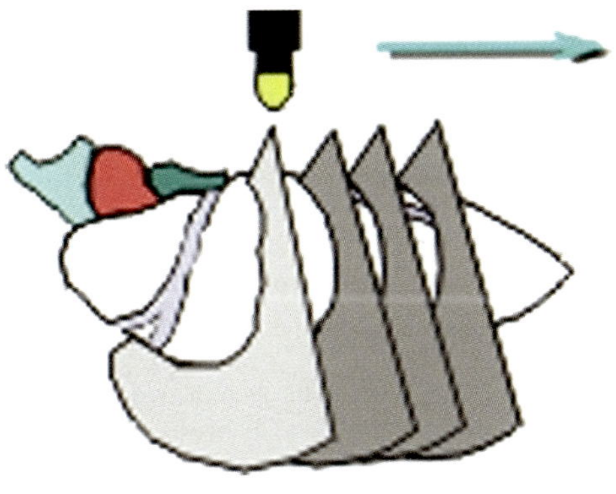

Fig. 3. Linear acquisition. Schematics of the sequential ultrasound images obtained by progressive linear, fanlike, and rotational motion of the transducer in a prespecified fashion. Images then were reconstructed offline.

The rotational device did not track the transducer in space, but rather assumed that (other than rotation) the transducer axis remained in one place throughout the scan. The rotational device was large, and as a result cumbersome; it came to be known, not necessarily in an affectionate way, as the bazooka (see Fig. 6A). This rotational device, as its name implied, rotated the transducer through a 180-degree arc and acquired an image (a complete heart cycle) every 3 to 5 degrees. For such an acquisition to be successful, a sonographer would have to hold the rotational device and the transducer within it as still as possible while the device rotated. Although clinically possible, a scan then required the standard echo machine and transducer, the rotational device, and the workstation. From a practical standpoint, such a three-piece system was not mobile and largely limited scanning to within the echo laboratory, or in some cases in the operating room; hence portable 3DE examinations became oxymoronic. In actuality, to be successful, this type of 3DE required a very skilled sonographer, a very cooperative patient, an echocardiographer physician or technician skilled with 3D reconstructions, and a little bit of luck. Ultimately, a rotational transducer was developed with the rotational mechanism contained within the transducer and the driving mechanism contained onboard the ultrasound system (see Fig. 6B). Although this apparatus was portable, as it was consolidated into the ultrasound machine, the image quality still was less than desirable except in pediatric patients, where it saw limited application. Although image quality was particularly suboptimal for smaller discrete structure analysis such as valvular structures, even at this time, ventricular volume assessment was useful.

Later, using the technology developed by Raab, free-hand scanning became commercially available from TomTec Imaging Systems and from 3D Echo Tech (Boulder, Colorado), acquired by GE Medical Systems. An electromagnetic transducer locator, an enhanced version of the device originally described by Raab, was used (see Fig. 7). As shown in the figure, a magnet enclosed in a plastic housing was placed in close proximity of the patient. The electromagnet was attached to the ultrasound machine, the transducer, and a separate computer. With freehand scanning, the electromagnet creates a highly sophisticated magnetic field that orients sequentially acquired 2DE images and their imaging planes by tracking the transducer through space as it is

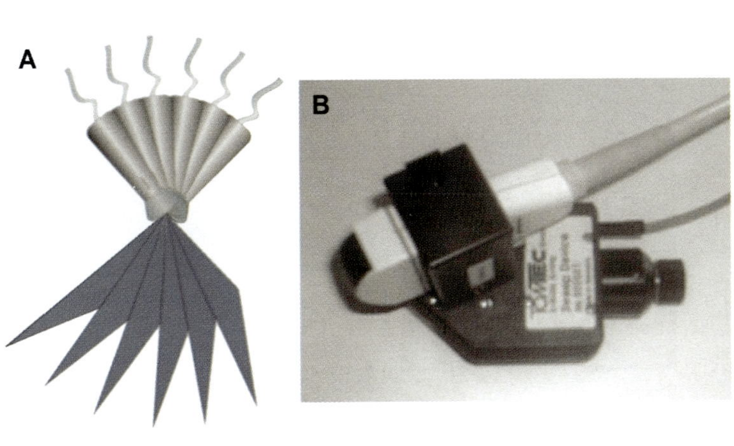

Fig. 4. (*A*, *B*) The actual hardware that was used for fanlike acquisition.

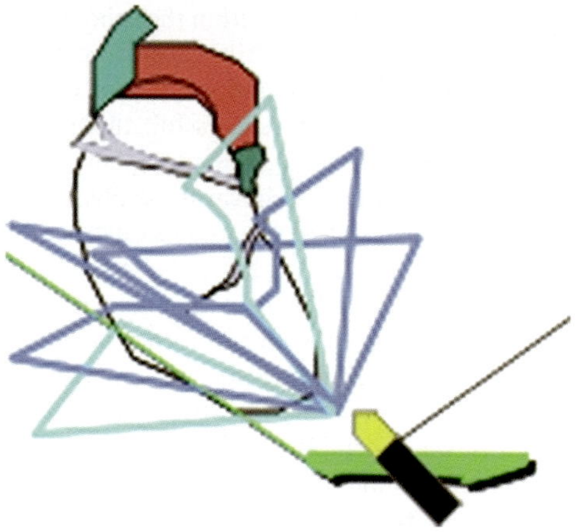

Fig. 5. Transesophageal echo (TEE) probe using rotational acquisition. The TEE probe was positioned in the esophagus in a position to visualize the heart. Then, the TEE probe was pulled back in a prescribed fashion using a stepper motor with ECG and respiratory cycle gating.

moved so by the sonographer. Therefore, at the end of the scan, the collection of images (typically 15 to 60 cardiac cycles, with 10 to 15 frames/cardiac cycle) can be oriented appropriately into a 3D data cube and ultimately rendered into a 3D image by placing each individual image in its appropriate plane relative to the others. This particular technology gained some popularity in the late 1990s and is still today used by some researchers [9]. It arguably was the most likely technology to make it to the clinical arena before the advent of RT3D imaging.

The reason why RT3D imaging took essentially three decades to be developed from the earliest forms of 3D is related simply to fact that adequate computing power did not exist to support the infrastructure needed for RT3D. In addition, transducer technology was not advanced enough to acquire a volume of data.

Integrated transesophageal echo methodology with rotational transducer

Initially 3D TEE was performed using an external computer and a TEE probe advanced in a parallel mode using a stepper motor (see Fig. 8). Then in a cooperative effort between Hewlett-Packard and TomTec in 1994, a TEE method of 3D acquisition with software onboard the ultrasound machine became commercially available. The multiplane TEE probe, invented by Hewlett-Packard in the early 1990s and sold commercially starting in 1992, provided a ready-made rotational device to couple with technology already used by TomTec in its transthoracic rotational device. That is the multiplane TEE probe had an inherent design for the ultrasound transducer at the tip of the probe to rotate within the TEE probe itself between 0 and 180 degrees (Fig. 9). Hence, all that had to be added was software and hardware onboard the ultrasound system itself that automatically drove the TEE probe through its 0- to 180-degree rotation, typically (although adjustable up or down by the user) through 3-degree increments, and acquired a complete 2D heart cycle. In addition, respiratory and cardiac cycle gating was added to assure uniformity to the 2D images. The result was 61 2D cardiac cycles that then were transferred to an offline PC and reconstructed into a cube of

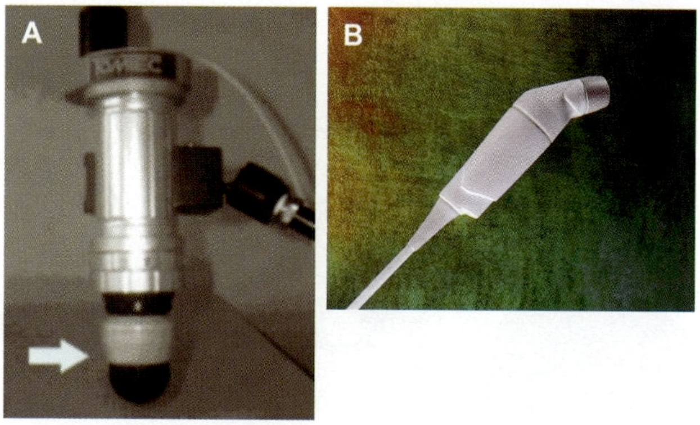

Fig. 6. (*A*) An early mechanical rotator that housed an external stepper motor that controlled transthoracic echocardiography (TTE) probe rotation. (*B*) A transducer with rotational capacity within the head of the transducer for transthoracic imaging.

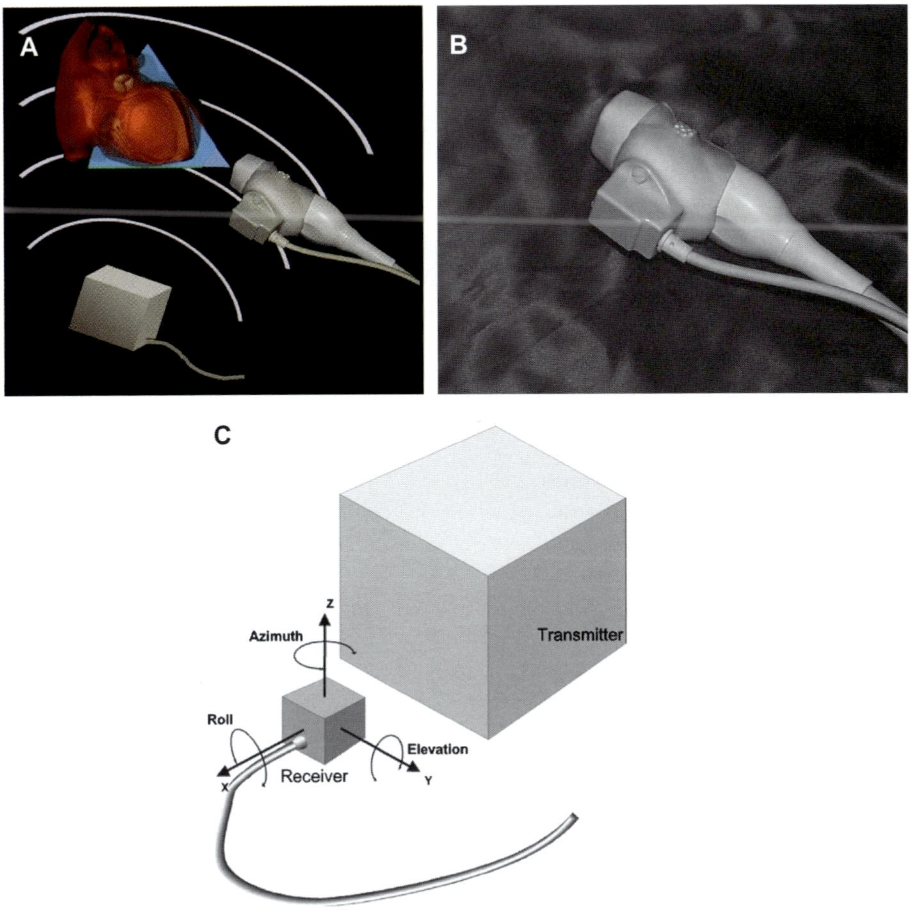

Fig. 7. (*A*, *B*) Freehand scanning. A modified ultrasound probe is tracked in 3D space using an electromagnetic field device; images then may be reconstructed off-line to create 3D data sets (*C*). Schematic of the receiver and transmitting device and the Cartesian coordinate system for tracking the location of the transducer. (*Courtesy of* TomTec Imaging Systems, Munïch, Germany; with permission.)

data and ultimately cropped into a 3D image. This type of 3DE was limited by the fact that it had to be reconstructed after the examination was completed, because the reconstruction process was not on the ultrasound system. It did, however, offer the tremendous advantage of working with high-quality 2D images, because they were obtained by means of TEE. During this time period (1994 to 2000), a solution for most multiplane TEE probes was available from TomTec using an external acquistion computer, but only Hewlett Packard integrated the acquisition software into the ultrasound system itself. In 1992, Nanda performed one of the first 3D reconstructions using a mutliplane TEE for acquistion [10]. It is notable that Chen and colleagues [11], at the Thorax center in Rotterdam, Netherlands, had developed their own apparatus for TEE acquisition, again using TomTec software for offline reconstruction. Finally it is also worth noting that in 2004 Siemens Ultrasound (Mountain View, California), in cooperation with TomTec, began offering a similar system with reconstruction (in addition to acquisition) possible onboard the ultrasound system, a clear advantage. However, it is clear that the advent of real-time 3D echo imaging has made any type of 3D echo that utilizes a reconstructive process obsolete.

Real-time 3D methods

RT3D first was developed by von Ramm at Duke University during the 1990s [10–13]. With RT3D, an entire volume of heart was obtained

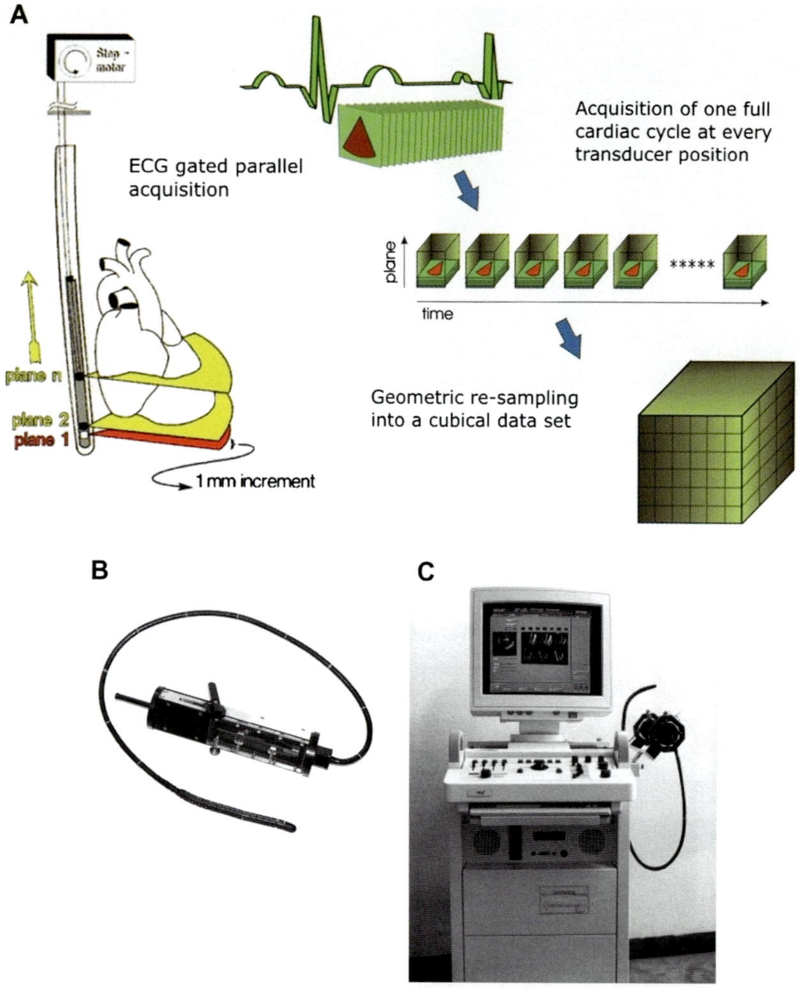

Fig. 8. The parallel acquisition of a 3D image by transesophageal echo (TEE) (*A*). The TEE probe in schematic and how it was advanced in the esophagus using a stepper motor (*B*). The actual TEE probe attached to the stepper motor, a device known as the lobster tail (*C*). The original TomTec Echo CT showing the computer that was used to drive the acquisition and the lobster tail in a carrier with the computer. (*Courtesy of* TomTec Imaging Systems, Munïch, Germany; with permission.)

using one cardiac cycle. This was of course a major transition from the thin slice sector imaging that 2D provided. And although it was a very positive development with the volumetric acquisition, the negative was that the images displayed were in fact 2D images. The 2D images were in fact derived from the 3D data but were displayed as 2D orthogonal planes. This was the major advent of the C scan (Fig. 10). An attempt was made to commercialize this product through the company Volumetrics (Chapel Hill, North Carolina). Although Volumetrics had an imaging system in production and commercially available for a few years (from 1997 to 2000), the system was large and not particularly versatile for also performing 2D imaging. Additionally, to derive true 3D images, an off-line workstation had to be used (TomTec, Echo-Scan). There were no truly RT3D images. Having said that, Volumetrics did show RT3D rendering at the 2000 American Heart Association meetings, but soon after that, the company folded never to be heard from again.

By the time that Volumetrics had shown its RT3D rendering, a similar, yet much more advanced product was already well into the development stage at Hewlett-Packard. Hewlett-Packard

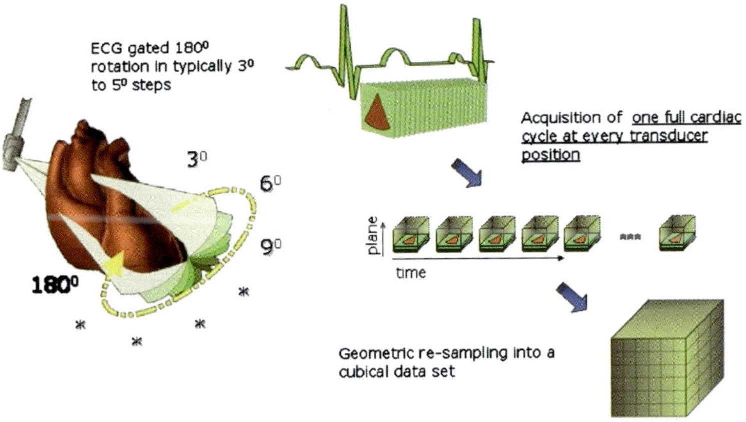

Fig. 9. Schematic of how 3D transesophageal echo (TEE) was acquired. The TEE probe is shown with its range of rotation from 180 degrees. Typically, a 2D image was acquired every 3 degrees. The relationship between the heart and the TEE rotation. (*Courtesy of* TomTec Imaging Systems, Munïch, Germany; with permission.)

began developing RT3DE in roughly 1996. The company had already been a force in the development of 3D TEE using the 2D reconstruction approach and had released that product for general consumption in 1995. By late 1998, Hewlett-Packard had a working prototype for transthoracic RT3D (RT3DE) and began showing it to luminary customers by 1999. A major development in the history of RT3D came in 1999 when Hewlett-Packard spun off its medical division and some other noncomputer divisions as Agilent Technologies (Andover, Massachusetts). One year later in 2000, this led to the purchase of the medical division of Agilent Technologies, including its medical ultrasound division, the most pertinent division for this discussion, by

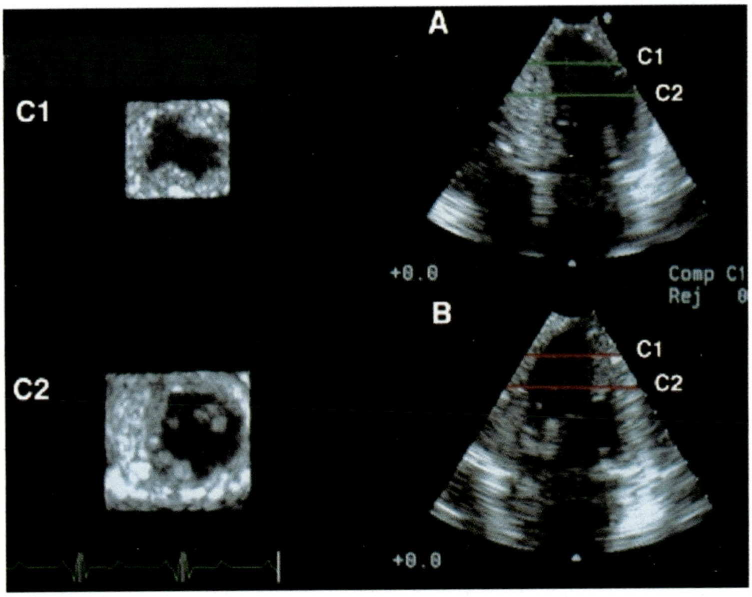

Fig. 10. Real-time 3D echocardiograph C-scan images, Volumetrics, Inc. The images shown are apical view of the heart on right, four chamber on top, and two chamber on the bottom. On the left are short axis or C scans of the LV derived from perpendicular cuts through the apical views on the right. (*Courtesy of* David Adams, RDCS, Durham, NC.)

Philips Medical Systems. As Philips Medical Systems (Bothell, Washington) had purchased another ultrasound company, Advanced Technology Laboratories (ATL), (Bothell, Washington), in 1998, the plan became for ATL and Agilent to merge their ultrasound knowledge to further develop this 3D technology. Hence, in November 2002, at the time of the American Heart Association meetings, Philips released the first generation of RT3DE. Two years later, at the 2004 American Heart Association meetings, General Electric Health Care (Chalfont St. Giles, United Kingdom) would follow-suit with its introduction of RT3D. At the 2007 American College of Cardiology Annual Scientific Sessions, New Orleans, Louisiana, Toshiba revealed its version of RT3D. Hence, currently, three of the four major ultrasound companies now have RT3D with the fourth, Siemens expected to soon have a version.

The major breakthrough that allowed quality real-time imaging was the development of a microbeam former. This was necessary, because the Matrix transthoracic imaging probe developed by von Ramm and commercialized by Volumetrics was a sparse array transducer (not all of the transducer head was used and connected to individual elements) (Fig. 11). That is because of earlier lack of miniaturization and the fact that only 128 channels can be connected to this array. This limits the beam-forming characteristics and hence image quality. When the entire crystal of the transducer head is sampled or covered with elements, the transducer is a dense array (Fig. 12). The microbeam former is required for this arrangement to provide a communication of all of the approximately 3000 elements to the ultrasound system. Although still only 128 channels are used on the ultrasound system, the 3000 elements are divided into subgroups, and each of the subgroups is attached to one of the 128 channels. This arrangement makes the beam steering very powerful, and this is how the image quality is maximized to result in a high-resolution, RT3D rendered image. More detail regarding the mechanism of operation of this transducer can be found in the article by Salgo elsewhere in this issue.

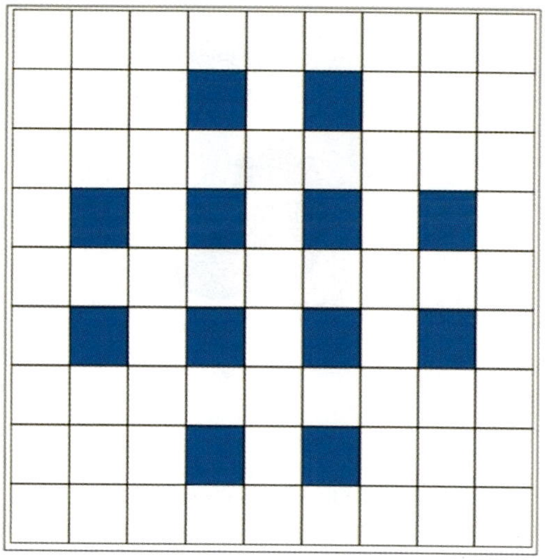

Fig. 11. Sparse array transducer. The diagram depicts the difference between a sparse array shown here and a dense array. Not all of the transducer head is connected to an element. This limits image quality. See discussion in text.

Since the initial release of RT3DE by Philips Medical Systems in 2002, much research has been performed on this system, and to a lesser degree on other systems. This research is summarized in the remainder of this edition. In November 2006, the second generation of RT3D imaging was released by Philips Medical Systems, again at the American Heart Association annual meeting. It is anticipated that GE soon will release a significant upgrade to its first generation of RT3D imaging. With these developments, RT3DE has become more commonplace throughout the United States and the world. In fact, technology in 3D has proliferated more throughout Europe and Asia than the United States. Proliferation of the technology continues as improved methods of image management and analysis are developed. In the United States, billing and reimbursement for RT3DE was instituted in 2005 using a general 3D radiology billing code. In January 2006, two new 3D ultrasound billing codes were introduced: RT3DE acquisition and analysis and off-line analysis. With the combination improved image quality, rapid image management and analysis, and reimbursement, it is likely the RT3D imaging will become a routine in most clinical echo laboratories in the near future. At this point, it is clear that the advent of RT3DE has transitioned 3DE from a relatively impractical research tool to a very user-friendly clinically applicable diagnostic test. Finally, all of the vendors for 3DE have developed practical software for quantification. This is important from the standpoint of moving 3DE from a qualitative pretty picture technology

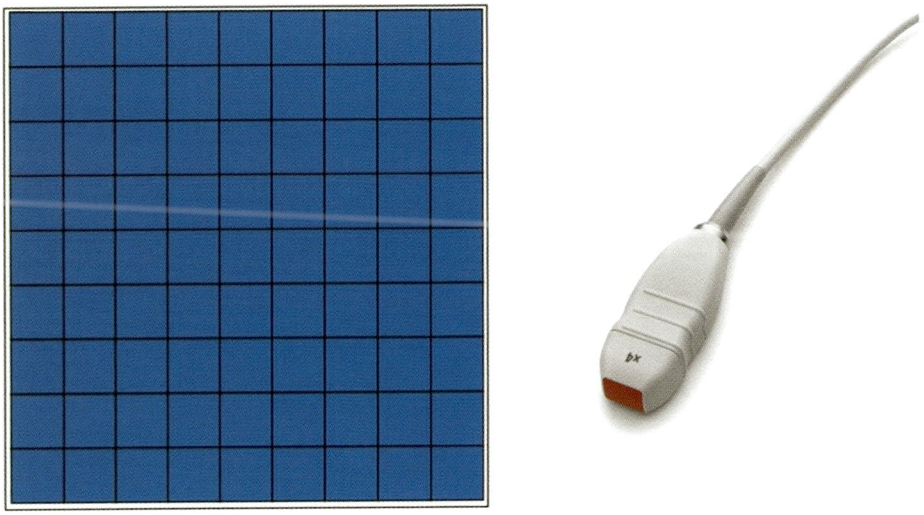

Fig. 12. Dense array transducer. Schematic shows that compared with Fig. 10, in this rendition, all of the squares on the transducer head are connected to one of the roughly 3000 elements. It is the microbeam former that allowed the utilization of the very large (3000) number of elements, the definition of dense array transducer.

to one of providing significant quantification, particularly of left ventricular function.

References

[1] Dekker DL, Piziali RL, Dong E Jr. A system for ultrasonically imaging the human heart in three dimensions. Comput Biomed Res 1974;7:544–53.

[2] Moritz WE, Shreve PL. A microprocessor-based spatial locating system for use with diagnostic ultrasound. IEEE Trans Biomed Eng 1976;64: 966–74.

[3] Geiser EA, Lypkiewicz SM, Christie LG, et al. A framework for three-dimensional time varying reconstruction of the human left ventricle: sources of error and estimation of their magnitude. Comput Biomed Res 1980;13:225–41.

[4] Matsumoto M, Matsuo H, Kitabatake A, et al. Three-dimensional echocardiographic images at desired planes by a computerized system. Ultrasound Med Biol 1977;3:163–78.

[5] Pearlman AS, Moritz WE, Medema DK, et al. Three-dimensional reconstruction of the formalin-fixed ventricle using nonparallel two-dimensional ultrasonic scans. Circulation 1981;64(Suppl IV): 65.

[6] Maurer G, Ghosh A, Nanda NC. Volume determination and three-dimensional reconstruction of echocardiographic images using rotation method. Circulation 1981;64(Suppl IV):206.

[7] Ghosh A, Nanda NC, Maurer G. Three-dimensional reconstruction of echocardiographic images using the rotation method. Ultrasound Med Biol 1982;8:655–61.

[8] Raab FH, Blood EB, Steiner TO, et al. Magnetic position and orientation tracking system. IEEE Trans Aerosp Electron Syst 1979;AES-15:709–18.

[9] Legget ME, Leotta DF, Bolson EL, et al. System for quantitative three-dimensional echocardiography of the left ventricle based on a magnetic field position and orientation sensing system. IEEE Trans Biomed Eng 1998;45:494–504.

[10] Nanda N, Pinheiro L, Sanyal R, et al. Multiplane transesophageal echocardiographic imaging and three-dimensional reconstruction. Echocardiography 1992;9:667–76.

[11] Chen Q, Hosir YF, Vletter WB, et al. Accurate assessment of MVA in patients with mitral stenosis by three-dimensional echocardiography. J Am Soc Echocardiogr 1997;10:133–40.

[12] von Ramm OT, Smith SW, Pavy HG Jr. High-speed ultrasound volumetric imaging system. Part II. Parallel processing and image display. IEEE Trans Ultrason Ferroelectr Freq Control 1991;38:109–15.

[13] von Ramm OT, Smith SW. Real time volumetric ultrasound imaging system. J Digit Imaging 1990;3: 261–6.

ELSEVIER
SAUNDERS

Cardiol Clin 25 (2007) 231–239

CARDIOLOGY
CLINICS

Three-Dimensional Echocardiographic Technology

Ivan S. Salgo, MD, MS

Cardiovascular Investigations, Ultrasound Research & Development, Philips Medical Systems, 3000 Minuteman Road, Andover, MA 01810, USA

Today echocardiography remains the most commonly requested imaging study of the heart. Moreover, recent insights into the understanding of the sophistication of the structural and functional mechanisms of the heart have come from advances in this area. Combined with portability, safety, low cost, and widespread availability, it is a tribute to the evolution of ultrasound technology that echocardiography's role in deciphering clinical problems in cardiac physiology has kept pace with the ever-increasing demands of a busy practice. This article addresses the current state of the art of technology in 3D echocardiography as it applies to transducer design, beam forming, display, and quantification. Because 3D echocardiography encompasses many technical and clinical areas, this article reviews its strengths and limitations and concludes with an analysis of what to use when. In this article, the author will be precise about the terminology related to 3D imaging and use dimension to refer to one, two, or three spatial dimensions.

Transducer design

The ultrasound transducer keeps echocardiography unique among it siblings in imaging technology. It converts electrical energy into mechanical vibrations and vice versa. To understand what sets 3D systems apart from conventional scanning systems, one needs to review some acoustic principles. Current 2D systems transmit and receive acoustic beams in a flat 2D scanning plane. As opposed to M mode (one spatial and one temporal dimension), 2D scanning systems sweep a scan line to and fro within this 2D imaging plane; the angular position of the beam is said to vary in the azimuthal dimension. Even though traditional, flat 2D scanning comprises two spatial dimensions plus one temporal dimension, this is not 3D imaging. The transducer itself consists of elements working in concert to create a scan line. Typically, a conventional transducer consists of 64 to 128 elements spaced according to the ultimate frequency (and hence wavelength) of the acoustic vibrations; these propagate radially along the direction of the scan line. This array of elements steers the outward ultrasound beam or scan line by using interference patterns generated by varying the spatiotemporal phase of each element's transmit event. These principles comprise the underpinnings of any phased array system.

Armed with this knowledge, one can survey the key differences pertinent to 3D ultrasound imaging. First, these 64 to 128 elements of a conventional cardiac transducer are historically arranged along a single row. Technically this is referred to as a one-dimensional array of elements. (Remember, the two spatial dimensions in the image come from sweeping the beam by firing along this row at different times.) Nonetheless, the world has three spatial dimensions. Note that this flat scanning plane of ultrasound energy is not perfectly flat in three dimensions, even though the image appears so on the scanning system. An innovation applied in the last decade was to take just five to seven rows of elements to keep the beam flatter. These few stacks of rows now comprise for example a 5 × 64 or 320 element or primitive matrix array transducer. These rows, however, were not electrically independent from each other. These primitive matrix array transducers thinned the beam by growing the

This work was supported in part by NIH grant RO1 HL073647.

E-mail address: ivan.salgo@philips.com

0733-8651/07/$ - see front matter
doi:10.1016/j.ccl.2007.05.002

aperture in the elevation dimension. They did not however, steer in the third dimension.

True 3D ultrasound steering has been the subject of much academic and industrial research that began in the 1980s. To actually steer an ultrasound beam, a 2D matrix array comprising as many elements in the elevational dimension as in the azimuthal dimension needed to be fabricated. To do this, a block of transducer material was diced by a diamond tipped saw to create each element (Fig. 1). Today's transducers comprise more than 3000 elements and can have row and column sizes greater than 60. Note that this is a 2D matrix array that generates 3D images. This concept was known for decades. The significant innovation that actually allows steering is making the elements electrically independent from each other. This allows generating a scan line that varies azimuthally and elevationally. Thus a true 3D scan line is born. Early transducers, while having electrically independent rows, did not have every element electrically active, as the technology to connect such a dense array was not known yet. Newer types of electrical circuitry connecting each element first were commercialized in 2002. Today, miniaturization has allowed fitting thousands of fully sampled elements into the tip of a transesophageal transducer (Fig. 2). It is important to realize that the physical aperture needs to be designed according to the application. The wider the aperture in each dimension, the better the scan line can be focused. Transthoracic and transesophageal imaging, however, is physically limited by the

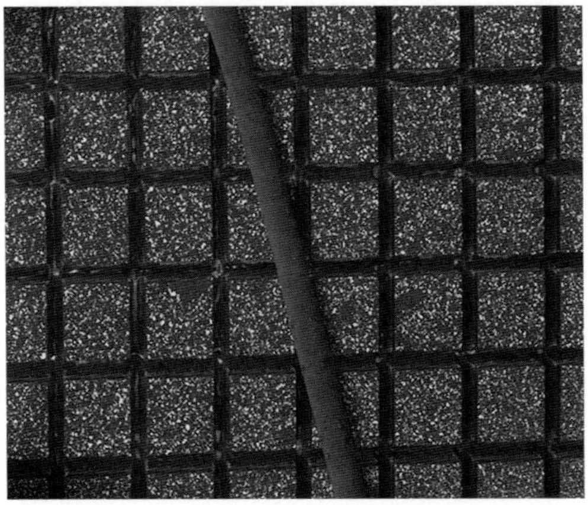

Fig. 1. Scanning electron micrograph of a fully sampled 2D matrix array used for 3D beam steering. A human hair is shown within the view for comparison.

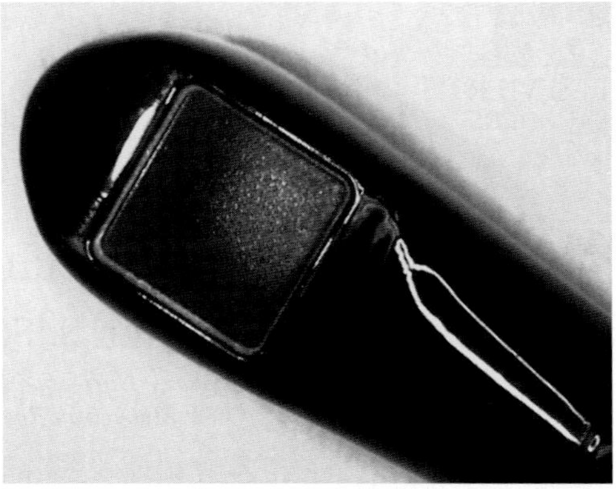

Fig. 2. A Matrix Array Transesophageal Transducer distal tip. The active aperture is 10 mm ×10 mm. Note that this supports 2D and 3D imaging, and spectral and color Doppler modes.

width and length of the transducer surface, and frequency aperture tradeoffs are taken into account when the transducer is designed for each application.

Modern 2D transducers therefore consist of thousands of electrically active elements that steer a scan line left and right as well as up and down. New materials that allow more bandwidth (simultaneous high and low frequencies) allow these matrix array transducers to obtain both penetration and high-resolution imaging.

Beam forming in three spatial dimensions

Beam forming constitutes the steering and focusing of transmitted and received scan lines. Because each element must have independent electrical control by the ultrasound system, a conventional cable that would be used to connect each element would make the transducer cable unwieldy. To reduce the size of the cable and reduce power consumption, a significant portion of the beam steering is done within the transducer in highly specialized integrated circuits. The main system steers at coarse angles, but the transducer circuits steer in fine increments in a process termed microbeam forming. Summing is the act of combining raw acoustic information from each element to generate a scan line and by summing these in a sequence (first in the transducer and then subsequently in the system). Both the transducer connectors and cable are reduced in size dramatically. The 3D beam former steers both in azimuth and elevation. This creates a 3D spherical wedge of acoustic information that subsequently is processed.

The radiofrequency (RF) data are summed and processed using various signal techniques and finally put into rectangular (Cartesian) space by a 3D scan converter. Note that this is an extension of the traditional phased array approach. Older 3D techniques used in the 1990s did not steer electronically but rather involved combining 45 to 100 cardiac loops and recombining them to create a 3D data set [1]. Although this works for static structures, irregular rhythms spell the downfall of gated reconstruction of many beats. Any transducer movement during acquisition of these many gates created artifacts and required a significant amount of smoothing of the data. Although this helped reduce attention to slippage or misalignment, it reduced the overall image quality if significant stitching needed to be done.

There are two major black and white modes run in an electronically steered 3D system. The first is a live mode where the system scans in real-time three dimensions. The test of this mode is as follows: if the transducer comes off the chest, the image disappears. As with sector scanning, the volume pyramid may be reduced to zoom in three dimensions. This is again a live mode. Today computer and beam forming processing power are not limiting for 3D ultrasound image generation; it is the speed of sound. Gating, this time only four to eight beats, allows a technique to generate wider volumes while maintaining frame rate. It is done by stitching four (or more) gates together in full-volume mode. This can generate greater than 90-degree scanning volumes at frame rates greater than 30 Hz. In patients who have arrhythmias, respiratory rate (RR) intervals that fall out of a set range cause the discard of the errant subvolume and the system scans again until all subvolumes are generated from suitable beat intervals. Thus in patients who have irregular intervals, as long as the average RR falls within a reasonable range, a full volume can be reconstructed. Because Doppler methods require many transmit events to be fired along a single path, color Doppler methods use gating. These multiple events are compared or cross-correlated to find the velocity of moving structures. The true 3D spatial modes may be summarized as follows (Figs. 3–5):

Live 3D mode–instantaneous
3D zoom–instantaneous
Full-volume–gated
3D color Doppler–gated

A variant of pyramidal 3D beam forming is to scan simultaneous planes in a process known as bi- and triplane imaging. Because this process requires firing fewer scan lines, frame rate is increased at the cost of spatial resolution. Here is a point worth emphasizing: all 3D echocardiography is subject to the laws of physics. Artifacts such as ringing, reverberations, shadowing, and attenuation occur in three and two dimensions. The system must play within these constraints. The numbers and densities of scan lines can be traded off to increase temporal resolution. The constraints of a 3D image are bounded by: (1) frame rate, (2) 3D volume size, and (3) image resolution. Increasing the requirement of one of these causes a drop in the other two, all things being equal. Systems can generate synthetic receive lines (four times, 16 times, or 32 times) for each transmit line by increasing beam forming parallelism. Note that as the interpolated receive line is steered farther and farther away from the transmitted scan line, the signal-to-noise ratio drops. Thus there is a practical limit to receive parallelism. The benefit is that it can increase the density of received lines, thereby improving resolution.

Display of 3D information

2D computer displays consist of rows and blocks of pixels (picture elements) that compromise a 2D image. A 3D data set consists of bricks of pixels called volume elements or voxels. Because the computer screen is only 2D in nature, perspective is used to simulate the appearance of 3D depth, as an object is virtually deeper or farther away from the viewing screen. Essentially the 3D data set (ie, collection of voxels) can be rotated with respect to the computer screen. Moreover, a process known as cropping can be used to cut into the volume and make some voxels invisible; for example, one can cut away the left atrium to see the mitral valve. After rotation and cropping, the remaining voxels are ready to be projected onto pixels in the same way as 3D objects in a room are projected onto the retina in two dimensions.

3D data sets of voxels are turned into 2D images in a process known as volume rendering. The 2D image appears in three dimensions because of perspective. There are several different algorithms to accomplish this conversion (eg, ray casting, shear-warp, and others), but they

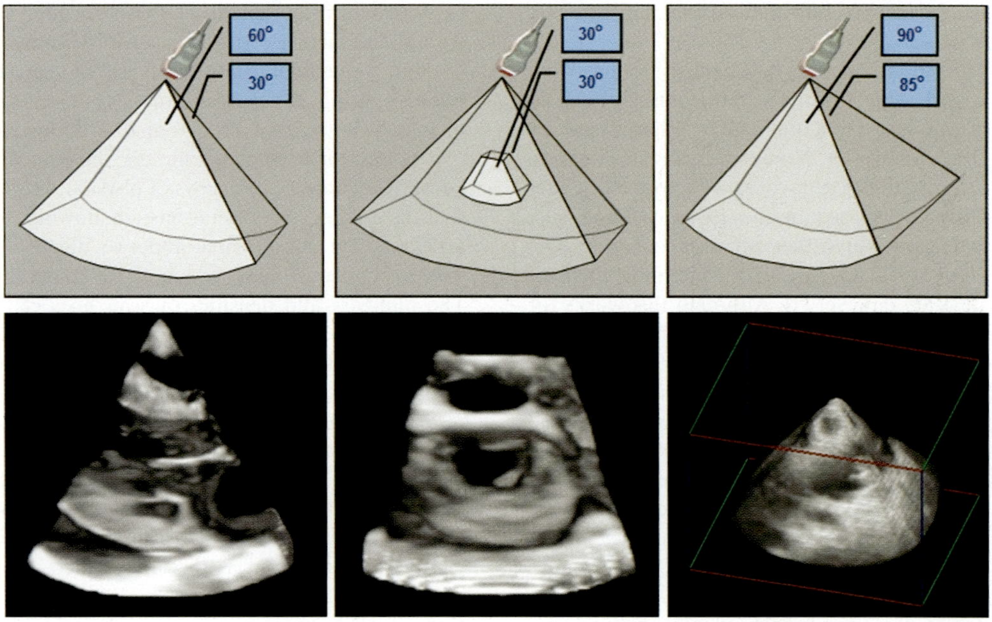

Fig. 3. 3D scanning volumes shown as volume rendering. These show the extent of the 2D scan line steering limits in each case. Ultimately, these will constitute a voxel data set. (*Courtesy of* the University of Chicago Medical Center, Chicago, IL; with permission.)

essentially cast a light beam through the collection of voxels. Either the light beam hits enough tissue so as to render it opaque (eg, tissue), or it keeps shining thought transparent voxels so as to render it transparent (eg, blood pool). Tissue surfaces derived from voxel data sets sometimes are termed surface rendering, but this is inaccurate terminology. Additional algorithms can be used to increase the perception of depth by applying different hues on the front (near the screen) of the data set as opposed to voxels far from the screen.

Quantification in three dimensions

Although visualization of anatomy in its true 3D state is important, many physicians believe that the most significant value 3D echocardiography

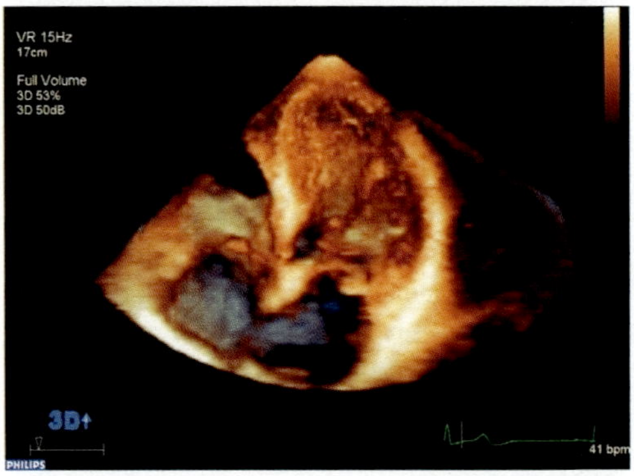

Fig. 4. Full volume acquisition encompassing the left ventricle. Depth-dependent dynamic colorization has been used to code hue according to depth perspective from the viewer. This adds visual cues to increase the "3D sense."

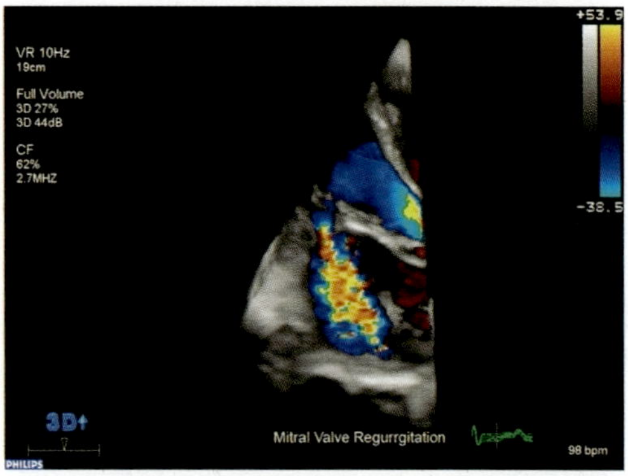

Fig. 5. Gated 3D color acquisition. A 3D jet of mitral regurgitation is shown. The classic 2D color map has been adapted to render color voxels showing the 3D nature of the jet.

has for adult echocardiography is quantification. True myocardial motion occurs in three dimensions, and traditional 2D scanning planes do not capture the entire motion of the heart or else move or slip while scanning. Quantifying implies segmenting structures of interest from the 3D voxel set. Although the voxels themselves can be tagged, for example coloring the right ventricular (RV) voxels separately from the left ventricular (LV) voxels, computer vision techniques frequently employ methods that define an interface (eg, the LV endocardial border). This interface typically is constructed as a mesh of points and lines and displayed in a process known as surface rendering (Fig. 6). Automobile, building, and engineering parts are rendered as meshes by surface rendering in computer-aided design tools.

3D quantification of the left ventricle typically employs a surface- rendered mesh. This allows accurate computation of volume, regional wall motion, and regional synchrony. Because the entire extent of the left ventricle is taken into account, no foreshortening errors or assumption of LV volume are generated [1,2]. Technically, a 3D deformable model is used to find the LV endocardial surface in three dimensions. This is the most accurate way to quantify LV volumes. Moreover, 3D LV remodeling can be displayed parametrically using differential geometry techniques (Fig. 7). Bi- and triplane methods help avoid foreshortening errors, but if an aneurysmal dilatation occurs between planes, the computed LV volumes will have some interpolation error. Quantification of LV synchrony is possible in

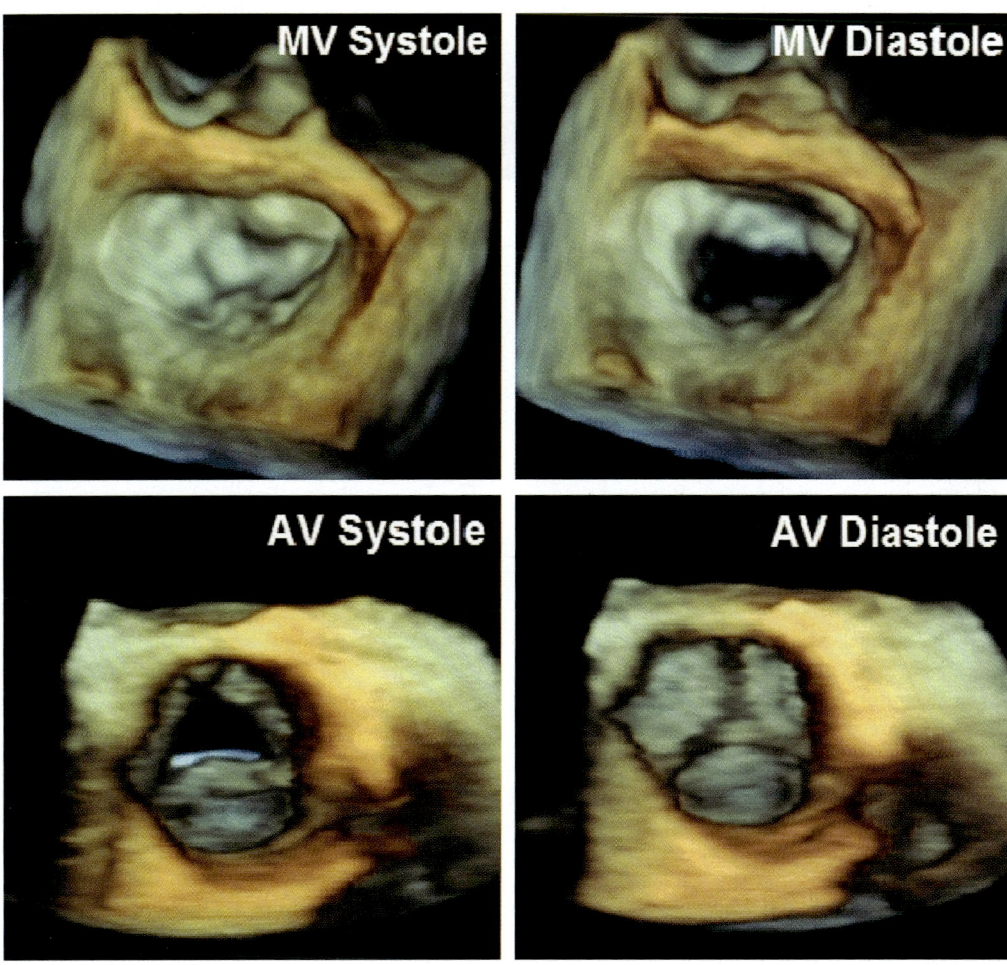

Fig. 6. 3D matrix TEE acquisitions of the aortic and mitral valves. (*Courtesy of* the University of Chicago Medical Center, Chicago, IL; with permission.)

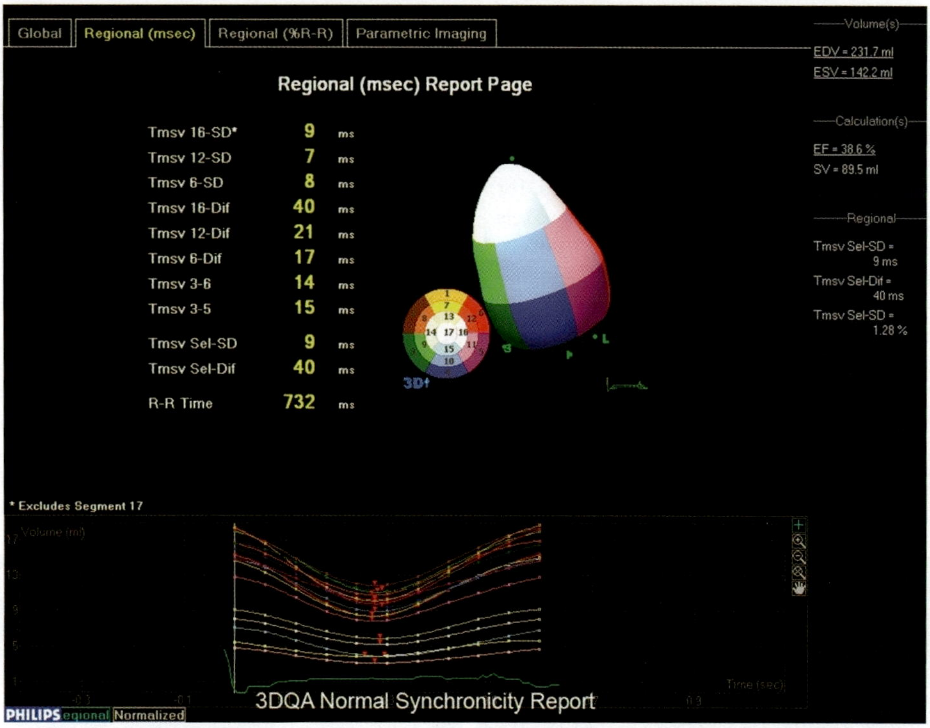

Fig. 7. 3D semi-automated border detection using surface rendering of the left ventricular shell to display its 3D nature in QLAB. Each segment has been analyzed for regional ejection, and segmental function is shown by the waveforms.

three dimensions also [3]. The required frame rate depends on the questions being asked. A frame rate of 30 Hz (33 milliseconds between frames) is inadequate to quantify intramyocardial motion; this is better suited to be studied by tissue Doppler or speckle tracking techniques. Regional synchrony, however, can be measured by three dimensions, because it assesses blood ejection not tissue motion. Because the ejection curve is naturally smooth, it requires less frame rate (has a lower band limit). Moreover, the Nyquist theorem frequently is misrepresented in this area. Some investigators argue that 20 millisecond phenomenon (eg, regional phase differences in peak ejection at different segments) cannot be quantified at 33 millisecond frame intervals. This is an incomplete statement. In fact, if the waveform's upper natural frequency limit reaches its maximum at 15 Hz (half the sampling frame rate) the waveform is fully determined. Thus increasing the frame rate to 100 Hz (10 millisecond intervals) would yield no additional information if the wave already was sampled fully at 30 Hz. This appears to be the case for many dyssynchrony patients and is why 3D echo stratifies dyssynchrony successfully.

New 3D electronically steered transesophageal transducers are yielding ultrasound images never before seen on the beating mitral valve (Fig. 8). This also allows the mitral apparatus to be segmented at end-systole with great accuracy. The true three dimensional nature of the mitral annulus, leaflets, and chordal apparatus can be measured. This further allows sophisticated analyses of the nonplanar shape of the mitral annulus [4,5]. These 3D measurements include: annular diameters, annular nonplanarity, commissural lengths, leaflet surface areas, aortic to mitral annular orientation.

Other areas subject to 3D quantification include quantifying volumes of all chambers of the heart (ie, the left and right atria and right ventricle). Quantification of 3D color flow is an active area of research [6]. One of the limitations for color flow quantification includes measuring unsteady flow (as in an intermittent jet of mitral regurgitation) that may not be sampled adequately by gated 3D color Doppler methods.

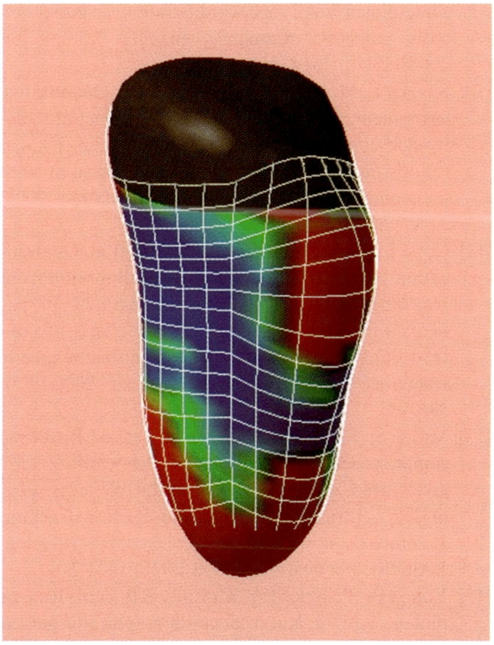

Fig. 8. 3D surface-rendered mesh from QLAB has been analyzed using principal curvature analysis. An aneurysmal portion of the anterior basal segment is shown in red. Note that the apex is normally red because of its high degree of curvature. Additionally, a set of white grid lines applying geodesic computation shows the bulge at the aneurysmal segment.

Patients who undergo mitral valve repair should have intraoperative transesophageal echo as part of their care. 3D methods now allow leaflet anatomy to be displayed functionally with resolution that was not possible before. Although conventional 2D echocardiography is likely sufficient for the detection of thrombus and vegetations, 3D echocardiography allows visualization and quantification of the mitral apparatus and tricuspid apparatus in their living 3D state [14,15]. Live 3D transesophageal echo (TEE) is especially useful in delineating areas of leaflet prolapse as in patients who have Barlow's disease. Moreover, 3D echo is useful is assessing the degree of leaflet restriction within the apparatus and annular changes (Fig. 9) [16,17]. Sophisticated changes in LV remodeling can be assessed in ischemic mitral regurgitation [18,19]. Changes of mitral leaflet systolic anterior motion can be assessed in hypertrophic cardiomyopathy [20].

3D visualization is especially useful in identifying intracardiac problems such as atrial septal defects. This is especially useful in identifying and characterizing congenital defects for children and the growing population of adults with congenital heart disease.

What to use when

As 3D technology increases in sophistication, so do the new physiologic parameters that can be measured [7]. It is important to begin with anatomic or physiologic questions and turn to 3D as needed to answer these questions with accuracy. The single most requested measurement for any indication for an echo examination is assessment of LV function and size. This should be measured by three dimensions, and techniques to assess LV endocardial volume, mass and regional function are readily available [8–10]. 3D techniques are more accurate than multiplane techniques, which more accurate than single plane methods. Echo contrast can be used to increase volume accuracy in patients who have poor acoustic windows [11]. Stress echo examinations can benefit from 3D or triplane methods [12,13]. This is because single plane scanning does not assure with quantitative certainty that the true apex of the heart is within the scanning volume. At this point, the application of 3D technology depends on the referring question.

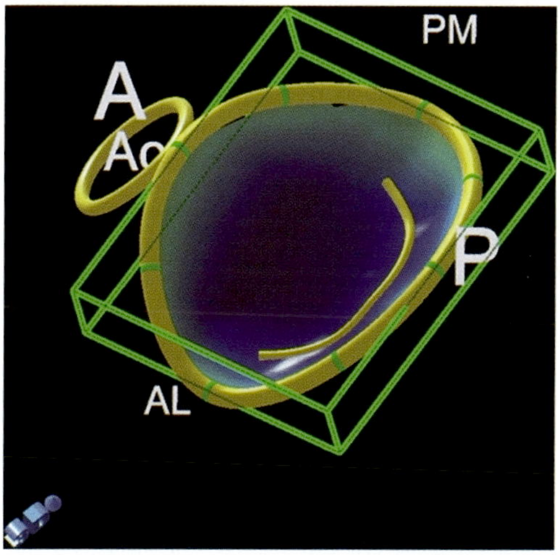

Fig. 9. 3D mitral valve quantification from matrix TEE images (QLAB). The mitral annulus in relation to the aortic annulus is shown. Additionally, coaptation from commissure to commissure is shown. Leaflet segmentation allows computation of leaflet restriction and prolapse area. The green box displays the nonplanarity of the mitral annulus in 3D space.

The future for 3D echocardiography looks bright. Advances in technology will allow larger scanning volumes and more sophisticated methods of quantification, such as 3D speckle tracking and analysis of LV torsion and mechanics. One of the most exciting areas includes the use of 3D echocardiography to guide intracardiac procedures without the need for cardiopulmonary bypass [21,22]. Placement of atrial septal defect (ASD) devices and percutaneous valve therapies likely will benefit from the live nature of 3D TEE imaging and broaden not only the diagnostic uses of 3D echocardiography but those used for therapy.

Acknowledgment

The author gratefully acknowledges the support and friendship of Bernard Savord and Karl Thiele in preparation of this manuscript.

References

[1] Salgo IS. Three-dimensional echocardiography. J Cardiothorac Vasc Anesth 1997;11(4):506–16.
[2] Gerard O, Billon AC, Rouet JM, et al. Efficient model-based quantification of left ventricular function in 3D echocardiography. IEEE Trans Med Imaging 2002;21(9):1059–68.
[3] Kapetanakis S, Kearney MT, Siva A, et al. Real-time three-dimensional echocardiography: a novel technique to quantify global left ventricular mechanical dyssynchrony. Circulation 2005;112(7):992–1000.
[4] Salgo IS, Gorman JH III, Gorman RC, et al. Effect of annular shape on leaflet curvature in reducing mitral leaflet stress. Circulation 2002;106(6):711–7.
[5] Watanabe N, Ogasawara Y, Yamaura Y, et al. Mitral annulus flattens in ischemic mitral regurgitation: geometric differences between inferior and anterior myocardial infarction: a real-time 3-dimensional echocardiographic study. Circulation 2005;112 (Suppl 9):I458–62.
[6] Pemberton J, Ge S, Thiele K, et al. Real-time three-dimensional color Doppler echocardiography overcomes the inaccuracies of spectral Doppler for stroke volume calculation. J Am Soc Echocardiogr 2006;19(11):1403–10.
[7] Lang RM, Mor-Avi V, Sugeng L, et al. Three-dimensional echocardiography: the benefits of the additional dimension. J Am Coll Cardiol 2006; 48(10):2053–69.
[8] Thomas JD, Popovi ZB, Thomas JD, et al. Assessment of left ventricular function by cardiac ultrasound. J Am Coll Cardiol 2006;48(10):2012–25.
[9] Mor-Avi V, Sugeng L, Weinert L, et al. Fast measurement of left ventricular mass with real-time three-dimensional echocardiography: comparison with magnetic resonance imaging. Circulation 2004;110(13):1814–8.
[10] Sugeng L, Mor-Avi V, Weinert L, et al. Quantitative assessment of left ventricular size and function: side-by-side comparison of real-time three-dimensional echocardiography and computed tomography with magnetic resonance reference. Circulation 2006; 114(7):654–61.
[11] Corsi C, Coon P, Goonewardena S, et al. Quantification of regional left ventricular wall motion from real-time 3-dimensional echocardiography in patients with poor acoustic windows: effects of contrast enhancement tested against cardiac magnetic resonance. J Am Soc Echocardiogr 2006;19(7): 886–93.
[12] Malm S, Frigstad S, Sagberg E, et al. Real-time simultaneous triplane contrast echocardiography gives rapid, accurate, and reproducible assessment of left ventricular volumes and ejection fraction: a comparison with magnetic resonance imaging. J Am Soc Echocardiogr 2006;19(12):1494–501.
[13] Yang HS, Pellikka PA, McCully RB, et al. Role of biplane and biplane echocardiographically guided 3-dimensional echocardiography during dobutamine stress echocardiography. J Am Soc Echocardiogr 2006;19(9):1136–43.
[14] Garcia-Orta R, Moreno E, Vidal M, et al. Three-dimensional versus two-dimensional transesophageal echocardiography in mitral valve repair. J Am Soc Echocardiogr 2007;20(1):4–12.
[15] Ton-Nu TT, Levine RA, Handschumacher MD, et al. Geometric determinants of functional tricuspid regurgitation: insights from 3-dimensional echocardiography. Circulation 2006;114(2):143–9.
[16] Watanabe N, Ogasawara Y, Yamaura Y, et al. Quantitation of mitral valve tenting in ischemic mitral regurgitation by transthoracic real-time three-dimensional echocardiography. J Am Coll Cardiol 2005;45(5):763–9.
[17] Yamaura Y, Watanabe N, Ogasawara Y, et al. Geometric change of mitral valve leaflets and annulus after reconstructive surgery for ischemic mitral regurgitation: real-time 3-dimensional echocardiographic study. J Thorac Cardiovasc Surg 2005; 130(5):1459–61.
[18] Hung J, Guerrero JL, Handschumacher MD, et al. Reverse ventricular remodeling reduces ischemic mitral regurgitation: echo-guided device application in the beating heart. Circulation 2002;106(20): 2594–600.
[19] Messas E, Yosefy C, Chaput M, et al. Chordal cutting does not adversely affect left ventricle contractile function. Circulation 2006;114(Suppl 1): I524–8.
[20] Song JM, Fukuda S, Lever HM, et al. Asymmetry of systolic anterior motion of the mitral valve in patients with hypertrophic obstructive cardiomyopathy: a real-time three-dimensional

echocardiographic study. J Am Soc Echocardiogr 2006;19(9):1129–35.

[21] Cannon JW, Stoll JA, Salgo IS, et al. Real-time three-dimensional ultrasound for guiding surgical tasks. Comput Aided Surg 2003;8(2):82–90.

[22] Suematsu Y, Takamoto S, Kaneko Y, et al. Beating atrial septal defect closure monitored by epicardial real-time three-dimensional echocardiography without cardiopulmonary bypass. Circulation 2003; 107(5):785–90.

ELSEVIER
SAUNDERS

Cardiol Clin 25 (2007) 241–251

CARDIOLOGY
CLINICS

Three-Dimensional Echocardiographic Evaluation of the Heart Chambers: Size, Function, and Mass

Victor Mor-Avi, PhD*, Roberto M. Lang, MD, FACC, FASE, FAHA

Section of Cardiology, Department of Medicine, University of Chicago, MC5084, 5841 S. Maryland Avenue, Chicago, IL 60637, USA

Over the past 3 decades, echocardiography has become a major diagnostic tool in the arsenal of clinical cardiology for real-time imaging of cardiac function. More and more, cardiologists' decisions are based on images created from ultrasound wave reflections. From the time ultrasound imaging technology provided the first insight into the human heart, our diagnostic capabilities have increased exponentially as a result of our growing knowledge and developing technology. One of the most significant developments of the past decades was the introduction of three-dimensional (3D) imaging and its evolution from slow and labor-intensive off-line reconstruction to real-time volumetric imaging. While continuing its meteoric rise instigated by constant technological refinements and continuing increase in computing power, this tool is guaranteed to be integrated into routine clinical practice in the near future. The major advantage of this technique is the improvement in the accuracy of the echocardiographic evaluation of cardiac chamber volumes, which is achieved by eliminating the need for geometric modeling and the errors caused by foreshortened 2D views. In this article, we review the literature that has provided the scientific basis for the clinical use of 3D ultrasound imaging of the heart in the assessment of cardiac chamber size, function, and mass, and discuss its potential future applications.

Historical perspective

Since the first successful attempts to interrogate organs and systems "hidden" inside the human body by reconstructing reflections along the ultrasound beam half a century ago, ultrasonography has evolved into a widely used imaging modality. With the important advantages of no ionizing radiation and unique real-time imaging capabilities, echocardiography has become the leading tool for the noninvasive assessment of cardiac anatomy and function. Over the years, the technological evolution has passed multiple milestones, including the transition from the one-dimensional M-mode imaging that provided limited "ice-pick views" to the dynamic 2D B-mode images of the beating heart created virtually in real time at increasingly growing frame rates. Another important milestone was the development of Doppler imaging, which depicts blood flow patterns in the heart chambers and vessels and continues to be a leading diagnostic tool for valvular and vascular pathologies. Whereas echocardiographic scanners have become an indispensable part of routine clinical cardiology practice anywhere from advanced medical centers in large urban areas to remote rural clinics, other more technologically complex and more costly, radiation-free imaging modalities, such as magnetic resonance, are still struggling today with multiple challenges on their ways to attain similar capabilities.

As huge a leap as live 2D imaging was from the M-mode, its limitations, when interrogating a 3D organ such as the heart, have become quickly recognized. Geometric modeling of ventricular volumes from one or two cross-sectional planes proved inaccurate in the presence of aneurysms or asymmetric ventricles [1–7]. Moreover, even in

* Corresponding author.
E-mail address: vmoravi@medicine.bsd.uchicago.edu (V. Mor-Avi).

0733-8651/07/$ - see front matter
doi:10.1016/j.ccl.2007.05.003

symmetric ventricles, the use of foreshortened views to improve endocardial definition turned out to be a major source of error in measuring ventricular volumes [4,8–12]. The potential of 3D imaging to overcome these limitations had become obvious in the early 1980s, when initial results of off-line 3D reconstruction from serial ECG-gated acquisitions of multiple 2D planes were reported [13–15]. This multiplane acquisition strategy was implemented in three different approaches based on parallel linear motion [16,17], rotation [18–20], and free-hand sectioning with electromagnetic or acoustic (spark-gap) locating devices capable of registering transducer position and spatial orientation [21–24]. While parallel linear motion was found less efficient because of the difficulties with maintaining adequate acoustic windows throughout the scan, rotation of the imaging plane from a fixed transducer position was implemented and widely used with transesophageal imaging. The free-hand scanning turned out to be a useful option for transthoracic imaging because it used commercially available transducers and allowed integrating information obtained from multiple acoustic windows from which the structures of interest could be optimally visualized. The main disadvantage of this latter approach is the portability difficulties associated with locator devices. Importantly, all multiplane acquisitions required ECG gating and relied on the assumption that all planes would be acquired at the same phase of the respiratory cycle to ensure identical shape and position of the heart within the chest for each consecutive acquisition.

Over the past decade, a different approach has been pursued to eliminate the need for tedious multiplane acquisition and time-consuming 3D reconstruction altogether. This approach is based on real-time volumetric imaging, which uses transducers containing arrays of piezoelectric elements capable of scanning pyramidal volumes (Fig. 1), rather than the conventional 2D phased-array transducers that scan a fan-shaped sector in a single plane. Initial reports on the use of sparse array transducers date back to the early 1990s [25,26]. Processing the information generated by these transducers required computational power that was orders of magnitude beyond what was available at the time. To overcome this limitation, a group of researchers and engineers at Duke University built a dedicated system based on parallel processing that allowed, for the first time, real-time 3D ultrasound imaging of the heart. A small number of such systems were used in several academic centers to demonstrate the added benefits of real-time 3D imaging in multiple clinical scenarios [27–32]. Importantly, real-time volumetric imaging allowed fast acquisition of pyramidal datasets during a single breath-hold without the need for off-line reconstruction, thus eliminating motion artifacts known to have adversely affected

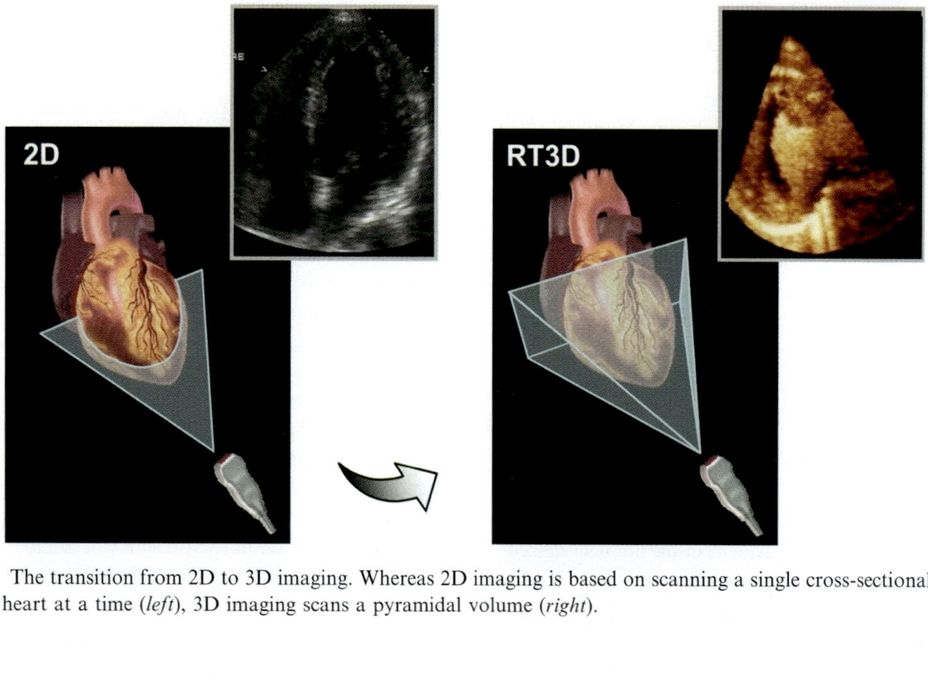

Fig. 1. The transition from 2D to 3D imaging. Whereas 2D imaging is based on scanning a single cross-sectional plane of the heart at a time (*left*), 3D imaging scans a pyramidal volume (*right*).

the multiplane acquisition and reconstruction methodology.

These earlier studies provided the scientific basis for further development of smaller matrix phased-array transducers with larger numbers of crystals and faster scanners based on modern digital processing and improved image formation algorithms to allow higher spatial and temporal resolution real-time volumetric imaging. Such systems have recently become commercially available and are currently offered by several major manufacturers. Their increasing availability gave rise to growing research efforts geared toward embracing this new modality. The large numbers of recent publications in this area reflect the rapidly growing body of knowledge necessary for accepting and incorporating this methodology into the arsenal of clinical cardiac imaging.

Clinical applications

Since the early 1990s, the usefulness of 3D echocardiography has been demonstrated in several areas. In this article, we focus on only a few major applications, including direct evaluation of cardiac chamber volumes without the need for geometric modeling and without the detrimental effects of foreshortened views [12,27–29,31,33–43], and direct 3D assessment of regional left ventricular wall motion aimed at objective detection of ischemic heart disease at rest [40,44–47] and during stress testing [48,49], as well as quantification of systolic asynchrony to guide ventricular resynchronization therapy [50–54].

Assessment of heart chamber volumes and function

One of the main reasons for requesting an echocardiogram in routine clinical practice is the assessment of global and regional left ventricular (LV) function. To date, this assessment is predominantly performed using visual interpretation or "eye-balling" of dynamic ultrasound images of the beating heart, which requires adequate training and experience to accurately estimate LV ejection fraction (EF) and evaluate wall motion. However, the limitations of this subjective interpretation have been long recognized, and consequently the use of quantitative techniques has been recommended. Thus, multiple methods to measure LV size and function have been developed, validated, and refined for both M-mode and 2D B-mode images, and subsequently for reconstructed 3D images and more recently for volumetric real-time 3D datasets. The relative inaccuracy of the one- and 2D echocardiographic approaches has been attributed to the need for geometric modeling of the ventricle. The "missing dimensions" have also been consistently referred to as the main source of the relatively wide intermeasurement variability of the echocardiographic estimates of ventricular size and function. In addition, the frequently encountered limitations in endocardial visualization, particularly in the apical-lateral segments of the left ventricle, are commonly compensated for by tilting the transducer. This maneuver generally improves endocardial visualization, but at the same time generates oblique or "foreshortened" views of the ventricle, resulting in even less accurate and reproducible measurements. In this regard, the biggest advantage of 3D echocardiography is the lack of dependence on geometric modeling and image plane positioning, which theoretically should result in more accurate chamber quantification.

Indeed, almost all studies that have directly compared the accuracy of 3D measurements of LV volumes and EF have demonstrated the superiority of the 3D approach over the 2D methodology, which was shown to consistently underestimate LV volumes. This superiority was demonstrated in both accuracy and reproducibility when compared against independent reference techniques, such as radionuclide ventriculography or MRI [11,12,22,31,37,38,48,55–59]. These improvements have been shown to occur irrespective of the 3D acquisition strategy employed. Whereas in earlier 3D studies, quantification of LV size and function relied on tedious, manual, or at best semi-automated tracing of endocardial boundaries in multiple planes, today it is based on near fully automated frame-by-frame detection of the 3D endocardial surface from real-time 3D datasets (Fig. 2). Recently a similar approach was implemented in commercial imaging systems, and is rapidly gaining widespread popularity because of its accuracy and ease of use [12], and is poised to become part of the mainstream assessment of LV function.

Similar results confirming improved accuracy and reproducibility of the 3D approach were reported by investigators who compared 2D and 3D echocardiographic measurements of left and right atrial volumes against an independent gold standard [22,42,60,61]. These findings may have

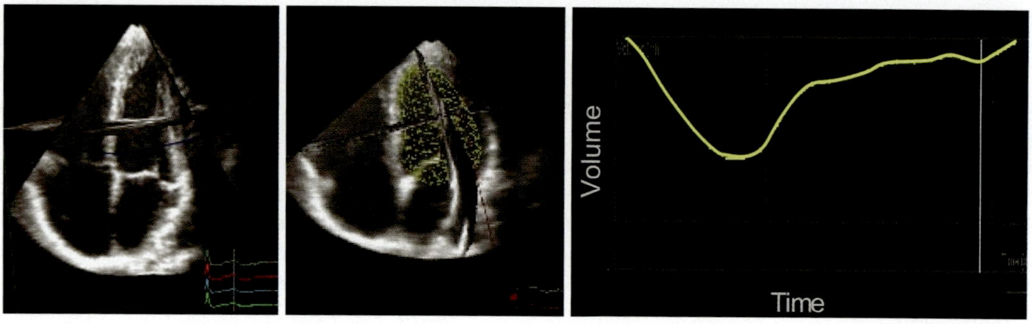

Fig. 2. Dynamic analysis of real-time 3D data. Biplane display (*left*) can be used to detect LV endocardial surface at each time point (*middle*), which allows the calculation of LV volume over time throughout the cardiac cycle (*right*).

important clinical implications on the diagnosis and management of patients with atrial fibrillation, diastolic dysfunction, and acute myocardial infarction.

Because of its complex geometrical crescent shape, the estimation of right ventricular volumes based on geometric modeling from 2D images has been extremely challenging. Thus, not surprisingly, the intrinsic ability of 3D imaging to directly measure right ventricular volumes without the need for geometrical modeling has resulted in significant improvements in accuracy and reproducibility compared with previously employed 2D techniques [27,34,62–64].

Assessment of left ventricular mass

Another clinically important variable that is frequently assessed by echocardiography is LV mass. Measurement of LV mass relies not only on endocardial but also epicardial visualization, which is known to be even more challenging because of the difficulties in identifying the epicardial border. This difficulty is in addition to the limitations previously discussed for the measurements of LV volumes such as inaccurate modeling and foreshortening. Again, the use of 3D images appears to have overcome these limitations, as several studies have reported significant improvements in the accuracy and reproducibility of 3D estimates of LV mass compared with their traditional M-mode and 2D counterparts (Fig. 3) [65–71].

Assessment of regional ventricular function

Diagnosis of regional wall motion abnormalities in echocardiographic studies is routinely performed by visually integrating regional endocardial motion and wall thickness. The reproducibility of this interpretation is limited because of its subjective nature, which is also extremely dependent on the experience of the reader. This is of particular concern in patients with suboptimal image quality that impedes endocardial visualization. Not only endocardial segments that are poorly visualized may be incorrectly interpreted as having abnormal wall motion, but also discrete areas of hypokinesis may be missed because they are simply not visualized in the standard imaging planes. It is not uncommon for an echocardiographer performing the test to slightly change transducer orientation to "better see" a specific myocardial segment. Such maneuvers can make a myocardial segment look like an area of hypokinesis or alternatively make an apparent wall motion abnormality disappear, and thus affect the diagnostic accuracy of the test. In this regard, volumetric imaging is different because the 3D dataset contains the complete dynamic information on LV chamber contraction and filling.

Importantly, such datasets are acquired virtually instantaneously, and any 2D view can be obtained from them simply by cropping out or "peeling off" the rest of the information. In addition, the function of any ventricular wall can be objectively assessed by measuring a variety of wall motion parameters (Fig. 4) [40]. For these reasons, 3D datasets are extremely appealing for the evaluation of regional LV function. Real-time 3D imaging has been recently used during dobutamine stress testing and found to be feasible and useful for the detection of stress-induced wall motion abnormalities (Fig. 5) [72]. Several other studies have explored the potential of quantitative evaluation of regional LV function based on segmental analysis of the dynamic 3D endocardial

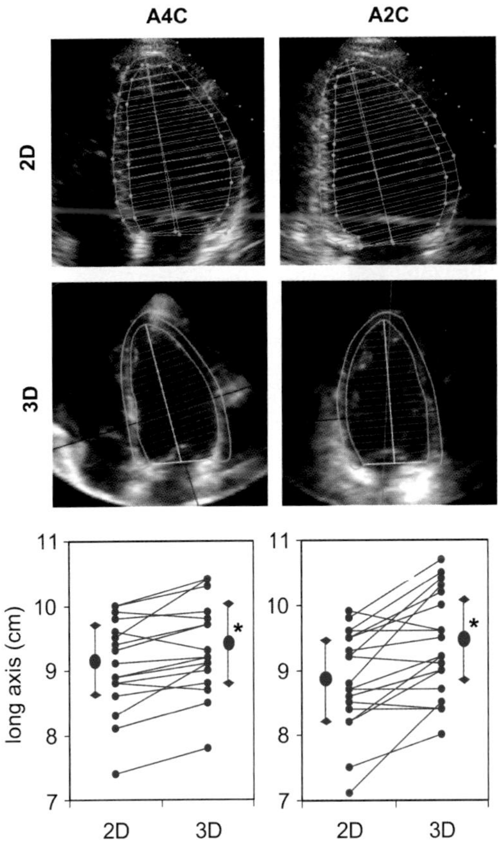

Fig. 3. Effects of volumetric imaging on the accuracy of LV mass measurements. End-diastolic apical four- and two-chamber views of the left ventricle obtained in a patient using conventional 2D imaging (*top*) and anatomically correct apical four- and two-chamber cut-planes selected from a real-time 3D dataset obtained in the same subject (*middle*). Manually traced endocardial and epicardial boundaries used to calculate LV mass are shown on the images. Left ventricular long axis dimension measured on such images in 19 patients (*bottom*). Note the increase in the length of the left ventricle in both apical views, as assessed by the 3D technique in most patients (large circles and error bars represent mean ± SD, $*P < .05$). (*Reproduced from* Mor-Avi V, Sugeng L, Weinert L, et al. Fast measurement of left ventricular mass with real-time 3D echocardiography; comparison with magnetic resonance imaging. Circulation 2004;110:1814–8; with permission.)

surface [40,44–47]. The use of this methodology in clinical practice requires further studies to be performed in larger groups of patients.

A clinically useful by-product of the 3D quantification of regional LV wall motion is the ability to quantify the temporal aspects of regional endocardial systolic contraction, which have been used for objective serial diagnosis of LV systolic asynchrony as a guide for resynchronization therapy [52,53], despite the relatively low temporal resolution of real-time 3D imaging. The standard deviation of the regional ejection times (interval between the R wave and peak systolic endocardial motion) has been used as an index of myocardial synchrony. This approach has been used to assess the short- and long-term benefits of biventricular pacing (Fig. 6). A recent study has shown a direct relationship between overall LV performance and synchronicity [54]. In this study, this approach has also been shown to be useful in identifying patients with severe heart failure and asynchronous LV contraction who could theoretically benefit from resynchronization therapy but would not be considered candidates based on their QRS duration [54]. Also, real-time 3D intracardiac imaging has been successfully used to guide the positioning of pacing catheters during interventional electrophysiology [51].

Contrast-enhanced 3D echocardiography

The ability of conventional contrast-enhanced echocardiographic imaging to provide accurate information on the extent and severity of either wall motion or perfusion abnormalities is also limited by its 2D nature. Despite the obvious appeal of the 3D imaging in this context, its use in humans has not been explored until recently. This is because this approach relied on off-line reconstruction from multiple planes, significantly complicating volumetric assessment of LV function. The feasibility of applying volumetric analysis to contrast-enhanced real-time 3D datasets obtained in patients with suboptimal image quality was recently tested. This approach allows quantification of global [73] as well as regional [74] LV function, when used with selective dual triggering at end-systole and end-diastole to reduce the destructive effects of ultrasound on contrast microbubbles.

Future directions

Future advances in transducer and computer technology will allow wider angle acquisition and color flow imaging to be completed in a single cardiac cycle, which will shorten data acquisition and eliminate stitching artifacts. The transducers will have a smaller footprint and weight with higher spatial and temporal resolution. In

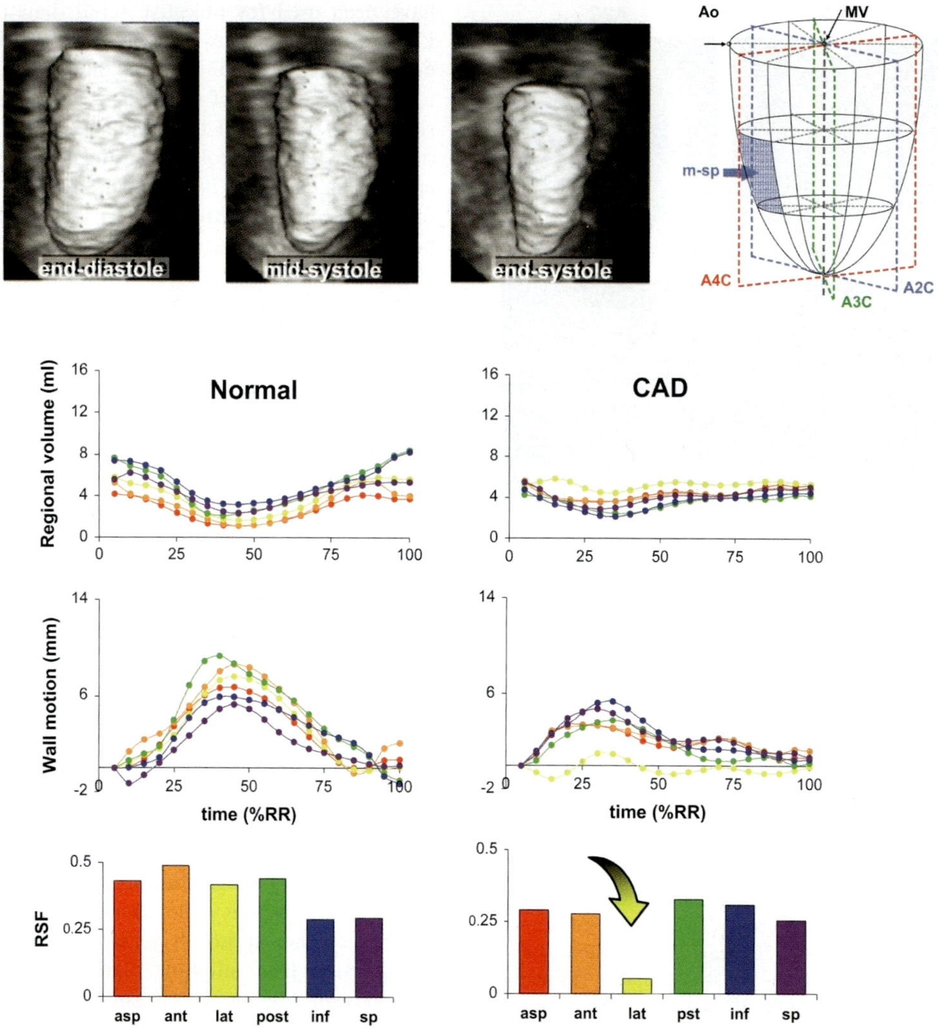

Fig. 4. Volumetric analysis of regional LV function. Example of LV endocardial surface detected from a 3D dataset at three different phases of the cardiac cycle, superimposed on cross-sectional long axis plane (*top left*). Schematic representation of the 3D segmentation model. A2C, A3C, and A4C, apical 2-, 3-, and 4-chamber planes; MV, central point of the mitral valve; Ao, central point of the aortic annulus (*top right*). Shaded area is an example of an LV endocardial surface segment representing the mid-septal (m-sp) wall. Below are examples of regional volume and wall motion time curves and regional shortening fraction (RSF) in six apical segments, obtained in a normal subject (*left*) and a patient with coronary artery disease (CAD, *right*) and hypokinesis in the lateral wall (*arrow*). (*Reproduced from* Corsi C, Lang RM, Veronesi F, et al. Volumetric quantification of global and regional left ventricular function from real-time 3D echocardiographic images. Circulation 2005;112:1161–70; with permission.)

addition, transducers capable of 2D imaging only will be gradually phased out and replaced by new probes that will be versatile in their capability of imaging in different modes, including 2D, 3D, color, and tissue Doppler. With these multitasking transducers, it may be possible to significantly reduce the number of steps required to complete an echocardiographic examination, and thus reduce the time of the test. For example, the standard 2D views could theoretically be obtained from a single volumetric dataset and used for diagnostic purposes assuming that both spatial and temporal resolution are sufficiently high. Significant improvements from the current state of the art are needed in the temporal resolution as well as in the spatial resolution in the far field. We

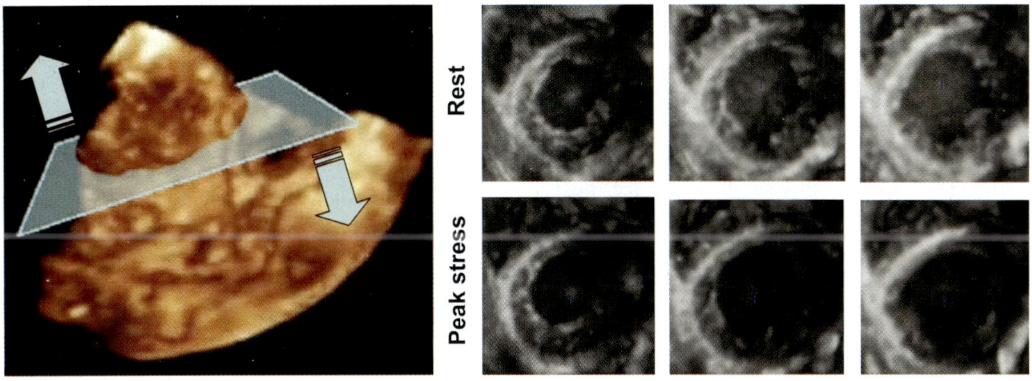

Fig. 5. Off-line viewing of real-time 3D data obtained during dobutamine stress test. These datasets can be used to extract multiple short-axis views at different levels of the left ventricle (*left*). Example of such views extracted from datasets obtained at rest and during peak dobutamine stress (*right*).

also anticipate that the quantification of all cardiac chambers, including flow dynamics, will be performed on the imaging system in an increasingly automated fashion, thus gradually eliminating the need for off-line analysis.

Summary

In the next years, we anticipate that real-time 3D imaging will continue to be integrated into the routine echocardiographic examination. Presently,

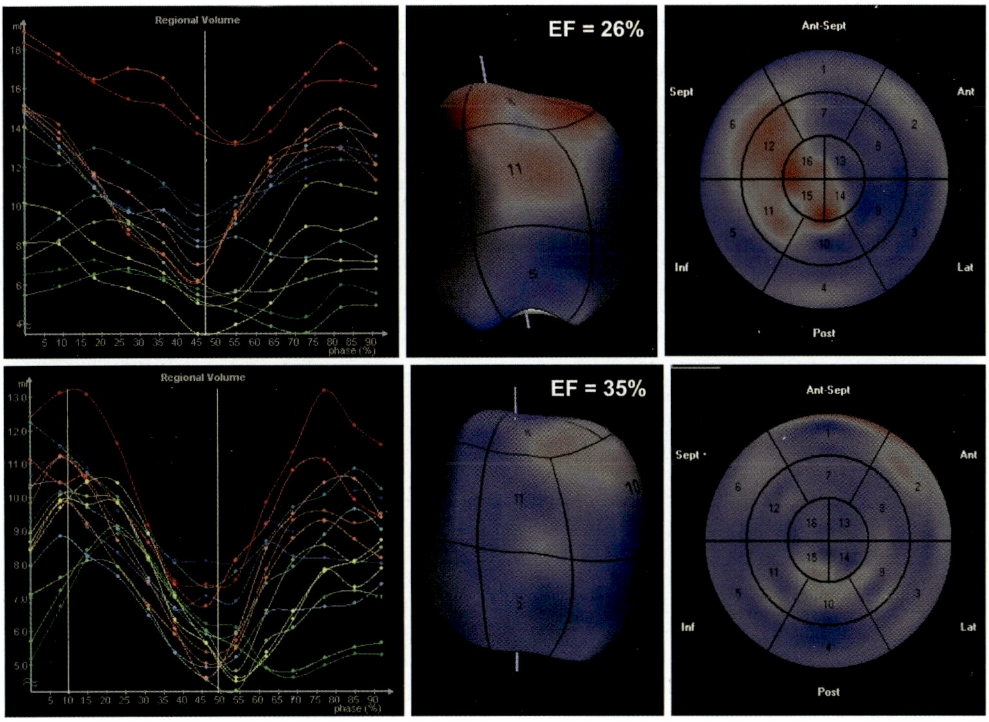

Fig. 6. Assessment of the improvement in synchrony of LV contraction with pacing. Regional volume time curves (*left*) obtained in a patient with LV dyssynchrony without (*top*) and with (*bottom*) biventricular pacing. Endocardial surfaces reconstructed from each dataset are shown with segmentation and color-coding according to regional time to end ejection (*middle*) along with the bull's eye representation of the same data (*right*). Note the changes in colors with pacing reflecting the effects of resynchronization therapy in this parametric display.

there is sufficient evidence to prove that 3D imaging is superior to the traditional 2D techniques and should be routinely used for the quantification of LV volume, EF, and mass. Future clinical applications of this technology are likely to include stress testing with real-time volumetric or simultaneous multiplane imaging from a single transducer position. Volumetric assessment of ventricular asynchrony will be used as an additional tool to guide resynchronization therapy. Also, miniaturization of the matrix-array transducer technology will enable the acquisition of real-time 3D transesophageal images.

References

[1] Parisi AF, Moynihan PF, Feldman CL, et al. Approaches to determination of left ventricular volume and ejection fraction by real-time two-dimensional echocardiography. Clin Cardiol 1979;2:257–63.

[2] Schiller NB, Acquatella H, Ports TA, et al. Left ventricular volume from paired biplane two-dimensional echocardiography. Circulation 1979;60: 547–55.

[3] Erbel R, Krebs W, Henn G, et al. Comparison of single-plane and biplane volume determination by two-dimensional echocardiography. 1. Asymmetric model hearts. Eur Heart J 1982;3:469–80.

[4] Schnittger I, Fitzgerald PJ, Daughters GT, et al. Limitations of comparing left ventricular volumes by two dimensional echocardiography, myocardial markers and cineangiography. Am J Cardiol 1982; 50:512–9.

[5] Weiss JL, Eaton LW, Kallman CH, et al. Accuracy of volume determination by two-dimensional echocardiography: defining requirements under controlled conditions in the ejecting canine left ventricle. Circulation 1983;67:889–95.

[6] Kuroda T, Seward JB, Rumberger JA, et al. Left ventricular volume and mass: comparative study of two-dimensional echocardiography and ultrafast computed tomography. Echocardiography 1994; 11:1–9.

[7] Bernard Y, Meneveau N, Boucher S, et al. Lack of agreement between left ventricular volumes and ejection fraction determined by two-dimensional echocardiography and contrast cineangiography in postinfarction patients. Echocardiography 2001;18: 113–22.

[8] Edelman SK, Rowe DW, Pechacek LW, et al. Left ventricular volumes and ejection fraction derived from apical two-dimensional echocardiography. Cardiovasc Dis 1981;8:344–54.

[9] Kan G, Visser CA, Lie KI, et al. Left ventricular volumes and ejection fraction by single plane two-dimensional apex echocardiography. Eur Heart J 1981;2:339–43.

[10] Gordon EP, Schnittger I, Fitzgerald PJ, et al. Reproducibility of left ventricular volumes by two-dimensional echocardiography. J Am Coll Cardiol 1983;2:506–13.

[11] Gopal AS, Keller AM, Rigling R, et al. Left ventricular volume and endocardial surface area by three-dimensional echocardiography: comparison with two-dimensional echocardiography and nuclear magnetic resonance imaging in normal subjects. J Am Coll Cardiol 1993;22:258–70.

[12] Jacobs LD, Salgo IS, Goonewardena S, et al. Rapid online quantification of left ventricular volume from real-time three-dimensional echocardiographic data. Eur Heart J 2006;27:460–8.

[13] Matsumoto M, Inoue M, Tamura S, et al. Three-dimensional echocardiography for spatial visualization and volume calculation of cardiac structures. J Clin Ultrasound 1981;9:157–65.

[14] Stickels KR, Wann LS. An analysis of three-dimensional reconstructive echocardiography. Ultrasound Med Biol 1984;10:575–80.

[15] McPherson DD, Skorton DJ, Kodiyalam S, et al. Finite element analysis of myocardial diastolic function using three-dimensional echocardiographic reconstructions: application of a new method for study of acute ischemia in dogs. Circ Res 1987;60: 674–82.

[16] Fulton DR, Marx GR, Pandian NG, et al. Dynamic three-dimensional echocardiographic imaging of congenital heart defects in infants and children by computer-controlled tomographic parallel slicing using a single integrated ultrasound instrument. Echocardiography 1994;11:155–64.

[17] Bartel T, Muller S, Erbel R. Dynamic three-dimensional echocardiography using parallel slicing: a promising diagnostic procedure in adults with congenital heart disease. Cardiology 1998;89:140–7.

[18] Ludomirsky A, Vermilion R, Nesser J, et al. Transthoracic real-time three-dimensional echocardiography using the rotational scanning approach for data acquisition. Echocardiography 1994;11:599–606.

[19] Roelandt J, Salustri A, Mumm B, et al. Precordial three-dimensional echocardiography with a rotational imaging probe: methods and initial clinical experience. Echocardiography 1995;12:243–52.

[20] Delabays A, Pandian NG, Cao QL, et al. Transthoracic real-time three-dimensional echocardiography using a fan-like scanning approach for data acquisition: methods, strengths, problems, and initial clinical experience. Echocardiography 1995;12: 49–59.

[21] Raichlen JS, Trivedi SS, Herman GT, et al. Dynamic three-dimensional reconstruction of the left ventricle from two-dimensional echocardiograms. J Am Coll Cardiol 1986;8:364–70.

[22] King DL, Harrison MR, King DL Jr, et al. Improved reproducibility of left atrial and left ventricular measurements by guided three-dimensional echocardiography. J Am Coll Cardiol 1992;20:1238–45.

[23] Sapin PM, Schroeder KD, Smith MD, et al. Three-dimensional echocardiographic measurement of left ventricular volume in vitro: comparison with two-dimensional echocardiography and cineventriculography. J Am Coll Cardiol 1993;22:1530–7.
[24] Siu SC, Rivera JM, Guerrero JL, et al. Three-dimensional echocardiography. In vivo validation for left ventricular volume and function. Circulation 1993; 88:1715–23.
[25] von Ramm OT, Smith SW. Real time volumetric ultrasound imaging system. J Digit Imaging 1990; 3:261–6.
[26] Sheikh K, Smith SW, von Ramm OT, et al. Real-time, three-dimensional echocardiography: feasibility and initial use. Echocardiography 1991;8:119–25.
[27] Ota T, Fleishman CE, Strub M, et al. Real-time, three-dimensional echocardiography: feasibility of dynamic right ventricular volume measurement with saline contrast. Am Heart J 1999;137:958–66.
[28] Schmidt MA, Ohazama CJ, Agyeman KO, et al. Real-time three-dimensional echocardiography for measurement of left ventricular volumes. Am J Cardiol 1999;84:1434–9.
[29] Shiota T, McCarthy PM, White RD, et al. Initial clinical experience of real-time three-dimensional echocardiography in patients with ischemic and idiopathic dilated cardiomyopathy. Am J Cardiol 1999;84:1068–73.
[30] Binder TM, Rosenhek R, Porenta G, et al. Improved assessment of mitral valve stenosis by volumetric real-time three-dimensional echocardiography. J Am Coll Cardiol 2000;36:1355–61.
[31] Qin JX, Jones M, Shiota T, et al. Validation of real-time three-dimensional echocardiography for quantifying left ventricular volumes in the presence of a left ventricular aneurysm: in vitro and in vivo studies. J Am Coll Cardiol 2000;36:900–7.
[32] Yalcin F, Shiota T, Odabashian J, et al. Comparison by real-time three-dimensional echocardiography of left ventricular geometry in hypertrophic cardiomyopathy versus secondary left ventricular hypertrophy. Am J Cardiol 2000;85:1035–8.
[33] Qin JJ, Jones M, Shiota T, et al. New digital measurement methods for left ventricular volume using real-time three-dimensional echocardiography: comparison with electromagnetic flow method and magnetic resonance imaging. Eur J Echocardiogr 2000;1:96–104.
[34] Schindera ST, Mehwald PS, Sahn DJ, et al. Accuracy of real-time three-dimensional echocardiography for quantifying right ventricular volume: static and pulsatile flow studies in an anatomic in vitro model. J Ultrasound Med 2002;21:1069–75.
[35] Sugeng L, Weinert L, Thiele K, et al. Real-time three-dimensional echocardiography using a novel matrix array transducer. Echocardiography 2003; 20:623–35.
[36] Zeidan Z, Erbel R, Barkhausen J, et al. Analysis of global systolic and diastolic left ventricular performance using volume-time curves by real-time three-dimensional echocardiography. J Am Soc Echocardiogr 2003;16:29–37.
[37] Arai K, Hozumi T, Matsumura Y, et al. Accuracy of measurement of left ventricular volume and ejection fraction by new real-time three-dimensional echocardiography in patients with wall motion abnormalities secondary to myocardial infarction. Am J Cardiol 2004;94:552–8.
[38] Jenkins C, Bricknell K, Hanekom L, et al. Reproducibility and accuracy of echocardiographic measurements of left ventricular parameters using real-time three-dimensional echocardiography. J Am Coll Cardiol 2004;44:878–86.
[39] Kuhl HP, Schreckenberg M, Rulands D, et al. High-resolution transthoracic real-time three-dimensional echocardiography: quantitation of cardiac volumes and function using semi-automatic border detection and comparison with cardiac magnetic resonance imaging. J Am Coll Cardiol 2004;43:2083–90.
[40] Corsi C, Lang RM, Veronesi F, et al. Volumetric quantification of global and regional left ventricular function from real-time three-dimensional echocardiographic images. Circulation 2005;112:1161–70.
[41] Fleming SM, Cumberledge B, Kiesewetter C, et al. Usefulness of real-time three-dimensional echocardiography for reliable measurement of cardiac output in patients with ischemic or idiopathic dilated cardiomyopathy. Am J Cardiol 2005;95:308–10.
[42] Jenkins C, Bricknell K, Marwick TH. Use of real-time three-dimensional echocardiography to measure left atrial volume: comparison with other echocardiographic techniques. J Am Soc Echocardiogr 2005;18:991–7.
[43] van den Bosch AE, Robbers-Visser D, Krenning BJ, et al. Real-time transthoracic three-dimensional echocardiographic assessment of left ventricular volume and ejection fraction in congenital heart disease. J Am Soc Echocardiogr 2006;19:1–6.
[44] Bashein G, Sheehan FH, Nessly ML, et al. Three-dimensional transesophageal echocardiography for depiction of regional left-ventricular performance: initial results and future directions. Int J Card Imaging 1993;9:121–31.
[45] Maehle J, Bjoernstad K, Aakhus S, et al. Three-dimensional echocardiography for quantitative left ventricular wall motion analysis: a method for reconstruction of endocardial surface and evaluation of regional dysfunction. Echocardiography 1994; 11:397–408.
[46] Bjornstad K, Maehle J, Aakhus S, et al. Evaluation of reference systems for quantitative wall motion analysis from three-dimensional endocardial surface reconstruction: an echocardiographic study in subjects with and without myocardial infarction. Am J Card Imaging 1996;10:244–53.
[47] Frielingsdorf J, Franke A, Kuhl HP, et al. Evaluation of regional systolic function in hypertrophic cardiomyopathy and hypertensive heart disease:

a three-dimensional echocardiographic study. J Am Soc Echocardiogr 1998;11:778–86.
[48] Ahmad M, Xie T, McCulloch M, et al. Real-time three-dimensional dobutamine stress echocardiography in assessment of ischemia: comparison with two-dimensional dobutamine stress echocardiography. J Am Coll Cardiol 2001;37:1303–9.
[49] Matsumura Y, Hozumi T, Arai K, et al. Non-invasive assessment of myocardial ischaemia using new real-time three-dimensional dobutamine stress echocardiography: comparison with conventional two-dimensional methods. Eur Heart J 2005;26: 1625–32.
[50] Sogaard P, Kim WY, Jensen HK, et al. Impact of acute biventricular pacing on left ventricular performance and volumes in patients with severe heart failure. A tissue Doppler and three-dimensional echocardiographic study. Cardiology 2001;95: 173–82.
[51] Smith SW, Light ED, Idriss SF, et al. Feasibility study of real-time three-dimensional intracardiac echocardiography for guidance of interventional electrophysiology. Pacing Clin Electrophysiol 2002; 25:351–7.
[52] Krenning BJ, Szili-Torok T, Voormolen MM, et al. Guiding and optimization of resynchronization therapy with dynamic three-dimensional echocardiography and segmental volume–time curves: a feasibility study. Eur J Heart Fail 2004; 6:619–25.
[53] van der Heide JA, Mannaerts HF, Spruijt HJ, et al. Noninvasive mapping of left ventricular electromechanical asynchrony by three-dimensional echocardiography and semi automatic contour detection. Am J Cardiol 2004;94:1449–53.
[54] Kapetanakis S, Kearney MT, Siva A, et al. Real-time three-dimensional echocardiography: a novel technique to quantify global left ventricular mechanical dyssynchrony. Circulation 2005;112: 992–1000.
[55] Schroder KM, Sapin PM, King DL, et al. Three-dimensional echocardiographic volume computation: in vitro comparison to standard two-dimensional echocardiography. J Am Soc Echocardiogr 1993;6: 467–75.
[56] Belohlavek M, Foley DA, Seward JB, et al. Diagnostic performance of two-dimensional versus three-dimensional transesophageal echocardiographic images of selected pathologies evaluated by receiver operating characteristic analysis. Echocardiography 1994;11:635–45.
[57] Altmann K, Shen Z, Boxt LM, et al. Comparison of three-dimensional echocardiographic assessment of volume, mass, and function in children with functionally single left ventricles with two-dimensional echocardiography and magnetic resonance imaging. Am J Cardiol 1997;80:1060–5.
[58] Buck T, Hunold P, Wentz KU, et al. Tomographic three-dimensional echocardiographic determination of chamber size and systolic function in patients with left ventricular aneurysm: comparison to magnetic resonance imaging, cineventriculography, and two-dimensional echocardiography. Circulation 1997; 96:4286–97.
[59] Gutierrez-Chico JL, Zamorano JL, de lsla LP, et al. Comparison of left ventricular volumes and ejection fractions measured by three-dimensional echocardiography versus by two-dimensional echocardiography and cardiac magnetic resonance in patients with various cardiomyopathies. Am J Cardiol 2005;95:809–13.
[60] Keller AM, Gopal AS, King DL. Left and right atrial volume by freehand three-dimensional echocardiography: in vivo validation using magnetic resonance imaging. Eur J Echocardiogr 2000;1: 55–65.
[61] Kawai J, Tanabe K, Wang CL, et al. Comparison of left atrial size by freehand scanning three-dimensional echocardiography and two-dimensional echocardiography. Eur J Echocardiogr 2004;5:18–24.
[62] Jiang L, Handschumacher MD, Hibberd MG, et al. Three-dimensional echocardiographic reconstruction of right ventricular volume: in vitro comparison with two-dimensional methods. J Am Soc Echocardiogr 1994;7:150–8.
[63] Dorosz JL, Bolson EL, Waiss MS, et al. Three-dimensional visual guidance improves the accuracy of calculating right ventricular volume with two-dimensional echocardiography. J Am Soc Echocardiogr 2003;16:675–81.
[64] Kjaergaard J, Petersen CL, Kjaer A, et al. Evaluation of right ventricular volume and function by 2D and 3D echocardiography compared to MRI. Eur J Echocardiogr 2005;7:430–8.
[65] Gopal AS, Keller AM, Shen Z, et al. Three-dimensional echocardiography: in vitro and in vivo validation of left ventricular mass and comparison with conventional echocardiographic methods. J Am Coll Cardiol 1994;24:504–13.
[66] Sapin PM, Gopal AS, Clarke GB, et al. Three-dimensional echocardiography compared to two-dimensional echocardiography for measurement of left ventricular mass anatomic validation in an open chest canine model. Am J Hypertens 1996;9:467–74.
[67] Rodevand O, Bjornerheim R, Kolbjornsen O, et al. Left ventricular mass assessed by three-dimensional echocardiography using rotational acquisition. Clin Cardiol 1997;20:957–62.
[68] Kuhl HP, Hanrath P, Franke A. M-mode echocardiography overestimates left ventricular mass in patients with normal left ventricular shape: a comparative study using three-dimensional echocardiography. Eur J Echocardiogr 2003;4:312–9.
[69] Mor-Avi V, Sugeng L, Weinert L, et al. Fast measurement of left ventricular mass with real-time three-dimensional echocardiography: comparison with magnetic resonance imaging. Circulation 2004;110: 1814–8.

[70] Caiani EG, Corsi C, Sugeng L, et al. Improved quantification of left ventricular mass based on endocardial and epicardial surface detection with real time three dimensional echocardiography. Heart 2006; 92:213–9.

[71] van den Bosch AE, Robbers-Visser D, Krenning BJ, et al. Comparison of real-time three-dimensional echocardiography to magnetic resonance imaging for assessment of left ventricular mass. Am J Cardiol 2006;97:113–7.

[72] Takeuchi M, Otani S, Weinert L, et al. Comparison of contrast-enhanced real-time live 3-dimensional dobutamine stress echocardiography with contrast 2-dimensional echocardiography for detecting stress-induced wall-motion abnormalities. J Am Soc Echocardiogr 2006;19:294–9.

[73] Caiani EG, Coon P, Corsi C, et al. Dual triggering improves the accuracy of left ventricular volume measurements by contrast-enhanced real-time 3-dimensional echocardiography. J Am Soc Echocardiogr 2005;18:1292–8.

[74] Corsi C, Coon P, Goonewardena S, et al. Quantification of regional left ventricular wall motion from real-time 3-dimensional echocardiography in patients with poor acoustic windows: effects of contrast enhancement tested against cardiac magnetic resonance. J Am Soc Echocardiogr 2006;19: 886–93.

ELSEVIER
SAUNDERS

Cardiol Clin 25 (2007) 253–260

CARDIOLOGY
CLINICS

Intraventricular Dyssynchrony Assessment by Real-Time Three-Dimensional Echocardiography

Joseph A. Horstman, MD[a], Mark J. Monaghan, MD, PhD[b], Edward A. Gill, MD, FACC, FASE, FACP[c,*]

[a]*University of Washington School of Medicine, 325 Ninth Avenue, Seattle, WA 98104, USA*
[b]*King's College Hospital, Denmark Hill, London, UK*
[c]*Department of Medicine, Division of Cardiology, University of Washington School of Medicine, Harborview Medical Center, 325 Ninth Avenue, Box 359748, Seattle, WA 98104, USA*

Heart failure is extremely prevalent in the United States and worldwide, particularly in developed countries. In the United States, 4.7 million people or 2% of the population are affected by heart failure, and 550,000 new cases are diagnosed every year. Further, heart failure accounts for more than 45,000 United States deaths annually [1–3]. Heart failure is the single most frequent reason for hospitalization in the elderly [4,5]. Although there is considerable evidence that heart failure prognosis is improving, recent data from Sweden demonstrated that patients admitted to the hospital with the chief diagnosis of heart failure have a 25% 1-year mortality, an outcome worse than most cancers [6]. Moreover, mortality at 3 years remains greater than 25%, and 5-year mortality still approaches 50%. Based on heart failure patients' annual expenditures of $10,832, the annual expenditure for heart failure in the United States is as much as $48 billion [3]. Hence, it is clear that heart failure is a very significant problem, from morbidity, mortality, and cost standpoints. As technology and pharmaceutics provide more advanced treatments for heart failure, the cost obviously increases.

At least 40% of patients who have congestive heart failure have conduction system disease evidenced by a wide QRS on 12-lead ECG but only 30% have a QRS wider than 120 milliseconds [7–9]. Biventricular pacing has now become well established as an important therapy in patients suffering heart failure who remain symptomatic despite optimal medical therapy and who have evidence of dyssynchrony documented by a wide QRS duration. Indeed, biventricular pacing has been shown to increase functional capacity, improve quality of life, and even confer a mortality benefit, the latter based on the Cardiac Resynchronization in Heart Failure (CARE-HF) trial results [10]. Currently, only patients who have a QRS duration of 120 milliseconds or more are recommend for biventricular pacing. Paradoxically, mechanical asynchrony defined by echocardiographic parameters is present in up to 43% of heart failure patients who have a narrow QRS duration (<120 milliseconds) [11].

Correctly choosing the patients who will respond favorably to biventricular pacing has emerged as one of the important challenges for cardiologists and other physicians taking care of heart failure patients. This choice is difficult because the current selection criteria for dyssynchrony—a QRS of 120 milliseconds or greater—results in approximately 30% nonresponders. Paradoxically, 20% to 50% of patients who have a QRS less than 120 milliseconds have dyssynchrony documented by advanced echocardiography techniques. At least 45% of patients who have a narrow QRS and dyssynchrony apparently respond to therapy [11–13].

In fact, when dyssynchrony is well documented by all of the echocardiographic methods, the response to therapy tends to be favorable regardless

* Corresponding author.
E-mail address: eagill@u.washington.edu (E.A. Gill).

0733-8651/07/$ - see front matter
doi:10.1016/j.ccl.2007.05.004

of the QRS duration [14–19]. Therefore, it seems essential to develop more advanced techniques for defining dyssynchrony and to test those techniques for prediction of response to biventricular pacing. If such techniques truly define additional patients who respond to biventricular pacing, then the techniques need to be adopted by third-party payers, particularly CMS (Medicare) in the United States. More specifically, it is critical that such techniques more accurately identify those patients who would respond to biventricular pacing such that when compared with QRS duration, additional patients would be eligible for pacing and patients who currently do not respond to pacing would not be chosen such that the paradigm for this relatively expensive treatment is changed. It is clear, however, that despite substantial breakthroughs in the field, development of such an optimal test for biventricular pacing is a daunting task. In that regard, 3D echocardiography (3D echo) offers robust tomographic imaging of the left ventricle that may be capitalized on to provide a more accurate and reproducible index of left ventricular (LV) dyssynchrony than current techniques. In addition, 3D echo is unique in that it allows dyssynchrony comparison of all myocardial segments (including the apex) rather than those contained within a 2D scan plane.

Current techniques of dyssynchrony evaluation

Current techniques of echocardiography use regional velocity, strain, and strain rate using tissue Doppler, gray-scale tracking, or both. Currently, the time to maximum velocity of each of the 12 nonapical LV segments is typically analyzed. The SD of these 12 time increments has become arguably the most popular echocardiographic measure of dyssynchrony and also has the most robust compilation of verification data. In some circles, this approach is referred to as the Yu index because it was developed and largely validated by C. M. Yu [18]. Other methods include the opposing wall index, an index that uses the same data of time to peak systolic velocity, but instead of determining the SD, it compares the time to peak velocity between the anteroseptal and posterior, the anterior and inferior, and the septal and lateral walls. A difference of 65 milliseconds is considered consistent with dyssynchrony [15]. Regional strain and strain rate have also been used to evaluate dyssynchrony, but in most investigators hands, these rates have been inferior to tissue Doppler, mainly because the waveforms are relatively "noisy." The one clear exception has been strain determined by gray-scale speckle imaging, a technique that seems to correlate well with tissue Doppler–derived measures of dyssynchrony [20].

3D echo approach to dyssynchrony

3D echo offers a novel approach for identification of intraventicular dyssynchrony. Using semiautomated LV endocardial edge detection, or by partially automated tracing of multiple ventricular views, 3D echo allows functional assessment of all 16 individual segments of the left ventricle. By integrating the function of all the segments, a simple, reproducible method for quantifying global LV dyssynchrony was developed by Monaghan and colleagues [21].

The real-time 3D echo approach uses a dense-array 3D transducer such as the X4 matrix transducer used on the Philips ie33 (Philips Medical Systems, Bothel, Washington and Andover, Massachusetts). This transducer has roughly 3000 active elements that are continuously sending and receiving data, resulting in real-time 3D volume rendering. General Electric also manufactures a matrix transducer that reportedly is somewhat similar in design. This approach typically cannot capture the entire LV volume but captures a series of relatively narrow sector–width subvolumes (typically 30° × 50°). Between 4 and 7 of these subvolumes are "stitched" together to provide a full-volume dataset. The result is a pyramidal data set, technically a "frustum," because the far-field capture is curved (105° × 105°). These data can then be cropped to create orthogonal views equivalent to the apical four- and two-chamber views. From there, manual tracing or semiautomated endocardial border techniques are applied using software developed by TomTec (Munich, Germany) or Philips Medical Systems (Fig. 1). After application of the tracing or edge detection algorithm, an LV cast is created that shows the individual 16 segments of the left ventricle (Fig. 2). From this 16-segment cast of the LV cavity, individual pyramidal subvolumes are created using mathematic modeling, with a nonfixed centerline of the ventricle used as the starting point for the volumes. The pyramidal volumes then protrude outward from the centerline to the edge of the ventricle. By using these pyramidal subvolumes of the entire left ventricle, it is possible to display time–volume data that correspond to each of the 16 standard myocardial

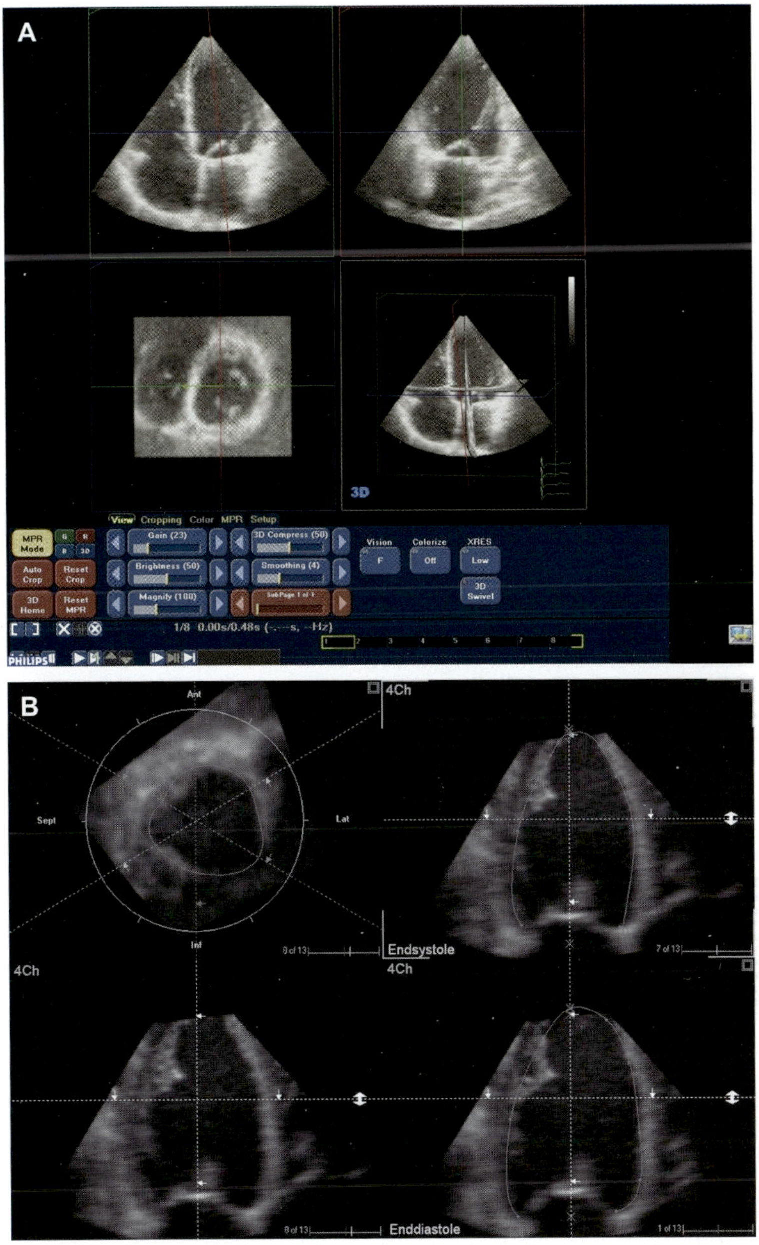

Fig. 1. A 3D data set is displayed after cropping. Cropping results in the display of three orthogonal planes of data. (*A*) Top left is the four-chamber view, top right is the two-chamber view, and bottom left is the short-axis view. The entire volume of the heart is shown in the bottom right view, with the partial cut-out showing the summarizing of the orthogonal views displayed in the other views. This data set is an example of cropping using Philips Q Lab. (*B*) A similar example using TomTec software for cropping. The orientation is different, with the short-axis view in the upper left and orthogonal apical views shown in the remaining views.

segments, as defined by the American Society of Echocardiography [22]. When all 16 segments reach minimum systolic volume at nearly the same time, synchrony is present. Conversely, when the points of minimum systolic volume show great variation (defined in the next section) between segments, there is intraventricular dyssynchrony (Fig. 3).

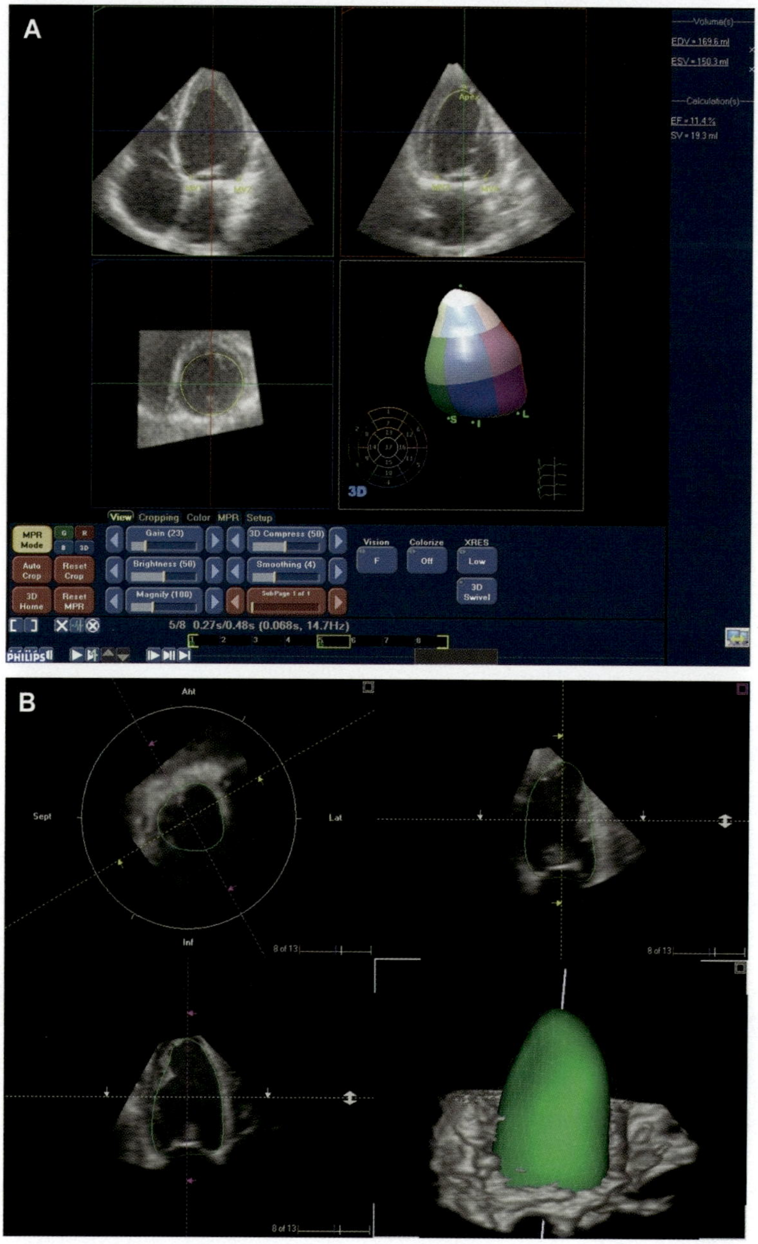

Fig. 2. A "cast" of the ventricle is displayed with the individual segments by Philips Q Lab (*A*) and without the individual segments with using TomTec software (*B*).

Development of an index to quantify left ventricular dyssynchrony with real-time 3D echocardiography

A dyssynchrony index has been devised by measuring the time from the onset of the cardiac cycle (defined as the start of the R wave) to the minimum systolic volume for each segment, and then calculating the SD. The systolic dyssynchrony index (SDI) is the SD expressed as a percentage of the duration of the entire cardiac cycle. Higher SDI levels represent higher levels of dyssynchrony, and vice versa. SDI can be expressed as a percentage of the cardiac cycle rather

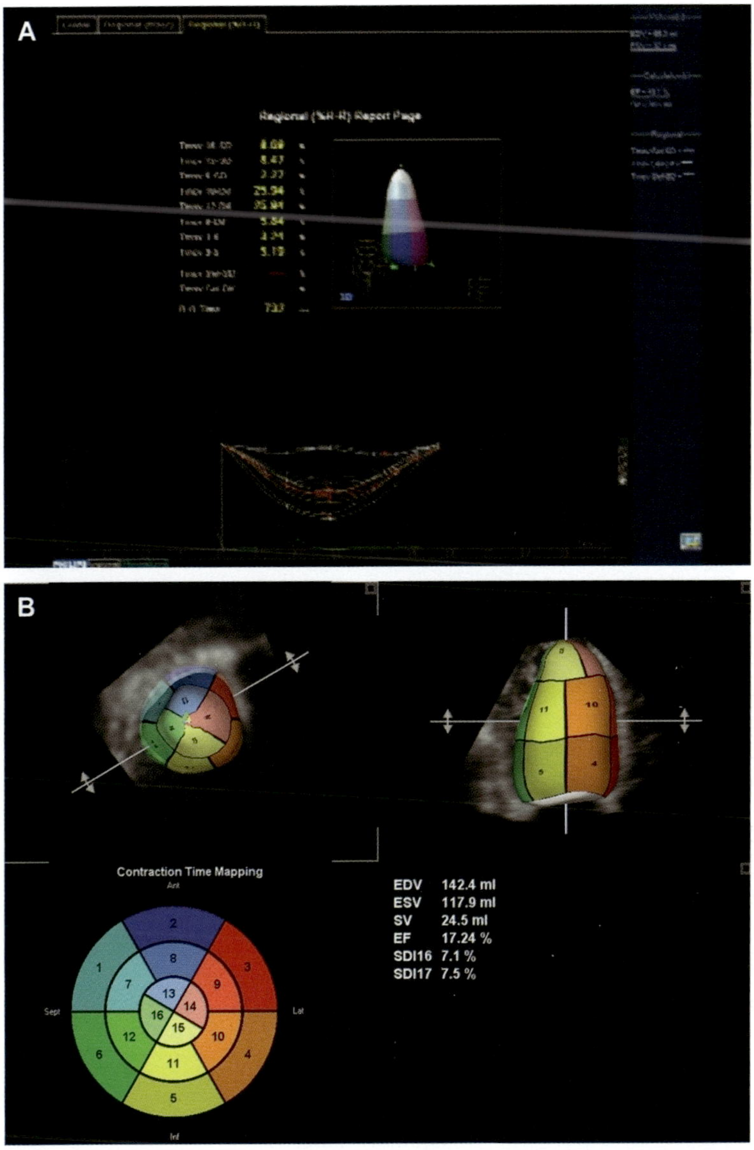

Fig. 3. (*A*) Normal synchrony, with time volume curves converging on a near-single time point. (*B–D*) Dyssynchrony, with the minimum volumes occurring at very different time frames for most segments. *A* and C are examples of analyzing the ventricle for dyssynchrony with Philips Q Lab and *B* and *D* are with TomTec software. Note that *B* shows the ability to calculate dyssynchrony by the 16- or 17-segment model.

than in milliseconds to allow comparisons between patients who have different heart rates.

Establishing a normal value for the systolic dyssynchrony index

A normal value for SDI was established based on the average for normal volunteers plus 3 SDs. Because healthy volunteers had an SDI of 3.5+/−, the normal was established as 8.3%. Note that the average for patients with normal left ventricular ejection fraction was 4.5±2.4%. Hence an alternate "normal" for patients might be considered to be 11.7 [21]. However, since it is now postulated that even patients with normal left ventricular systolic function may have dyssynchrony [23], the

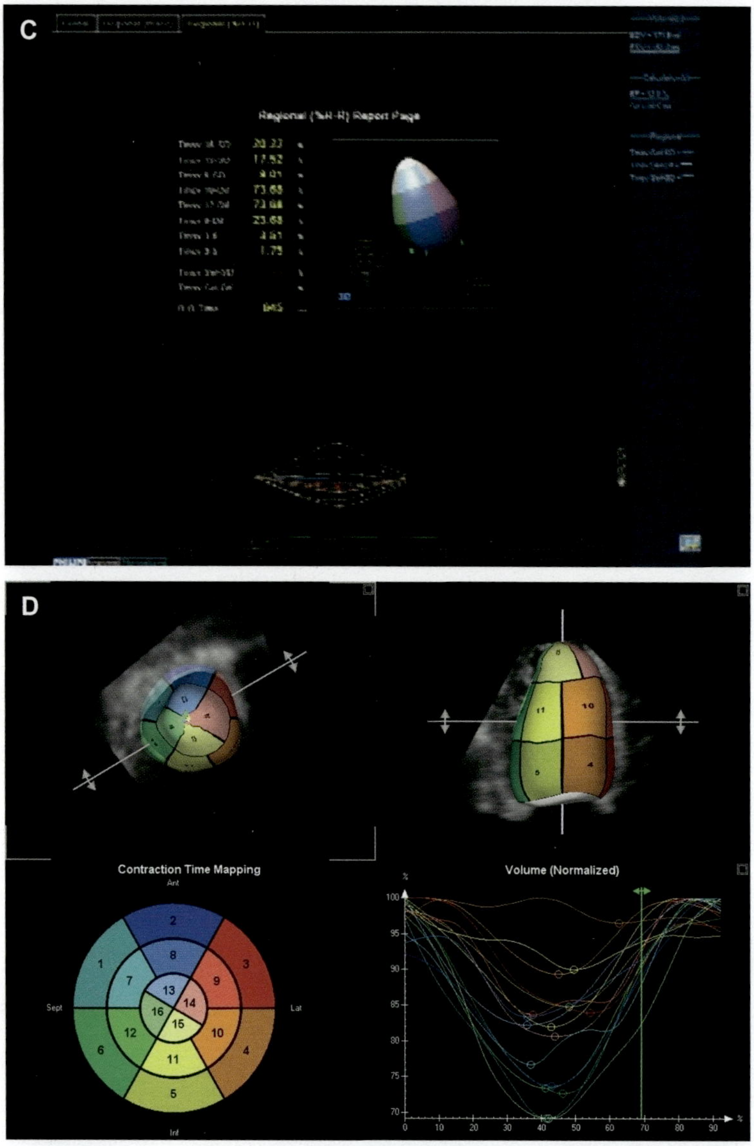

Fig. 3 (*continued*)

former normal value is likely more clinically applicable.

Response of the systolic dyssynchrony index to cardiac resynchronization therapy

The experience with SDI in response to biventricular pacing (cardiac resynchronization therapy [CRT]) is limited; however, in a small sample of patients (N = 26), Monaghan and colleagues reported significant improvement in SDI with CRT [21]. Yu and colleagues [18] saw improvement in the SDI when pacing was turned on versus turned off. Gill and colleagues (unpublished data, 2007) also found a significant improvement in a small group of patients. Clearly, a larger experience with CRT and SDI is needed to draw more concise conclusions. Of interest, Monaghan and colleagues [24] recently presented in abstract form a study of 81 patients before and after CRT by real-time 3D echo, with similar results as reported in their initial study [21].

Systolic dyssynchrony index compared with other indices of dyssynchrony

Monaghan and colleagues [24] compared the SDI to the SD of time to peak systolic velocity by tissue Doppler developed by Yu; there was little correlation, with an *r* value of 0.26 (nonsignificant *P* value). In data compiled in the authors' laboratory (Gill and colleagues, unpublished data, 2007), an essentially identical *r* value was found, but with tighter SD (significant *P* value). This result is in marked contrast to recent data by Takeuchi and colleagues [25]. As noted earlier, Yu and colleagues [18,20] evaluated SDI when CRT was turned off and compared it to when patients had CRT turned on. They found the 16-segment SD to be 70 ± 19 (CRT off) versus 46 ± 14 (CRT on). Notable is that although these investigators used the SDI not corrected for R-R interval, their SDI values correlated much better than the authors' values with the 12-segment SD ($r = 0.739$).

Correlation with maximum opposing wall difference was also minor. In fact, SDI correlated best with variables of ventricular systolic function, specifically the ejection fraction, fractional shortening, and wall motion score index. These data are summarized in Tables 1 and 2.

Table 1
Correlations of SDI with other echocardiography parameters and QRS

Parameters	*r*	*P*
LVEF	0.794	<.0001
FS	0.635	<.0001
WMSI	0.547	<.0001
MPI	0.520	<.0001
SPWMD	0.406	<.0001
EDV	0.580	<.0001
QRS	0.264	.0005
SD-Ti	0.330	.0205
SD-Ts	0.264	.0640
SD-Te	0.169	.2466
SD-Ta	0.334	.203
SD- T€	0.470	.0021

Abbreviations: EDV, end diastolic volume; FS, fractional shortening; LVEF, left ventricular ejection fraction; MPI, Myocardial Performance Index; SPWMD, difference between maximal excursion of the septal and posterior wall by M mode; SD-T€, SD of time to minimum strain; SD-Ta, SD of time to late diastolic peak velocity; SD-Te, SD of time to early diastolic peak velocity; SD-Ti, SD of time to isometric contraction; SD-Ts, SD of time to maximum systolic velocity; WMSI, wall motion score index.

Data from Kapetanakis S, Kearney MT, Siva A. Real-time 3D echocardiography: a novel technique to quantify global left ventricular mechanical dyssynchrony. Circulation 2005;112:992–1000.

Table 2
Correlations of SDI with other echocardiography parameters and QRS

Parameters	*r*	*P*
LVEF	0.71	<.001
SPWMD	0.377	.0013
QRS	0.46	<.001
SD-Ts	0.26	.022
SD-Te	0.185	.11
SD- T€	0.07	.54

Abbreviations: LVEF, left ventricular ejection fraction; SPWMD, difference between maximal excursion of the septal and posterior wall by M mode; SD-T€, SD of time to minimum strain; SD-Te, SD of time to early diastolic peak velocity; WMSI, wall motion score index.

Summary

Real-time 3D echo is a feasible, relatively easy, and reproducible method to evaluate LV systolic function and intraventricular dyssynchrony. Correlation with tissue Doppler indices has been modest in the authors' experience, but other investigators have found more robust correlation [25]. Dyssynchrony by 3D echo inversely correlates with ejection fraction in a tight manner. Additional studies are needed to further correlate the 3D index of intraventricular dys-snchrony with responders to biventricular pacing. Particularly, more patients need to be followed with 3D echo before and after biventricular pacing is instituted. In addition, follow-up of biventricular pacing beyond 6 months will establish the longevity of benefit from biventricular pacing and the longevity of the 3D index over time. At this point, there are two significantly different algorithms for calculating the dyssynchrony index by 3D echo. Both are now largely automated but result in somewhat different results. Again, more studies are necessary to further establish the reliability of the two indices.

References

[1] Ghali JK, Cooper R, Ford E. Trends in hospitalization rates for heart failure in the United States 1973–1986: evidence for increasing population prevalence. Arch Inten Med 1990;150:769–73.

[2] Jessup M. The less familiar face of heart failure. J Am Coll Cardiol 2003;41:224–6.

[3] Liao L, Anstrom KJ, Gottdiener JS, et al. Long-term costs and resource use in elderly participants with congestive heart failure in the Cardiovascular Health Study. Am Heart J 2007;153(2):245–52.
[4] Croft JB, Giles WH, Pollard RA, et al. National trends in the initial hospitalization for heart failure. J Am Geriatr Soc 1997;45:270–5.
[5] Schulman KA, Mark DB, Califf RM, et al. Outcomes and costs within a disease management program for advanced congestive heart failure. Am Heart J 1998;135:S285–92.
[6] Schaufelberger M, Swedberg K, Koster M, et al. Decreasing one-year mortality and hospitalization rates for heart failure in Sweden: data from the Swedish Hospital Discharge Registry 1988 to 2000. Eur Heart J 2004;25:300–7.
[7] Bader H, Garrigue S, Lafitte S, et al. Intra-left ventricular electromechanical asynchrony. J Am Coll Cardiol 2004;43:248–56.
[8] Freudenberger R, Sikora JA, Fisher M, et al. Electrocardiogram and clinical characteristics of patients referred for cardiac transplantation: implications for pacing in heart failure. Clin Cardiol 2004; 27:151–3.
[9] Kashani A, Barold SS. Significance of QRS complex duration in patients with heart failure. J Am Coll Cardiol 2005;46:2183–92.
[10] Cleland JG, Daubert JC, Erdmann E. The effect of cardiac resynchronization on morbidity and mortality in heart failure. N Engl J Med 2005;352(15): 1539–49.
[11] Yu C-M, Chan Y-S, Zhang Q, et al. Benefits of cardiac resynchronization therapy for heart failure patients with narrow QRS complexes and coexisting systolic asynchrony by echocardiography. J Am Coll Cardiol 2006;48:2251–7.
[12] Bleeker GB, Holman ER, Steendijk P. Cardiac resynchronization therapy in patients with a narrow QRS complex. J Am Coll Cardiol 2006;48:2243–50.
[13] Bentkover JD, Dorian P, Thibault B, et al. Economic analysis of a randomized trial of biventricular pacing in Canada. Pacing Clin Electrophysiol 2007; 30(1):38–43.
[14] Bax JJ, Marwick TH, Molhoek SG, et al. Left ventricular dyssynchrony predicts benefit of cardiac resynchronization therapy in patients with end-stage heart failure before pacemaker implantation. Am J Cardiol 2003;92:1238–40.
[15] Bax JJ, Bleeker GB, Marwick TH, et al. Left ventricular dyssynchrony predicts response and prognosis after cardiac resynchronization therapy. J Am Coll Cardiol 2004;44:1834–40.
[16] Bordachar P, Lafitte S, Reuter S, et al. Echocardiographic parameters of ventricular dyssynchrony validation in patients with heart failure using sequential biventricular pacing. J Am Coll Cardiol 2004;44:2157–65.
[17] Breithardt OA, Stellbrink C, Kramer AP, et al. Echocardiographic quanitification of left ventricular asynchrony predicts an acute hemodynamic benefit of cardiac resynchronization therapy. J Am Coll Cardiol 2002;40:536–45.
[18] Yu CM, Fung WH, Lin H, et al. Predictors of left ventricular reverse remodeling after cardiac resyncrhonization therapy for heart failure secondary to idiopathic dilated or ischemic cardiomyopathy. Am J Cardiol 2003;91:684–8.
[19] Zhang Q, Yu CK, Fung JWH, et al. Assessment of the effect of cardiac resynchronization therapy on intraventricular mechanical synchronicity by regional volumetric changes. Am J Cardiol 2005; 95:126–9.
[20] Suffoletto MS, Dohi K, Cannesson M, et al. Novel speckle-tracking radial strain from routine black-and-white echocardiographic images to quantify dyssynchrony and predict response to cardiac resyncrhonization therapy. Circulation 2006;113:960–8.
[21] Kapetanakis S, Kearney MT, Siva A. Real-time three-dimensional echocardiography: a novel technique to quantify global left ventricular mechanical dyssynchrony. Circulation 2005;112:992–1000.
[22] Lang RM, Bierig M, Devereaux RB, et al. Recommendations for chamber quantification: a report from the American Society of Echocardiography's Guidelines and Standards Committee and the Chamber Quantification Writing Group, developed in conjunction with the European Association of Echocardiography, a branch of the European Society of Cardiology. J Am Soc Echocardiogr 2005; 18(12):1440–63.
[23] Wang J, Kurrelmeyer KM, Torre-Amione G, et al. Systolic and diastolic dyssynchrony in patients with diastolic heart failure and the effect of medical therapy. J Am Coll Cardiol 2007;49:88–96.
[24] Monaghan MJ, et al. ACC abstracts, 2007.
[25] Takeuchi M, Sugeng L, Nishikage T, et al. Assessment of left ventricular dyssynchrony with real time 3-dimensional echocardiography: comparison with tissue Doppler imaging. J Am Soc Echocardiogr, in press.

ELSEVIER
SAUNDERS

Cardiol Clin 25 (2007) 261–265

CARDIOLOGY
CLINICS

Real-Time Three-Dimensional Echocardiography in Stress Testing: Bi- and Triplane Imaging for Enhanced Image Acquisition

Andreas Franke, MD*

Medical Clinic I, RWTH University Hospital, Paulwelsstr 30, D52057 Aachen, Germany

Stress echocardiography has become a widely used technique in the hands of the clinical cardiologist for diagnosis and risk stratification of patients who have suspected or known coronary artery disease.

There are still numerous methodological limitations, however, so that it remains difficult to acquire high-quality data and to reproducibly analyze the images. These limitations result in reduced test accuracy and a lack of ability to detect regional myocardial ischemia. Main limitations for conventional 2D stress echocardiography are problems during acquisition on one hand and of data analysis on the other hand. Data acquisition may be impaired by

- Probe positioning errors resulting in inadequate image planes
- A reduced image quality during transthoracic scanning with poor visualization of left ventricular (LV) walls
- The time-consuming serial acquisition of different image planes—the set of different 2D cut planes (parasternal short and long axis, apical four and two-chamber view as well as apical long axis) has to be acquired in a narrow time window during peak stress while wall motion abnormalities exist

Regarding data analysis, subjectivity of image interpretation remains the major problem, which leads to poor interobserver agreement and causes a relevant examiner dependency [1].

Over the last two decades, several attempts have been undertaken to make stress echo easier and less problematic. The use of pharmacological approaches (dobutamine plus atropine) instead of physical stress/exercise may improve image quality and increase the available time for peak level image acquisition. Harmonic imaging with and without contrast enhancement of LV cavity has been demonstrated to improve the endocardial visibility. Thus it will influence the image quality and test accuracy. Other advanced modalities such as tissue Doppler imaging, strain analysis, and color-coded wall motion tracking may facilitate or even replace subjective interpretation in the future. They provide more objective and quantifiable information on wall motion abnormalities. Although promising, because of their complexity, most of these techniques have not made their way into clinical routine. Besides these more technical approaches a human factor may improve test accuracy. Training and higher experience of the examiner lowers interobserver variability and increases test sensitivity, as does a common definition of what wall motion pattern is pathological.

Each of these different approaches was reported to increase stress echo test accuracy. Yet, already the variety of attempts demonstrates that today's 2D stress echocardiography obviously is not perfect.

The development of matrix array transducers and their commercial availability again create new technical possibilities: the simultaneous acquisition of two or three image planes (bi- or triplanar imaging) or even the acquisition of

* Medizinische Klinik I, Universitätsklinikum der RWTH Aachen, Pauwelsstr. 30, D52057 Aachen, Germany.

E-mail address: afranke@ukaachen.de

doi:10.1016/j.ccl.2007.05.007

a complete pyramidal volume data set dramatically decreases the number of serially acquired heart beats. Several of the previously mentioned limitations of conventional 2D stress echo can be solved using this technique. One clear advantage of the bi- and triplane imaging modalities is that intravenous contrast still can be used easily with the conventional 2D harmonic contrast settings. On the other hand, complete pyramidal volume data sets make the use of contrast more complex as the settings in the 3D rendering mode are being worked out.

Method

Matrix array transducers allow different approaches to perform a stress echocardiography. Two (biplanar, orthogonal or in any desired angle) or three triplanar, mostly in 60-degree increments) image planes can be acquired simultaneously (Fig. 1; videos 1 and 2). Bi- and triplanar techniques may serve as a first step toward complete 3D stress echocardiography.

(Access Biplanar stress and echocardiography and Triplanar stress echocardiography in the online version of this article at: http://www.cardiology.theclinics.com.)

The acquisition of wide-angle 3D data sets (so-called full-volume 3D) is based on the serial recording of four narrow subvolumes in consecutive heart beats. Immediately after acquisition, the subsegments are combined to a pyramidal 3D data set with an overall angle of about 80 by 80 degrees, which can comprise a complete LV cavity. Although theoretically more desirable because of complete LV coverage with a full volume, this type of acquisition is not feasible using exercise for stress because of the variable heart rate immediately following stress. Hence, this limitation makes the bi- and triplane imaging modes more desirable. In addition, in the particularly dilated hearts, even using the now-available wider 105 by 105 acquisition pyramid, sometimes not all of the heart can be acquired. Although this too is a problem for 2D echo, it is less so.

Like conventional 2D techniques, 3D echo during the stress echo workflow then is performed at rest, at low and peak stress, and during recovery. Both physical stress (either bicycle or treadmill exercise) and pharmacological stress (mainly dobutamine plus atropine) have been used in combination with 3D techniques. Left heart contrast agents can be applied for better endocardial delineation.

Once the 3D data set is acquired, image planes can be created in every desired orientation. Besides the extraction of conventional two-, three- and four-chamber-views, multiple parallel short axis slices can be used for systematic analysis of regional wall motion analysis. These slices can be extracted manually (Fig. 2) or semiautomatically, as it is meanwhile possible in several commercially available 3D echo machines (Fig. 3; video 3). The last step of stress echo analysis is a side-by-side analysis of the extracted image planes at different stress/exercise levels still is based on subjective interpretation of wall motion abnormalities.

(Access Nine-slices-technique in the online version of this article at: http://www.cardiology.theclinics.com.)

Clinical studies on 3D stress echo

Early studies using first-generation 3D equipment in the late 1990s already demonstrated that

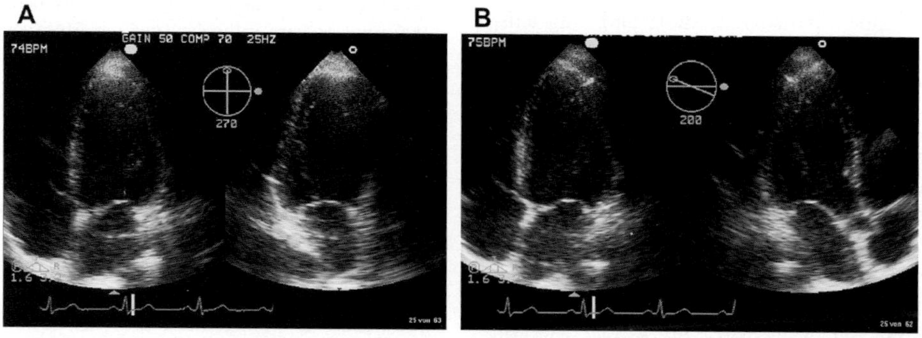

Fig. 1. Biplanar stress echocardiography. Stop frame images demonstrate the image orientation from an apical echo window. Four-chamber view is always shown at the left side, on the right side in (*A*): two-chamber view, in (*B*): apical long axis.

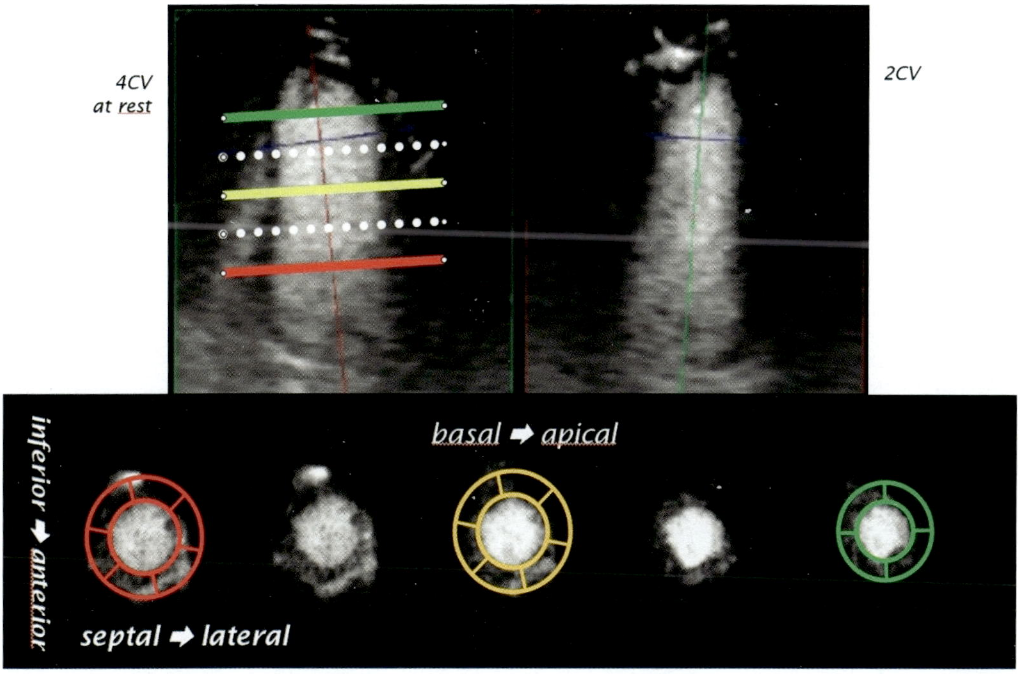

Fig. 2. Cut plane images from a contrast-enhanced 3D data set. Two representative long axis planes (upper panels: four-chamber view, 4CV and two-chamber view, 2CV) and a set of parallel short axis planes from the base (*left*) to the apex (*right lower panel*).

3D volumetric imaging can be used to analyze regional left ventricular wall motion [2]. Other studies even claimed a high sensitivity and superiority over conventional 2D stress echocardiography [3,4]. Overall poor image quality and other technical limitations of the purely 3D dedicated echo system, however, prevented this first approach from widespread clinical use.

Since the advent of the next generation of matrix array transducers, several groups used bi- and triplanar techniques as a first step toward complete 3D stress echo and performed comparative studies versus conventional 2D echo and nuclear imaging [5,6]. The main difference between both stress echo techniques was a significantly shorter scanning time to acquire a triplanar data set covering the complete LV (one loop from an apical window) compared with the serial scanning of three different 2D image planes. Importantly, the shorter scanning time did not reduce test accuracy.

Meanwhile, several recent studies on the use of full-volume 3D stress echocardiography [7–10] also found a good correlation between conventional 2- and 3D stress echo with a nearly identical sensitivity, specificity, and accuracy. The major difference between 2- and 3D echo techniques was a dramatically shorter scanning time to acquire a 3D data set covering the complete LV compared with the serial scanning of three or more different 2D image planes.

As a consequence of these first studies, a possible question of clinical cardiologists will be: If sensitivity and specificity are equivalent, why should one use a matrix array transducer at all and not continue to use a 2D stress echo? There are, however, more advantages of 3D imaging during stress echo workflow than only a shorter scanning time.

First, there is no need to change the transducer position during apical scanning once the echo window is found. This makes acquisition easier and faster for both beginners and expert echocardiographers. Furthermore, image plane positioning errors leading to false-positive or negative 2D stress echo examinations might be avoided.

Second, the narrow time window at peak stress—especially in physical exercise echo—can be used much more effectively when acquiring a complete 3D data set. Another recent publication on biplanar stress echo [5] has demonstrated that this results in a higher heart rate during exercise stress acquisition, a prerequisite for ischemia

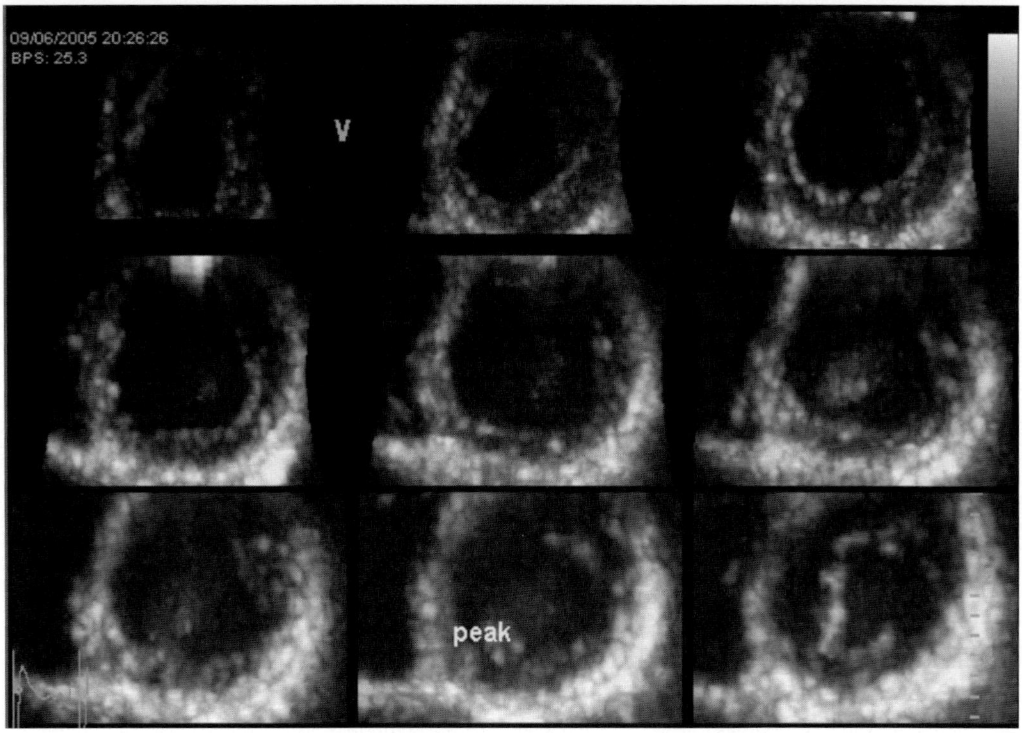

Fig. 3. Modern real-time 3D equipment allows the rapid semiautomatic generation of a set of parallel short axis slices of the LV (nine-slices technique), which makes the interpretation of wall motion abnormalities faster and easier. Stop frame image of nine simultaneously acquired and equidistant short axis slices during peak dobutamine stress. Most apical slice in the upper left corner, most basal slice in the lower right corner.

detection. A shorter time needed for scanning at peak stress and a more complete monitoring (more segments can be observed on-line during stress testing) also reduces the potential risk of prolonged myocardial ischemia for the individual patient. Moreover, reduction of stress echo duration on the long run also may reduce costs and increase throughput in the stress echo laboratory.

Finally, besides the advantages during image acquisition, there seem to be advantages analyzing regional LV wall motion abnormalities in short axis slices instead of long axis planes (see example in videos 4 and 5).

(Access Analyzing Regional LV Wall Motion Abnormalities in Short Axis Slices and 2D Stress Echo in the online version of this article at: http://www.cardiology.theclinics.com.)

Limitations

Despite all enthusiasm about a new and revolutionary imaging modality, there are also some limitations of 3D stress echo. Image quality using matrix array transducers still is worse than with high-end 2D equipment. This is because of a decreased line density and because of the mechanical limitation of a relatively large probe that interferes with narrow intercostal spaces. Some authors therefore claim that left heart contrast enhancement is mandatory for adequate endocardial delineation when acquiring full-volume 3D data [9], although most of the recent studies used no contrast. As previously mentioned, the settings used for contrast in 3D acquisitions are being worked out, and as a result, image enhancement is typically not as robust with full-volume 3D imaging as it is with conventional 2D imaging. Temporal resolution is limited to about 40 to 50 ms, which especially during peak stress influences tests sensitivity and remains unsatisfactory. Meanwhile, potential solutions for this problem are on their way. In addition, the limited sector width sometimes is not wide enough to encompass the complete left ventricle in the ultrasound sector. This is especially true in patients where follow-up of LV function is crucial, those who have an apical aneurysm or dilated ventricles. Even off-axis scanning sometimes cannot circumvent this problem.

Summary

3D stress echo has been demonstrated to be feasible, resulting in a test accuracy comparable to conventional 2D techniques. Besides the advantages during image acquisition, there are potential advantages to analyzing regional LV wall motion abnormalities in short axis slices instead of long axis planes. 3D stress echo is an important step forward on the way to solving the old dilemma in stress echo: reducing the scanning time and covering the complete left ventricle without loosing image quality. At the end of the day, real-time 3D stress echo without any doubt will be the fastest and probably sometime the best way to perform a stress echo. Because bi- and triplane imaging offer 2D quality imaging while simultaneously saving acquisition time, this is arguably the preferred method of using the matrix transducer during stress echo over full-volume acquisition.

References

[1] Hoffmann R, Lethen H, Marwick T, et al. Analysis of interinstitutional observer agreement in interpretation of dobutamine stress echocardiograms. J Am Coll Cardiol 1996;27:330–6.

[2] Collins M, Hsieh A, Ohazama CJ, et al. Assessment of regional wall motion abnormalities with real-time 3-dimensional echocardiography. J Am Soc Echocardiogr 1999;12:7–14.

[3] Ahmad M, Xie T, McCulloch M, et al. Real-time three-dimensional dobutamine stress echocardiography in assessment stress echocardiography in assessment of ischemia: comparison with two-dimensional dobutamine stress echocardiography. J Am Coll Cardiol 2001;37:1303–9.

[4] Zwas DR, Takuma S, Mullis-Jansson S, et al. Feasibility of real-time 3-dimensional treadmill stress echocardiography. J Am Soc Echocardiogr 1999; 12:285–9.

[5] Sugeng L, Kirkpatrick J, Lang RM, et al. Biplane stress echocardiography using a prototype matrix array transducer. J Am Soc Echocardiogr 2003;16: 937–41.

[6] Eroglu E, D'hooge J, Herbots L, et al. Comparison of real-time triplane and conventional 2D dobutamine stress echocardiography for the assessment of coronary artery disease. Eur Heart J 2006;27:1719–24.

[7] Matsumura Y, Hozumi T, Arai K, et al. Noninvasive assessment of myocardial ischaemia using new real-time three-dimensional dobutamine stress echocardiography: comparison with conventional two-dimensional methods. Eur Heart J 2005;26: 1625–32.

[8] Pulerwitz T, Hirata K, Abe Y, et al. Feasibility of using a real-time 3-dimensional technique for contrast dobutamine stress echocardiography. J Am Soc Echocardiogr 2006;19:540–5.

[9] Takeuchi M, Otani S, Weinert L, et al. Comparison of contrast-enhanced real-time live 3-dimensional dobutamine stress echocardiography with contrast 2-dimensional echocardiography for detecting stress-induced wall-motion abnormalities. J Am Soc Echocardiogr 2006;19:294–9.

[10] Yang HS, Pellikka PA, McCully RB, et al. Role of biplane and biplane echocardiographically guided 3-dimensional echocardiography during dobutamine stress echocardiography. J Am Soc Echocardiogr 2006;19:1136–43.

ELSEVIER
SAUNDERS

Cardiol Clin 25 (2007) 267–272

CARDIOLOGY
CLINICS

Three-Dimensional Stress Testing: Volumetric Acquisitions

Masaaki Takeuchi, MD[a,*],
Roberto M. Lang, MD, FACC, FASE, FAHA[b]

[a]*Department of Cardiology, Tane General Hospital, 1-2-31 Sakaigawa, Nishi-ku, Osaka 550-0024, Japan*
[b]*Cardiac Imaging Center, Department of Medicine and Radiology, University of Chicago, 5841 S. Maryland Avenue, MC5084, Chicago, IL 60637, USA*

2D stress echocardiography is a versatile and established technique for diagnosing coronary artery disease [1–3]. Exercise stress echocardiography (ESE) provides not only functional information about the severity of coronary artery stenosis, but also additional physiologic information on exercise capacity and blood pressure response during exercise [4]. Dobutamine stress echocardiography (DSE) should be used in patients who are unable to exercise adequately because of advanced age, orthopedic disease, and/or peripheral vascular disease [2]. Although exercise provides the most physiologic type of stress, DSE has the major advantage of a more controlled setting. It is more ideal for acquisition of multiple images and is particularly optimal for acquisition of full-volume 3D data sets. Both types of stress testing are useful for the detecting myocardial viability and are reliable predictors of future cardiac events [1–5]. Although second harmonic imaging and intravenous ultrasound contrast agents have improved image quality and reduced the number of uninterpretable myocardial segments, 2D stress echocardiography continues to be limited. Conventional wall motion assessment from the four standard imaging planes (parasternal long and short-axis and apical four- and two-chamber views) at times fails to display all left ventricular (LV) segments, with the potential risk of missing stress-induced wall motion abnormalities that could have been delineated using nontraditional off-axis views. Inadequate visualization of the true LV apex and malalignment of the standard imaging planes frequently result in erroneous interpretations.

Over the last decade, the rapid development of technological and engineering refinements have made the routine clinical application of real-time 3D (RT3D) echocardiography possible [6,7]. Acquisition of full-volume 3D datasets from a single acoustic window allows visualization of multiple imaging planes after cropping the dataset. These characteristics are valuable for stress echocardiography, because:

- Single volumetric acquisitions reduce the recording time and delay from peak stress, thus enhancing the detection rate of transient ischemia.
- Full-volume datasets incorporate the entire left ventricle.
- Alignment and cropping datasets enable visualization of the true apex, which frequently becomes hypokinetic with ischemia originating in the left anterior descending coronary artery.
- Alignment of equivalent views acquired at baseline and peak stress, and off-axis visualization of regional wall motion by cropping full-volume datasets could provide enhanced interpretation of wall motion abnormalities.

Accurate interpretation of stress echocardiography highly depends on image quality. One of the current limitations of RT3D echocardiography is the relatively poor image quality and low frame rate obtained compared with 2D imaging. These limitations could result in poor visualization of

* Corresponding author.
E-mail address: masaaki_takeuchi@hotmail.com (M. Takeuchi).

0733-8651/07/$ - see front matter
doi:10.1016/j.ccl.2007.05.008

subtle wall motion abnormalities. These issues should be taken into account when performing RT3D stress echocardiography.

Imaging modes

RT3D echocardiography currently allows two types of imaging modes useful for stress echocardiography. These are full-volume mode and multiplane (biplane or triplane) imaging mode.

Full-volume mode

Full-volume datasets usually are acquired during four or seven consecutive cardiac cycles from the apical transducer position. Because of variability in heart rate that occurs immediately following exercise, this mode is not suitable for exercise echocardiography (ie, treadmill echocardiography); therefore full-volume acquisitions are most suitable for DSE. The acquired RT3D echocardiography data are cropped using the software integrated in the 3D operating software (QLAB; Philips Medical Systems, Andover, Massachusetts) (Fig. 1). After alignment of the LV long axis, each pyramidal data set is cropped from apex to base to create multiple short-axis images. Long-axis assessment with multiple apical views is also possible. A side-by-side comparison of wall motion then is performed at the similar cut plane of the baseline and peak stress loops.

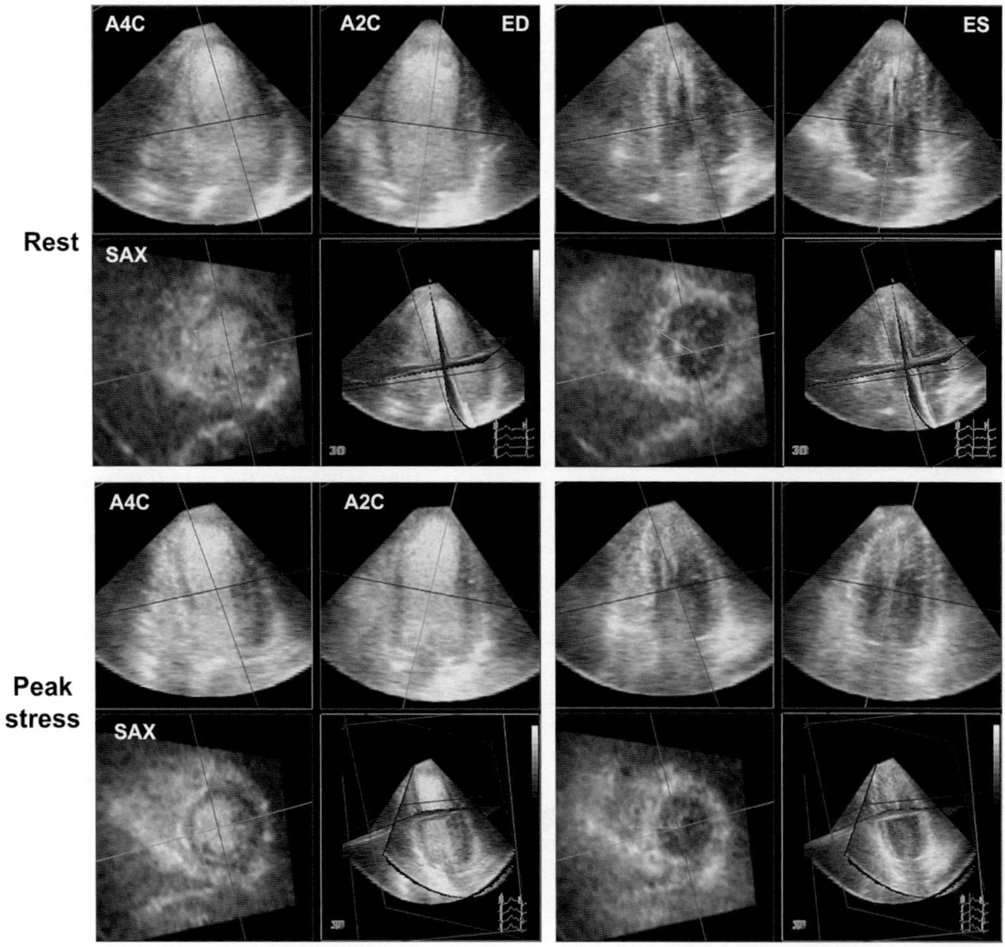

Fig. 1. Cropped image from full-volume datasets obtained during dobutamine stress echocardiography. Upper panels show baseline images, while the lower panels depict images obtained during peak dobutamine infusion. Simultaneous multiple cut plane images (apical four-chamber, two-chamber, and short-axis views) can be cropped from the full-volume datasets (left, end-diastole; right, end-systole).

In addition to manual editing, multiple short-axis 2D views can be created from full-volume datasets (iSlice in Philips Medical Systems, 9 slice in GE Healthcare, Milwaukee, Wisconsin, Fig. 2). With full-volume assessment, the individual wall segments (either 16 or 17 segments) can be divided more precisely and scored at both stress and rest. Finally, even LV dyssynchrony can be evaluated at rest and stress using QLAB or software available from TomTec (Unterschleisheim, Germany).

Biplane or triplane mode

The matrix-array transducer is also capable of imaging in biplane (Philips) or triplane (GE) modes, thus allowing simultaneous display of two or three imaging planes (Fig. 3). The real-time simultaneous acquisition of two or three planes from one acoustic window rather than LV full-volume mode reduces the acquisition time without a significant loss of image quality. This mode is particularly useful for exercise echocardiography.

3D exercise echocardiography

Few studies have reported on the clinical usefulness of RT3D echocardiography during exercise treadmill testing [8,9]. Irrespective of whether a first- or second-generation three-dimension echo machine was used, multiplane exercise echocardiography results in shorter acquisition times with post-treadmill images recorded at higher heart rates without a significant reduction in image quality. Although reduction of the time required to the completion of image acquisition at peak exercise could improve the sensitivity of exercise stress echocardiography, this hypothesis remains to be proven.

3D dobutamine stress echocardiography

The clinical usefulness of RT3D echocardiography during DSE first was reported using first-generation RT3D echocardiography [10]. Good correlation of segmental wall motion assessment between RT3D and conventional 2D techniques was noted at baseline and at peak stress. The diagnostic accuracy for detecting significant coronary stenosis was slightly higher in RT3D echocardiography (88%) compared with 2D echocardiography (80%). Although encouraging initial results were reported, relatively poor image quality because of the use of sparse-array transducers coupled with tedious off-line processing did not allow RT3D echocardiography to be embraced as the new reference imaging modality for stress echocardiography. Recently, the advent of second-generation RT3D echocardiography and commercially available 3D analysis software has facilitated the application of this technique during DSE in routine clinical setting. Several studies have addressed comparable diagnostic accuracy between RT3D and 2D echocardiography for detecting myocardial ischemia and coronary artery stenosis (Table 1) [11–15]. The use of intravenous ultrasound contrast agents has been shown to further improve endocardial border

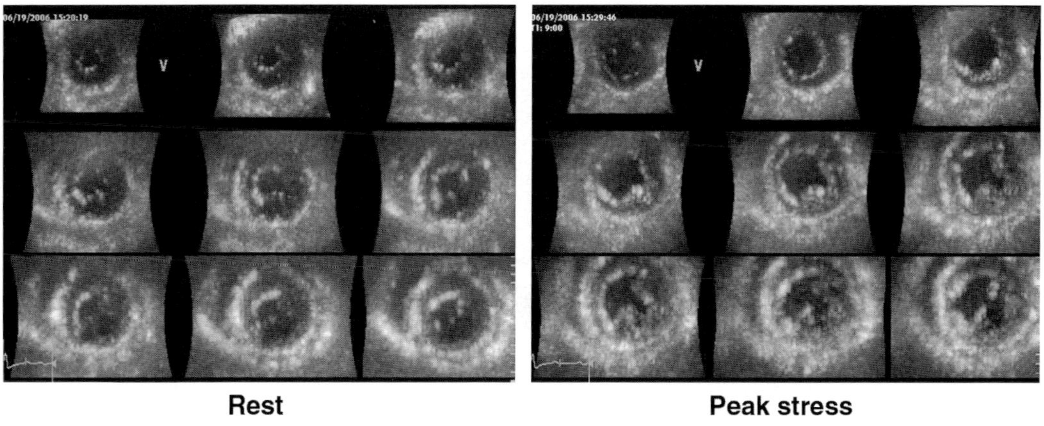

Fig. 2. Multiple 2D short-axis views (nine-slice) from full-volume datasets during dobutamine stress echocardiography. By cropping full-volume datasets, multiple 2D short-axis views from apex to the basal part of the heart can be obtained. These short-axis views obtained at end-systolic frame clearly show cavity dilatation at peak stress (*right panel*), suggesting the presence of multivessel disease. Coronary angiography confirmed the presence of triple vessel disease.

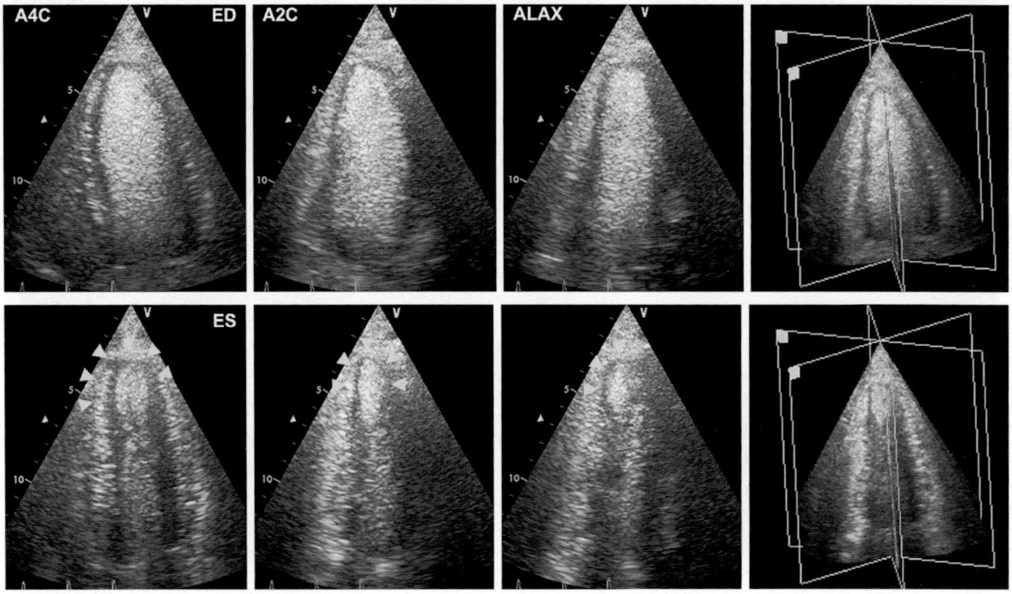

Fig. 3. Stress-induced apical wall motion abnormalities with triplane dobutamine stress echocardiography. Real-time triplane echocardiography from the apical window allows simultaneous visualization of apical four-, two- and long-axis views. The relative angles between the three images can be adjusted. Upper panels show end-diastolic triplane images obtained at peak stress. Lower panels show end-systolic images. Apical wall motion abnormalities are shown clearly, and their extent can be evaluated.

delineation and decrease the number of uninterpretable segments during 3D DSE [12,14]. Despite these excellent results, several limitations of RT3D DSE should be mentioned [13,14,16]. These include:

- Low frame rates
- The large matrix array transducer footprint results at times in poor image quality, particularly in patients who have narrow intercostals spaces.
- Contrast stitch artifacts
- Low frame rates and stitch artifacts originating from the wedge-shaped subvolume acquisitions may result in false-positive interpretations because of the erroneous diagnosis of inhomogeneous contraction and relaxation patterns.

Image quality of the matrix transducer is still not as good as that generated by conventional 2D transducer, even with the use of contrast agents. Despite the potential advantage of acquisition of a full-volume data set in terms of complete coverage of the left ventricle, the sensitivity, specificity, and accuracy remain less than ideal and not particularly better than conventional 2D methods [11–15].

The feasibility of real-time triplane DSE has been addressed in a recent study [17]. This study also reported that real-time triplane DSE appeared to be equally sensitive and specific as 2D DSE for assessing coronary artery disease. Although the triplane methodology has not been compared directly with full-volume acquisition, the sensitivity in this study was higher than reported in similar studies using the full-volume acquistion [10–15]. Clearly there are major discrepancies between these studies. Some use coronary angiography as their reference standard [10,15]; one used single photon emission computed tomography (SPECT) [11], and one used 2D DSE [13]. Whether ultrasound contrast agents could improve diagnostic accuracy of multiplane DSE further remains to be determined.

Future direction

In the future, technological transducer developments should improve the diagnostic yield of 3D stress echocardiography further. A single-beat acquisition of the full-volume datasets could avoid stitch artifacts and reduce acquisition time, thus allowing acquisition of full-volume datasets during exercise stress echocardiography.

Table 1
Feasibility and diagnostic accuracy of real-time 3D dobutamine stress echocardiography

Type	Author	Number of patients	Feasibility: Segments visible with conventional imaging	Feasibility: Segments visible with contrast imaging	Concordance rate (two-dimensional [2D] versus two-dimensional [3D]) (%)	Gold (reference) standard	Sensitivity (%)	Specificity (%)	Accuracy (%)
Full-volume	Ahmad, et al [10]	253	92%	NA	84 (baseline) 89 (peak)	CAG n = 90 (36%)	3D: 88 2D: 79	3D: 88 2D: 81	3D: 88 2D: 80
Full-volume	Matsumura, et al [11]	56	89%	NA		Tl SPECT n = 56 (100%)	3D: 86 2D: 86	3D: 80 2D: 83	3D: 82 2D: 84
Full-volume	Takeuchi, et al [13]	78	NA	97%	69 (pt) 88 (Vasc)	2D DSE n = 78 (100%)	Pt: 58 Vasc: 66	Pt: 75 Vasc: 92	Pt: 69 Vasc: 88
Full-volume	Pulerwitz, et al [12]	14	75%–87%	97%–99%					
Full-volume	Nemes, et al [14]	36	76%	90%					
Full-volume	Aggeli, et al [15]	56	NA	NA	98 (baseline) 82 (peak)	CAG N = 56 (100%)	3D: 84 2D: 82	3D: 72 2D: 83	3D: 80 2D: 82
Triplane	Eroglu, et al [17]	36	97%	98%		CAG n = 36 (100%)	3D: 96 2D: 93	3D: 78 2D: 78	3D: 92 2D: 89

Abbreviations: CAG, coronary angiography; NA, not available; pt, patient; T1 SPECT, thallium single photon emission computed tomography; Vasc, vascular territory.

Introduction of matrix transducers with smaller footprints will enhance lateral image quality. Increases in the frame rate will avoid the false interpretation of inhomogeneous contraction and relaxation patterns currently seen at higher heart rates.

Summary

Although several preliminary clinical studies have been shown that RT3D echocardiography has tremendous promise on stress echocardiography, further technological refinements and larger size clinical studies will be required for the widespread application of volumetric 3D stress echocardiography.

References

[1] Armstrong W, Zoghbi W. Stress echocardiography: current methodology and clinical applications. J Am Coll Cardiol 2005;45:1739–47.

[2] Geleijnse M, Fioretti P, Roelandt J. Methodology, feasibility, safety, and diagnostic accuracy of dobutamine stress echocardiography. J Am Coll Cardiol 1997;30:595–606.

[3] Marwick T. Stress echocardiography. Heart 2003; 89:113–8.

[4] Roger VL, Pellikka PA, Oh JK, et al. Stress echocardiography. Part I. Exercise echocardiography: techniques, implementation, clinical applications, and correlations. Mayo Clin Proc 1995;70:5–15.

[5] Marwick T, Case C, Sawada S, et al. Prediction of mortality using dobutamine echocardiography. J Am Coll Cardiol 2001;37:754–60.

[6] Hung J, Lang R, Flachskampf F, et al. 3D echocardiography: a review of the current status and future directions. J Am Soc Echocardiogr 2007;20:213–33.

[7] Lang R, Mor-Avi V, Sugeng L, et al. Three-dimensional echocardiography: the benefits of the additional dimension. J Am Coll Cardiol 2006;48: 2053–69.

[8] Sugeng L, Kirkpatrick J, Lang R, et al. Biplane stress echocardiography using a prototype matrix array transducer. J Am Soc Echocardiogr 2003;16: 937–41.

[9] Zwas D, Takuma S, Mullis-Jansson S, et al. Feasibility of real-time 3-dimensional treadmill stress echocardiography. J Am Soc Echocardiogr 1999;12: 285–9.

[10] Ahmad M, Xie T, McCulloch M, et al. Real-time three-dimensional dobutamine stress echocardiography in assessment stress echocardiography in assessment of ischemia: comparison with two-dimensional dobutamine stress echocardiography. J Am Coll Cardiol 2001;37:1303–9.

[11] Matsumura Y, Hozumi T, Arai K, et al. Noninvasive assessment of myocardial ischaemia using new real-time three-dimensional dobutamine stress echocardiography: comparison with conventional two-dimensional methods. Eur Heart J 2005;26: 1625–32.

[12] Pulerwitz T, Hirata K, Abe Y, et al. Feasibility of using a real-time 3-dimensional technique for contrast dobutamine stress echocardiography. J Am Soc Echocardiogr 2006;19:540–5.

[13] Takeuchi M, Otani S, Weinert L, et al. Comparison of contrast-enhanced real-time live 3-dimensional dobutamine stress echocardiography with contrast 2-dimensional echocardiography for detecting stress-induced wall motion abnormalities. J Am Soc Echocardiogr 2006;19:294–9.

[14] Nemes A, Geleijnse M, Krenning B, et al. Usefulness of ultrasound contrast agent to improve image quality during real-time three-dimensional stress echocardiography. Am J Cardiol 2007;99:275–8.

[15] Aggeli C, Giannopoulos G, Misovoulos P, et al. Real-time three-dimensional dobutamine stress echocardiography for coronary artery disease diagnosis—validation with coronary angiography. Heart 2007;93:672–5.

[16] Geleijnse M, Nemes A, Vletter W. Response to: "Contrast-enhanced real-time 3-dimensional dobutamine stress echocardiography". J Am Soc Echocardiogr 2006;19:1076.

[17] Eroglu E, D'hooge J, Herbots L, et al. Comparison of real-time triplane and conventional 2D dobutamine stress echocardiography for the assessment of coronary artery disease. Eur Heart J 2006;27: 1719–24.

ELSEVIER
SAUNDERS

Cardiol Clin 25 (2007) 273–282

CARDIOLOGY
CLINICS

Three-Dimensional Echocardiographic Evaluation of Myocardial Perfusion

Victor Mor-Avi, PhD*, Roberto M. Lang, MD, FACC, FASE, FAHA

The Cardiac Imaging Center, Departments of Medicine and Radiology, University of Chicago MC5084, 5841 S. Maryland Avenue, Chicago, IL 60637, USA

One of the most intriguing developments in ultrasound imaging of the heart that brought about a 2-decade-long combination of expectations and disappointments was the introduction of echocardiographic contrast agents. Despite repeated waves of controversy regarding the readiness of this technology for clinical use, it is widely accepted that echocardiographic contrast is a powerful tool that improves our ability to evaluate left ventricular (LV) function and allows differential diagnosis of thrombi and intravascular masses. Another use of echocardiographic contrast media, which has sparked tremendous interest and over the years generated a significant body of research, is the assessment of myocardial perfusion. Nevertheless, to date, the assessment of myocardial perfusion by contrast echocardiography is not as well established as the use of LV opacification. There is still a fair amount of debate in the attempt to establish standardized techniques and clinically usable protocols. While the vast majority of published work has been based on the use of contrast for two-dimensional (2D) perfusion imaging, there are a small number of recent studies aimed at exploring the idea of three-dimensional (3D) assessment of myocardial perfusion, which has the potential to overcome many of the limitations of the 2D methodology. In this article, we provide a brief overview of the 2D work that provided the scientific basis for the emerging 3D methodology and discuss the unique features and promises as well as the challenges posed by this novel approach.

* Corresponding author.
E-mail address: vmoravi@medicine.bsd.uchicago.edu (V. Mor-Avi).

History of 2D perfusion imaging

Although 2D echocardiographic imaging has been playing a pivotal role in the clinical assessment of cardiac function for several decades, its ability to assess myocardial perfusion is not as well established. Since the early reports of successful visualization of myocardial perfusion in the mid 1980s [1–5], a large number of research studies and scientific publications have been dedicated to this cause. A quick literature search on this subject today will result in over a thousand published papers. These studies have been instigated by multiple technological breakthroughs in both the development of improved contrast agents and imaging technologies, such as the development of contrast-targeted modes specifically "tailored" to improve the contrast-enhancing effects of these agents. Among these contrast-targeted techniques, the most widely used are pulse inversion and power modulation, both currently available in commercial scanners. These techniques selectively enhance microbubble-generated reflections, while simultaneously suppressing reflections originating from cardiac structures and tissues, thus resulting in better visualization of intramyocardial contrast.

For more than 2 decades, the evaluation of myocardial perfusion has been frequently referred to as the "holy grail" of contrast echocardiography. The different aspects of this "crusade" have been previously discussed by different authors in over a hundred review papers in the English language alone [6–20]. Thus, it is difficult to briefly review the published work on myocardial contrast echocardiography without unjustly omitting many important studies. Generally speaking, published papers ranged from

doi:10.1016/j.ccl.2007.05.005

attempts to simply visualize intramyocardial contrast and thus detect perfusion defects using different imaging techniques [1,3,21–30] to methodologically more complex approaches aimed at the quantification of myocardial tissue blood flow [31–44].

With the steady improvements in stability and uniformity of contrast agents as well as the development of more robust imaging techniques, the qualitative perfusion imaging studies have progressively showed incremental improvements in the ability to visualize myocardial contrast, resulting in a steady increase in the confidence of the interpretation of perfusion images. Whereas many of these studies reached clinically acceptable levels of diagnostic accuracy, these levels remained at best only modest in multicenter trials. It is likely that this hurdle mostly reflects the subjective nature of the interpretation and its reliance on the experience of the reader necessary to differentiate between true perfusion abnormalities and attenuation-related artifacts that are more severe in the presence of highly echogenic contrast materials.

The more objective, quantitative perfusion techniques rely on measuring beat-by-beat changes in myocardial contrast, such as contrast inflow or washout following bolus injections [32,34–37,39], or, alternatively, its replenishment after destructive high-energy ultrasound pulses delivered during contrast infusion [14,40,45–47]. Although it is well understood that these changes are essential for the assessment of tissue blood flow dynamics, each specific maneuver has its advantages and disadvantages in terms of ease of use and reliability of information yielded [45,48,49]. As a result, there is no consensus on the specific technique that would be preferable for routine clinical use. Also, quantification offers little if anything in terms of dealing with image artifacts and cardiac translation, which may affect quantitative techniques even more than intelligent visual interpretation capable of immediately recognizing these issues [43].

Importantly, myocardial contrast echocardiography, with or without quantification, proved useful in multiple clinical scenarios. Beyond the obvious detection of resting perfusion defects [1,3,21–30] and evaluation of severity and extent of perfusion deficit [24,30,50–54], it was found useful in detecting stress-induced myocardial ischemia [55–60] and diagnosing acute coronary events in patients presenting with atypical chest pain in the emergency department [61–63], as well as evaluation of myocardial reperfusion after coronary revascularization [56,64–67].

From 2D to 3D perfusion imaging

Nevertheless, it has been recognized that the ability of conventional contrast-enhanced echocardiographic imaging to provide accurate information on the extent and severity of perfusion abnormalities is limited by its 2D nature, similar to the assessment of LV volume and function (see the article on chamber quantification elsewhere in this issue). Despite the appeal of 3D imaging in this context, its use in humans has not been explored until recently. This is because the 3D approach has required off-line reconstruction from multiple planes, significantly complicating the volumetric evaluation. As a result, 3D assessment of myocardial perfusion remained limited to occasional reports on the visualization of perfusion defects in animals undergoing experimental coronary occlusion or the quantification of the perfusion defect size [68,69] using repeated boluses of contrast media during consecutive acquisitions of multiple planes (Fig. 1). These studies demonstrated that the location and extent of perfusion defects measured on contrast-enhanced 3D images correlated closely with the location and extent of the infarct as assessed by tissue staining. The use of bulls-eye displays generated from these 3D images of the myocardium

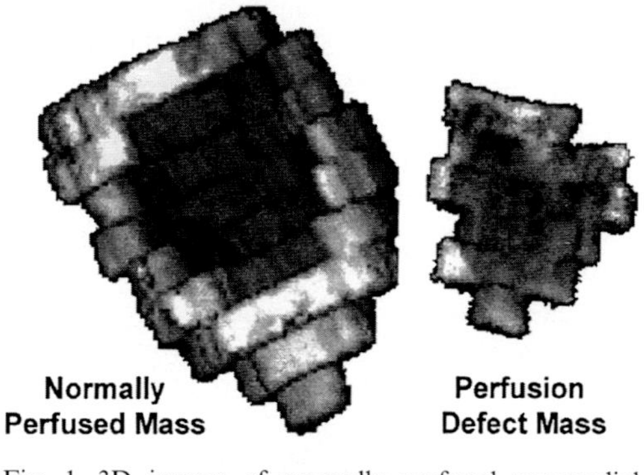

Fig. 1. 3D images of normally perfused myocardial mass and perfusion defect mass reconstructed by manually contouring the above regions in multiple short-axis slices of the left ventricle derived from a contrast-enhanced 3D data set. (*Reproduced from* Yao J, De CS, Delabays A, et al. Bulls-eye display and quantitation of myocardial perfusion defects using 3D contrast echocardiography. Echocardiography 2001;18:581–8; with permission.)

allowed easy visualization of perfusion defects without the need to compensate for the adjacent highly contrasted LV cavity (Fig. 2).

From multiple planes to volume acquisitions

Volumetric quantification of tissue blood flow would require repeated contrast maneuvers, such as bolus injections, that are necessary to assess flow dynamics for each imaging plane, thus rendering this methodology clinically inapplicable. The development of matrix array transducers that allow real-time volumetric imaging has obviated the need for repeated contrast maneuvers since the entire volume is captured during a single maneuver without reconstruction from multiple planes. This major conceptual change has opened new possibilities for the quantitative 3D assessment of myocardial perfusion. The initial experience with real-time perfusion imaging was obtained in an open-chest sheep model of acute ischemia using epicardial imaging with a sparse array transducer (Fig. 3) [70]. This methodology allowed accurate delineation of perfusion defects in close agreement with tissue-staining anatomic reference [70]. These findings were subsequently confirmed in animals undergoing open-chest coronary occlusion using epicardial imaging with a fully sampled matrix array transducer that yielded an incremental improvement in image quality [71,72]. These studies suggested that noninvasive volumetric assessment of perfusion defects may eventually be feasible in patients with suspected coronary artery disease.

From manual tracing to automated myocardial segmentation

The quantification of tissue blood flow in a certain area of the myocardium, either as absolute values in mL/min/g or as quantitative indices calculated from contrast intensity time curves, requires the definition of a myocardial region of interest (ROI) in which dynamic changes in contrast intensity are then analyzed. Traditionally, quantitative 2D analysis of myocardial perfusion has been based on manual tracing of ROIs in a single imaging plane and frame-by-frame realignment of these ROIs to compensate for cardiac translation. Although this methodology is subjective and time-consuming, it is relatively straightforward and easy to implement in software. In contrast, drawing ROIs in 3D space, a prerequisite for volumetric perfusion analysis, is significantly more complex, both conceptually and from the point of view of implementation. Needless to say, realignment of 3D ROIs throughout the image sequence to compensate for cardiac translation is not simple.

To overcome these limitations, we initially developed a technique for automated identification of myocardial regions of interest for fast, translation-free analysis of myocardial contrast enhancement from 2D images [73]. Our approach

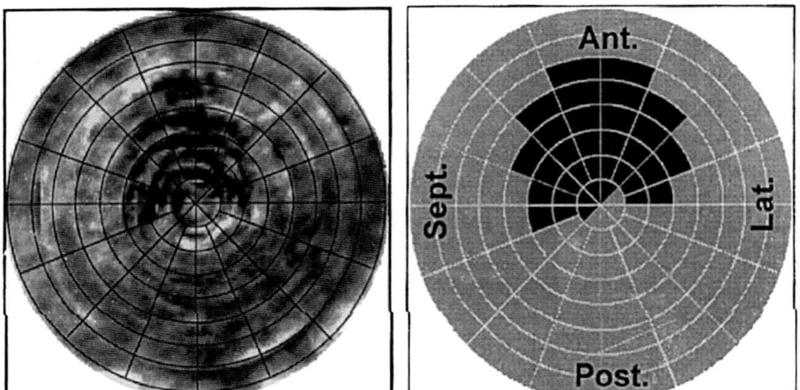

Fig. 2. Bulls-eye image formed from a contrast-enhanced 3D data set (*left*) and the corresponding binary image showing underperfused sectors (*right*). (*Reproduced from* Yao J, De CS, Delabays A, et al. Bulls-eye display and quantitation of myocardial perfusion defects using 3D contrast echocardiography. Echocardiography 2001;18:581–8; with permission.)

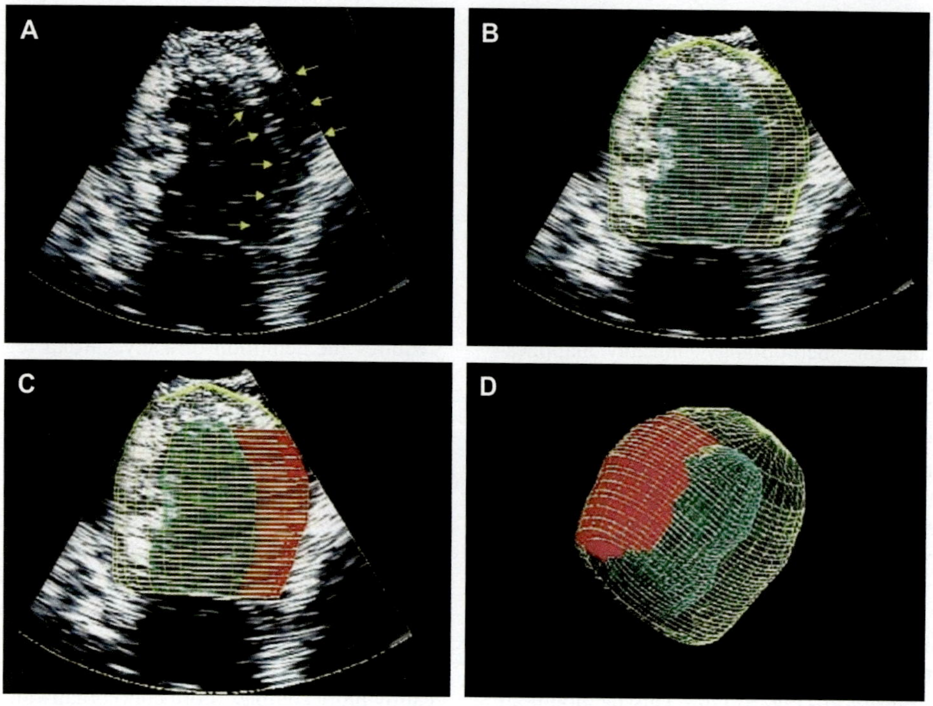

Fig. 3. Representative example of methodology used to quantitatively assess mass of underperfused myocardium from RT3D images in sheep with acute occlusion of circumflex coronary artery. (*A*) Tomographic view derived from volumetric image showing area of myocardium devoid of contrast opacification (*arrows*). (*B*) 3-dimensional rendering of left ventricular (LV) endocardial (in green) and epicardial (in yellow) surfaces generated by computer, based on operator's tracing. Area between both surfaces corresponds to myocardial volume, which is used to calculate myocardial mass. (*C*) Rendering of LV region without contrast opacification generated by computer, based on operator's tracing of corresponding endocardial surface. Red area represents volume used to calculate mass of underperfused myocardium. After tracing is completed, volumetric image can be freely rotated to examine 3-dimensional appearance of LV endocardial and epicardial surfaces and underperfused myocardium, as shown in (*D*). (*Reproduced from* Camarano G, Jones M, Freidlin RZ, et al. Quantitative assessment of left ventricular perfusion defects using real-time 3D myocardial contrast echocardiography. J Am Soc Echocardiogr 2002;15:206–13; with permission. Copyright © 2002, American Society of Echocardiography.)

was based on automated detection of the endocardial boundaries, which are relatively easy to detect in the presence of contrast in the LV cavity, followed by outward expansion into the myocardium and segmentation (Fig. 4). We tested this approach on power modulation images obtained in pigs undergoing coronary occlusions, and found that it allowed automated translation-free quantification of regional myocardial perfusion, without the need for ROI tracing [73]. More recently, we extended this concept to 3D images by automatically detecting LV endocardial surface and then defining and segmenting the 3D myocardial shell to allow automated volumetric analysis of myocardial perfusion without ROI tracing. Importantly, since the detection of LV myocardium is automated, it can be performed quickly on every consecutive frame, thus providing an ultimate solution for the problem of myocardial translation.

From manual boluses to alternative maneuvers

Another important challenge on the way to quantitative evaluation of myocardial perfusion is the choice of the contrast maneuver that would provide access to information about tissue blood flow. Because the effects of contrast boluses on echocardiographic images are difficult to predict, and "on-the-flight" optimization of gain setting for a short-lived bolus is virtually impossible, it has been long recognized that bolus injections are hardly the solution for either 2D or 3D perfusion quantification. The alternative approach, based on the use of continuous contrast infusion and

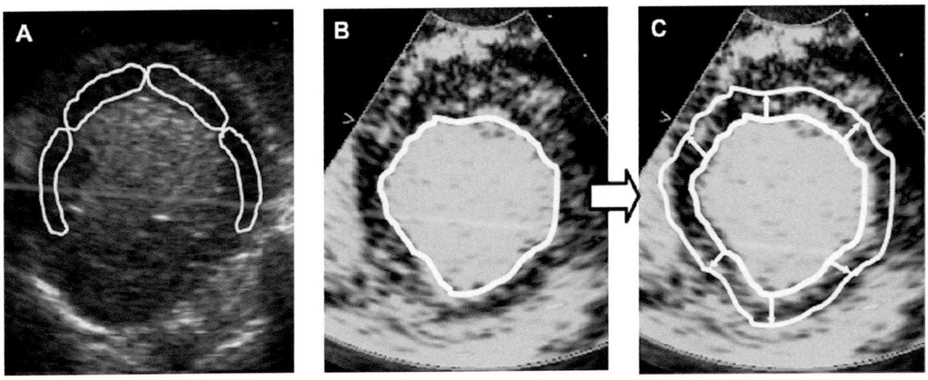

Fig. 4. Regional contrast is usually assessed by manually tracing myocardial regions of interest (*A*). High-contrast LV cavity is suitable for automated endocardial border detection (*B*), which allows automated identification of the myocardium (*C*) in each consecutive end-systolic frame, as a basis for automated, translation-free perfusion analysis. (*Reproduced from* Caiani EG, Lang RM, Caslini S, et al. Quantification of regional myocardial perfusion using semiautomated translation-free analysis of contrast-enhanced power modulation images. J Am Soc Echocardiogr 2003;16:116–123; with permission. Copyright © 2003, American Society of Echocardiography.)

high-energy ultrasound pulses that is widely used for 2D perfusion evaluation [14,40,45–47], is not available because of the excessive energy required for microbubble destruction in the entire heart.

We recently described an alternative contrast maneuver that could be safely used to quantify perfusion from real-time 3D echocardiographic images. This approach uses continuous infusion of contrast and thus allows ample time to optimize imaging settings. It does not require microbubble destruction by high-energy pulses, but instead uses a brief infusion interruption, which effectively

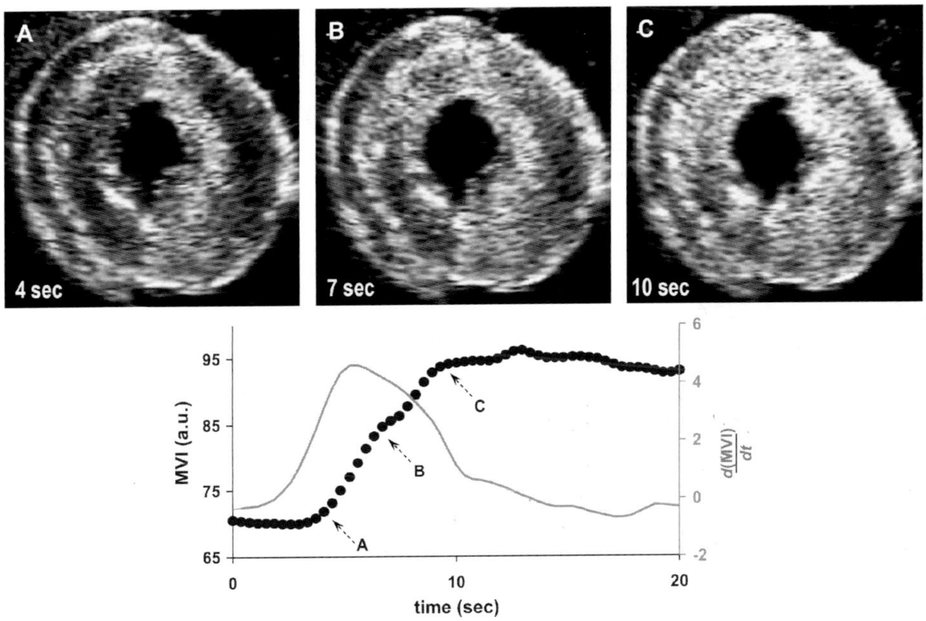

Fig. 5. (*Top*) Example of short-axis images of the isolated rabbit heart, which are part of a sequence acquired during brief interruption of contrast infusion: (*A*) at peak contrast clearance, (*B*) during contrast wash-in, and (*C*) after reestablishing steady-state enhancement. (*Bottom*) Myocardial video intensity time curve and its time derivative, which is used to calculate peak contrast inflow rate, a quantitative index of perfusion. Labels *A* through *C* depict the time points in the sequence at which the three images in the top panels were obtained.

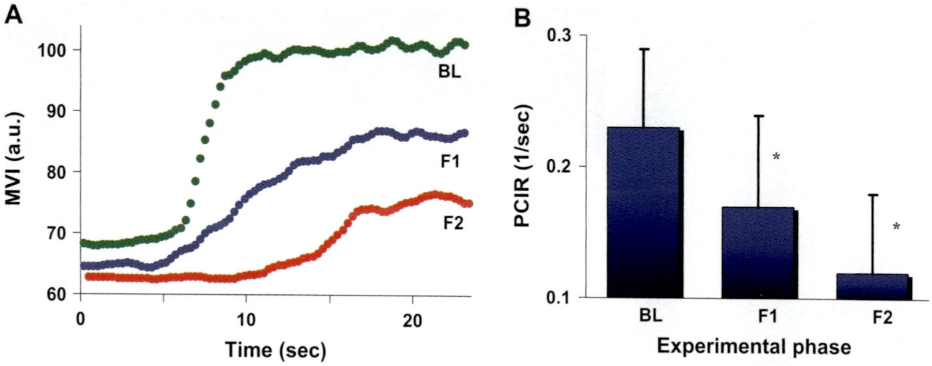

Fig. 6. (*A*) Myocardial video intensity (MVI) time curves obtained from a 3D slice of an isolated rabbit heart at three levels of coronary flow. BL, baseline; F1, 40% to 60%; F2, 10% to 20% of baseline flow. (*B*) Average values of myocardial peak contrast inflow rates (PCIR; $*P < .01$ versus BL).

results in a "negative bolus" of contrast [44,49]. We found that in human subjects, the transition from no enhancement to steady-state enhancement occurred within less than 45 seconds, which can be captured in a single data acquisition [44]. Quantitative analysis of image sequences obtained during the replenishment phase of this "bolus" results in peak contrast inflow rate, an index of myocardial perfusion (Fig. 5). This approach was initially tested and optimized with 2D perfusion imaging and was found to be more reproducible, less affected by noise, and more sensitive to changes in myocardial perfusion than the standard analysis of postpulse contrast replenishment using exponential fitting [49]. Subsequently, we used analysis of contrast inflow in conjunction with real-time 3D echocardiographic images, including graded perfusion alterations in an isolated rabbit heart (Fig. 6), localized myocardial ischemia in closed-chest pigs (Fig. 7), and global alterations in myocardial perfusion in humans induced by infusion of adenosine [74].

From fundamental imaging to contrast-targeted modes

Another important recent technological development was the incorporation of harmonic imaging and later power modulation imaging [40] into real-time 3D imaging. Despite the lower spatial resolution, these contrast-targeted modes resulted in incremental improvements in the ability to

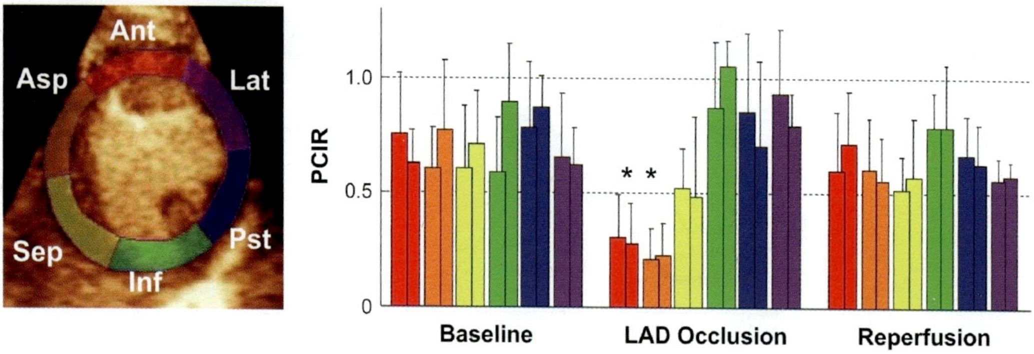

Fig. 7. (*Left*) En-face view of a short-axis slice of a pig heart with the myocardium divided into six segments. Ant, anterior; Asp, anteroseptal; Int, inferior; Lat, lateral; Pst, posterior, Sep, septal. (*Right*) Regional PCIR calculated at baseline, during partial LAD occlusion and reperfusion, averaged over all animals ($*P < .05$ versus baseline). The two bars of each color represent adjacent slices. LAD, left anterior descending coronary artery. (*Reproduced from* Toledo E, Lang RM, Collins KA, et al. Imaging and quantification of myocardial perfusion using real-time 3D echocardiography. J Am Coll Cardiol 2006;47:146–54; with permission. Copyright © 2006, American College of Cardiology Foundation.)

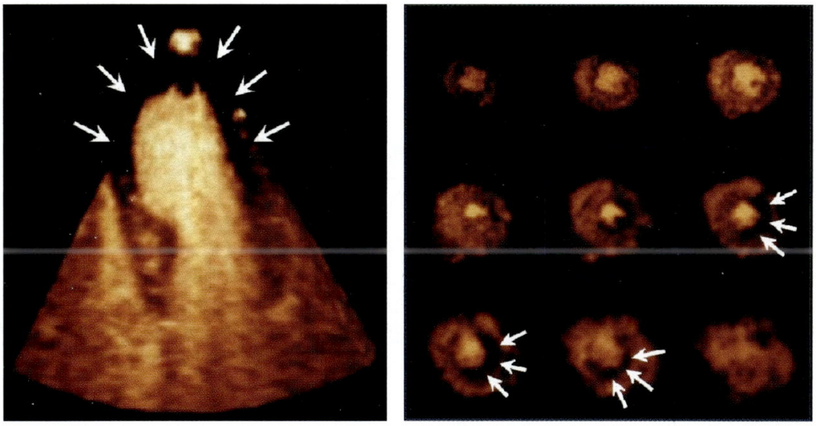

Fig. 8. (*Left*) RT3DE dataset obtained in a patient with LAD stenosis. Part of the septum lacks contrast enhancement indicating a perfusion defect. (*Right*) Short-axis slices at different levels of the left ventricle from apex to base extracted from a RT3DE dataset obtained in a patient with 90% stenosis in the proximal left circumflex coronary (LCX) artery. Note the perfusion defect in the LCX territory (*arrows*).

visualize intramyocardial contrast. The lower temporal resolution, which is an intrinsic property of the multipulse power modulation technique, is not a real limitation in the context of perfusion imaging since only one frame per cardiac cycle is required for perfusion analysis. Our initial experience with the use of this methodology in conjunction with adenosine stress testing in patients with suspected coronary artery disease indicates that it is possible to visualize and quantify myocardial perfusion abnormalities using contrast-enhanced real-time 3D echocardiographic imaging (Fig. 8). We studied a small group of patients with suspected coronary artery disease and found that the presence, location, and severity of perfusion abnormalities detected using this methodology are in agreement with the findings of coronary angiography.

Summary

Real-time 3D echocardiographic imaging allows visualization of myocardial perfusion in any arbitrary slice of the left ventricle and its volumetric quantification using a single contrast maneuver, which is necessary for the assessment of tissue blood flow dynamics. The use of this methodology in humans needs to be validated against accepted techniques for the evaluation of myocardial perfusion, such as positron emission tomography. Its potential clinical value for noninvasive diagnosis of coronary artery disease will need to be established in large groups of patients undergoing coronary angiography. This methodology may well prove to be a valuable addition to the noninvasive diagnostic cardiac imaging arsenal and become part of the routine cardiology practice.

Acknowledgments

We acknowledge the invaluable contribution of Eran Toledo, PhD, and Enrico G. Caiani, PhD, to this work. We also are thankful to Patrick D. Coon, RDCS, for his help with the images.

References

[1] Tei C, Sakamaki T, Shah PM, et al. Myocardial contrast echocardiography: a reproducible technique of myocardial opacification for identifying regional perfusion deficits. Circulation 1983;67:585–93.

[2] Santoso T, Roelandt J, Mansyoer H, et al. Myocardial perfusion imaging in humans by contrast echocardiography using polygelin colloid solution. J Am Coll Cardiol 1985;6:612–20.

[3] Lang RM, Feinstein SB, Feldman T, et al. Contrast echocardiography for evaluation of myocardial perfusion: effects of coronary angioplasty. J Am Coll Cardiol 1986;8:232–5.

[4] Feinstein SB, Lang RM, Dick C, et al. Contrast echocardiography during coronary arteriography in humans: perfusion and anatomic studies. J Am Coll Cardiol 1988;11:59–65.

[5] Cheirif J, Zoghbi WA, Raizner AE, et al. Assessment of myocardial perfusion in humans by contrast echocardiography. I. Evaluation of regional coronary reserve by peak contrast intensity. J Am Coll Cardiol 1988;11:735–43.

[6] Vandenberg BF. Myocardial perfusion and contrast echocardiography: review and new perspectives. Echocardiography 1991;8:65–75.
[7] Rovai D, Lombardi M, Distante A, et al. Myocardial perfusion by contrast echocardiography. From off-line processing to radio frequency analysis. Circulation 1991;83:III97–103.
[8] Feinstein SB. Myocardial perfusion: contrast echocardiography perspectives. Am J Cardiol 1992;69: 36H–41H.
[9] Kaul S. Myocardial contrast echocardiography in coronary artery disease: potential applications using venous injections of contrast. Am J Cardiol 1995;75: 61D–8D.
[10] Main ML, Grayburn PA. Clinical applications of transpulmonary contrast echocardiography. Am Heart J 1999;137:144–53.
[11] Mulvagh SL, DeMaria AN, Feinstein SB, et al. Contrast echocardiography: current and future applications. J Am Soc Echocardiogr 2000;13: 331–42.
[12] Porter TR, Cwajg J. Myocardial contrast echocardiography: a new gold standard for perfusion imaging? Echocardiography 2001;18:79–87.
[13] Villanueva FS. Myocardial contrast echocardiography in acute myocardial infarction. Am J Cardiol 2002;90:38J–47J.
[14] Wei K. Assessment of myocardial blood flow and volume using myocardial contrast echocardiography. Echocardiography 2002;19:409–16.
[15] Zoghbi WA. Evaluation of myocardial viability with contrast echocardiography. Am J Cardiol 2002;90: 65J–71J.
[16] Kaul S. Instrumentation for contrast echocardiography: technology and techniques. Am J Cardiol 2002; 90:8J–14J.
[17] Monaghan MJ. Stress myocardial contrast echocardiography. Heart 2003;89:1391–3.
[18] Monaghan MJ. Contrast echocardiography: from left ventricular opacification to myocardial perfusion. Are the promises to be realised? Heart 2003;89:1389–90.
[19] Senior R. Role of myocardial contrast echocardiography in the clinical evaluation of acute myocardial infarction. Heart 2003;89:1398–400.
[20] Lepper W, Belcik T, Wei K, et al. Myocardial contrast echocardiography. Circulation 2004;109: 3132–5.
[21] Armstrong WF, Mueller TM, Kinney EL, et al. Assessment of myocardial perfusion abnormalities with contrast-enhanced two-dimensional echocardiography. Circulation 1982;66:166–73.
[22] Keller MW, Glasheen W, Teja K, et al. Myocardial contrast echocardiography without significant hemodynamic effects or reactive hyperemia: a major advantage in the imaging of regional myocardial perfusion. J Am Coll Cardiol 1988;12:1039–47.
[23] Reisner SA, Ong LS, Lichtenberg GS, et al. Myocardial perfusion imaging by contrast echocardiography with use of intracoronary sonicated albumin in humans. J Am Coll Cardiol 1989;14:660–5.
[24] Cheirif J, Desir RM, Bolli R, et al. Relation of perfusion defects observed with myocardial contrast echocardiography to the severity of coronary stenosis: correlation with thallium-201 single-photon emission tomography. J Am Coll Cardiol 1992;19: 1343–9.
[25] Villanueva FS, Glasheen WP, Sklenar J, et al. Assessment of risk area during coronary occlusion and infarct size after reperfusion with myocardial contrast echocardiography using left and right atrial injections of contrast. Circulation 1993;88:596–604.
[26] Meza MF, Mobarek S, Sonnemaker R, et al. Myocardial contrast echocardiography in human beings: correlation of resting perfusion defects to sestamibi single photon emission computed tomography. Am Heart J 1996;132:528–35.
[27] Firschke C, Lindner JR, Wei K, et al. Myocardial perfusion imaging in the setting of coronary artery stenosis and acute myocardial infarction using venous injection of a second-generation echocardiographic contrast agent. Circulation 1997;96:959–67.
[28] Porter TR, Li S, Kilzer K, et al. Effect of significant two-vessel versus one-vessel coronary artery stenosis on myocardial contrast defects observed with intermittent harmonic imaging after intravenous contrast injection during dobutamine stress echocardiography. J Am Coll Cardiol 1997;30:1399–406.
[29] Marwick TH, Brunken R, Meland N, et al. Accuracy and feasibility of contrast echocardiography for detection of perfusion defects in routine practice: comparison with wall motion and technetium-99m sestamibi single-photon emission computed tomography. The Nycomed NC100100 Investigators. J Am Coll Cardiol 1998;32:1260–9.
[30] Masugata H, Cotter B, Peters B, et al. Assessment of coronary stenosis severity and transmural perfusion gradient by myocardial contrast echocardiography: comparison of gray-scale B-mode with power Doppler imaging. Circulation 2000;102:1427–33.
[31] Maurer G, Ong K, Haendchen R, et al. Myocardial contrast two-dimensional echocardiography: comparison of contrast disappearance rates in normal and underperfused myocardium. Circulation 1984; 69:418–29.
[32] Kaul S, Kelly P, Oliner JD, et al. Assessment of regional myocardial blood flow with myocardial contrast two-dimensional echocardiography. J Am Coll Cardiol 1989;13:468–82.
[33] Kemper AJ, Nickerson D, Boyle CC III, et al. Quantifying changes in regional myocardial perfusion with aortic contrast echocardiography. J Am Soc Echocardiogr 1989;2:36–47.
[34] Vandenberg BF, Kieso R, Fox-Eastham K, et al. Quantitation of myocardial perfusion by contrast echocardiography: analysis of contrast gray level appearance variables and intracyclic variability. J Am Coll Cardiol 1989;13:200–6.

[35] Keller MW, Spotnitz WD, Matthew TL, et al. Intraoperative assessment of regional myocardial perfusion using quantitative myocardial contrast echocardiography: an experimental evaluation. J Am Coll Cardiol 1990;16:1267–79.
[36] Mor-Avi V, David D, Akselrod S, et al. Myocardial regional blood flow: quantitative measurement by computer analysis of contrast enhanced echocardiographic images. Ultrasound Med Biol 1993;19: 619–33.
[37] Skyba DM, Jayaweera AR, Goodman NC, et al. Quantification of myocardial perfusion with myocardial contrast echocardiography during left atrial injection of contrast. Implications for venous injection. Circulation 1994;90:1513–21.
[38] Lindner JR, Villanueva FS, Dent JM, et al. Assessment of resting perfusion with myocardial contrast echocardiography: theoretical and practical considerations. Am Heart J 2000;139:231–40.
[39] Leistad E, Ohmori K, Peterson TA, et al. Quantitative assessment of myocardial perfusion during graded coronary artery stenoses by intravenous myocardial contrast echocardiography. J Am Coll Cardiol 2001;37:624–31.
[40] Mor-Avi V, Caiani EG, Collins KA, et al. Combined assessment of myocardial perfusion and regional left ventricular function by analysis of contrast-enhanced power modulation images. Circulation 2001;104:352–7.
[41] Bae RY, Belohlavek M, Greenleaf JF, et al. Rapid quantitative assessment of myocardial perfusion: spectral analysis of myocardial contrast echocardiographic images. J Am Soc Echocardiogr 2002;15: 63–8.
[42] Yu EH, Skyba DM, Leong-Poi H, et al. Incremental value of parametric quantitative assessment of myocardial perfusion by triggered low-power myocardial contrast echocardiography. J Am Coll Cardiol 2004; 43:1807–13.
[43] Lindner JR, Sklenar J. Placing faith in numbers: quantification of perfusion with myocardial contrast echocardiography. J Am Coll Cardiol 2004;43: 1814–6.
[44] Toledo E, Lang RM, Collins KA, et al. Quantitative echocardiographic evaluation of myocardial perfusion using interrupted contrast infusion technique: in vivo validation studies and feasibility in human beings. J Am Soc Echocardiogr 2005;18:1304–11.
[45] Pelberg RA, Wei K, Kamiyama N, et al. Potential advantage of flash echocardiography for digital subtraction of B-mode images acquired during myocardial contrast echocardiography. J Am Soc Echocardiogr 1999;12:85–93.
[46] Dijkmans PA, Knaapen P, Sieswerda GT, et al. Quantification of myocardial perfusion using intravenous myocardial contrast echocardiography in healthy volunteers: comparison with positron emission tomography. J Am Soc Echocardiogr 2006;19:285–93.
[47] Jeetley P, Hickman M, Kamp O, et al. Myocardial contrast echocardiography for the detection of coronary artery stenosis: a prospective multicenter study in comparison with single-photon emission computed tomography. J Am Coll Cardiol 2006;47:141–5.
[48] Wiencek JG, Feinstein SB, Walker R, et al. Pitfalls in quantitative contrast echocardiography: the steps to quantitation of perfusion. J Am Soc Echocardiogr 1993;6:395–416.
[49] Toledo E, Collins KA, Williams U, et al. Interrupted infusion of echocardiographic contrast as a basis for accurate measurement of myocardial perfusion: ex vivo validation and analysis procedures. J Am Soc Echocardiogr 2005;18:1312–20.
[50] Kaul S, Pandian NG, Okada RD, et al. Contrast echocardiography in acute myocardial ischemia: I. In vivo determination of total left ventricular "area at risk." J Am Coll Cardiol 1984;4:1272–82.
[51] Kemper A, Force T, Gilfoil M, et al. Topographic correspondence of contrast echocardiographic perfusion mapping and myocardial infarct extent after varying durations of coronary occlusion. J Am Soc Echocardiogr 1988;1:104–13.
[52] Cheirif J, Narkiewicz-Jodko JB, Hawkins HK, et al. Myocardial contrast echocardiography: relation of collateral perfusion to extent of injury and severity of contractile dysfunction in a canine model of coronary thrombosis and reperfusion. J Am Coll Cardiol 1995;26:537–46.
[53] Leong-Poi H, Le E, Rim SJ, et al. Quantification of myocardial perfusion and determination of coronary stenosis severity during hyperemia using real time myocardial contrast echocardiography. J Am Soc Echocardiogr 2001;14:1173–82.
[54] Masugata H, Lafitte S, Peters B, et al. Comparison of real-time and intermittent triggered myocardial contrast echocardiography for quantification of coronary stenosis severity and transmural perfusion gradient. Circulation 2001;104:1550–6.
[55] Porter TR, Xie F, Kilzer K, et al. Detection of myocardial perfusion abnormalities during dobutamine and adenosine stress echocardiography with transient myocardial contrast imaging after minute quantities of intravenous perfluorocarbon-exposed sonicated dextrose albumin. J Am Soc Echocardiogr 1996;9:779–86.
[56] Meza MF, Ramee S, Collins T, et al. Knowledge of perfusion and contractile reserve improves the predictive value of recovery of regional myocardial function postrevascularization: a study using the combination of myocardial contrast echocardiography and dobutamine echocardiography. Circulation 1997;96:3459–65.
[57] Oraby MA, Hays J, Maklady FA, et al. Assessment of myocardial perfusion during pharmacologic contrast stress echocardiography. Am J Cardiol 2002;89:640–4.
[58] Elhendy A, O'Leary EL, Xie F, et al. Comparative accuracy of real-time myocardial contrast perfusion

imaging and wall motion analysis during dobutamine stress echocardiography for the diagnosis of coronary artery disease. J Am Coll Cardiol 2004; 44:2185–91.

[59] Moir S, Haluska BA, Jenkins C, et al. Myocardial blood volume and perfusion reserve responses to combined dipyridamole and exercise stress: a quantitative approach to contrast stress echocardiography. J Am Soc Echocardiogr 2005;18:1187–93.

[60] Tsutsui JM, Elhendy A, Anderson JR, et al. Prognostic value of dobutamine stress myocardial contrast perfusion echocardiography. Circulation 2005;112:1444–50.

[61] Kontos MC, Hinchman D, Cunningham M, et al. Comparison of contrast echocardiography with single-photon emission computed tomographic myocardial perfusion imaging in the evaluation of patients with possible acute coronary syndromes in the emergency department. Am J Cardiol 2003;91: 1099–102.

[62] Rinkevich D, Kaul S, Wang XQ, et al. Regional left ventricular perfusion and function in patients presenting to the emergency department with chest pain and no ST-segment elevation. Eur Heart J 2005;26:1606–11.

[63] Tong KL, Kaul S, Wang XQ, et al. Myocardial contrast echocardiography versus thrombolysis in myocardial infarction score in patients presenting to the emergency department with chest pain and a nondiagnostic electrocardiogram. J Am Coll Cardiol 2005;46:920–7.

[64] deFilippi CR, Willett DL, Irani WN, et al. Comparison of myocardial contrast echocardiography and low-dose dobutamine stress echocardiography in predicting recovery of left ventricular function after coronary revascularization in chronic ischemic heart disease. Circulation 1995;92:2863–8.

[65] Perchet H, Dupouy P, Duval-Moulin AM, et al. Improvement of subendocardial myocardial perfusion after percutaneous transluminal coronary angioplasty. A myocardial contrast echocardiography study with correlation between myocardial contrast reserve and Doppler coronary reserve. Circulation 1995;91:1419–26.

[66] Lepper W, Hoffmann R, Kamp O, et al. Assessment of myocardial reperfusion by intravenous myocardial contrast echocardiography and coronary flow reserve after primary percutaneous transluminal coronary angioplasty in patients with acute myocardial infarction. Circulation 2000;101: 2368–74.

[67] Biagini E, van Geuns RJ, Baks T, et al. Comparison between contrast echocardiography and magnetic resonance imaging to predict improvement of myocardial function after primary coronary intervention. Am J Cardiol 2006;97:361–6.

[68] Bae RY, Belohlavek M, Tanabe K, et al. Rapid three-dimensional myocardial contrast echocardiography: volumetric quantitation of nonperfused myocardium after intravenous contrast administration. Echocardiography 1999;16:357–65.

[69] Yao J, De CS, Delabays A, et al. Bulls-eye display and quantitation of myocardial perfusion defects using three-dimensional contrast echocardiography. Echocardiography 2001;18:581–8.

[70] Camarano G, Jones M, Freidlin RZ, et al. Quantitative assessment of left ventricular perfusion defects using real-time three-dimensional myocardial contrast echocardiography. J Am Soc Echocardiogr 2002;15:206–13.

[71] Chen LX, Wang XF, Nanda NC, et al. Real-time three-dimensional myocardial contrast echocardiography in assessment of myocardial perfusion defects. Chin Med J (Engl) 2004;117:337–41.

[72] Pemberton J, Li X, Hickey E, et al. Live real-time three-dimensional echocardiography for the visualization of myocardial perfusion—a pilot study in open-chest pigs. J Am Soc Echocardiogr 2005;18: 956–8.

[73] Caiani EG, Lang RM, Caslini S, et al. Quantification of regional myocardial perfusion using semiautomated translation-free analysis of contrast-enhanced power modulation images. J Am Soc Echocardiogr 2003;16:116–23.

[74] Toledo E, Lang RM, Collins KA, et al. Imaging and quantification of myocardial perfusion using real-time three-dimensional echocardiography. J Am Coll Cardiol 2006;47:146–54.

ELSEVIER
SAUNDERS

Cardiol Clin 25 (2007) 283–295

CARDIOLOGY
CLINICS

Three-Dimensional Echo for the Assessment of Valvular Heart Disease

Bernhard Mumm, MS*, Rolf Baumann, MS, Martin Hyca, MD, MS

TomTec Imaging Systems GmbH, Edisonstraße 6, Unterschleissheim 85716, Germany

Three-dimensional echocardiography (3DE) has been developed during the last 15 to 20 years. Within the last 10 years its clinical value has been proven in many publications around the world [1,2]. The technological improvements in computer speed, transducer technology, and the integration into the ultrasound systems have increased the clinical role of 3DE significantly. Started mainly as a qualitative technology, 3DE more and more has become a precise quantitative tool.

One important application of 3DE is its use for assessing valvular structures [3–5]. Especially in valvular heart disease it is important to understand the complex spatial geometry of the valves [6] and the subvalvular apparatus with its chordae and papillary muscles. Without 3DE, this assessment needs to be done as a kind of mental 3D reconstruction based on 2D echocardiography [2]. 3DE does not require such a mental 3D reconstruction process and is not based on any geometrical assumptions. In addition, it greatly helps to communicate the echocardiographic findings to the cardiac surgeon.

Technical background

The acquisition of 3DE data sets for valvular assessment today is done in two different ways: (1) with 3D TEE multiplane probes using the gating or reconstruction technique or (2) with matrix array transthoracic transducers (TTE) in real time (RT3DE). Both 3DE acquisition methods are commercially available for several ultrasound systems from various vendors. Recent transducer developments have been done to miniaturize the matrix array real-time transducer into a transesophageal echo (TEE) endoscope (Philips mTEE probe, Andover, Massachusetts) [7].

The 3DE American Society of Echocardiography position paper [1] published in March of this year describes how to assess the valvular morphology in a complete 3DE protocol by acquiring a wide-angle RT3DE data set, starting from a parasternal long-axis view, including RT3DE color interrogation of the aortic, mitral, tricuspid, and pulmonary valve. In addition, another RT3DE data set starting from an apical four-chamber window for the aortic, mitral, and tricuspid valve shall be acquired.

Although RT3DE can provide a real-time 3D reconstruction or display of the beating heart and its valvular structures during the acquisition, 3DTEE based on the gating technique first needs to complete the acquisition process. The average reported acquisition time ranges from 3 to 8 minutes. After that, the 3D reconstruction, display, manipulation, and quantification tools are more or less identical. To visualize an inner structure of the heart like the mitral valve in three dimensions, the heart needs to be sliced or unroofed with a cut plane. Unique en face views of a valve from above (looking down from the atrium like surgical views) and below (looking up from the apex) can be generated in real time (Fig. 1). Besides such 3D displays, oblique cut planes (anyplane echocardiography [8]) or so-called MPRs (multiplanar reconstructions) can be generated easily. For example three different cut planes, a sagittal (corresponds to a long axis view), a coronal (four-chamber view), and a

* Corresponding author. TomTec Imaging Systems GmbH, Edisonstraße 6, Unterschleissheim 85716, Germany.

E-mail address: bmumm@tomtec.de (B. Mumm).

0733-8651/07/$ - see front matter
doi:10.1016/j.ccl.2007.06.002

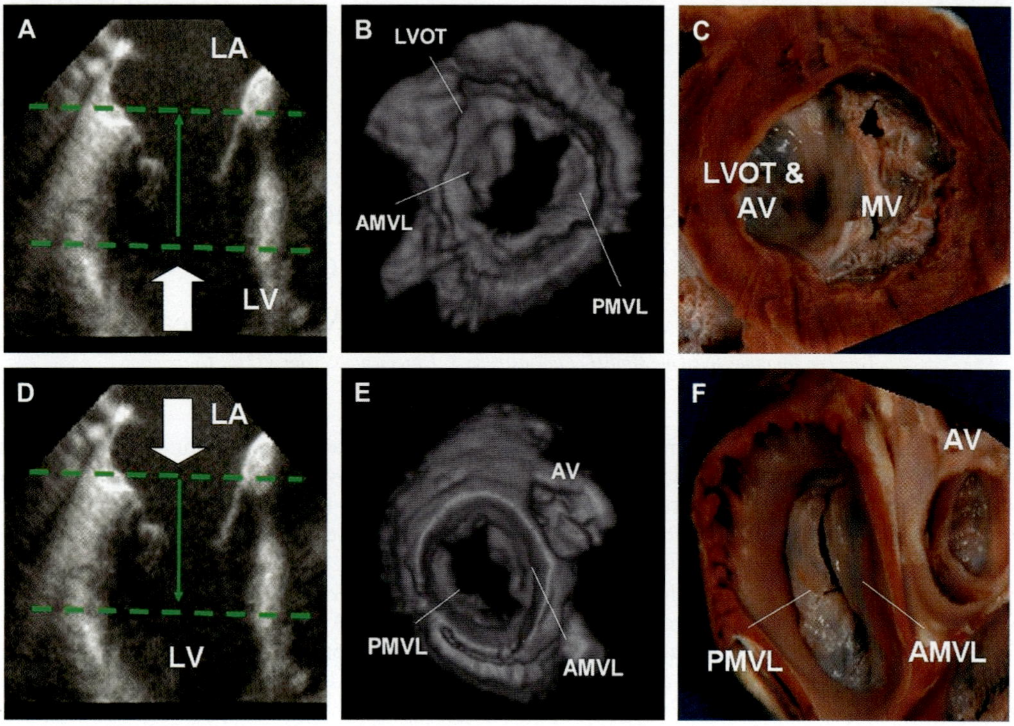

Fig. 1. Assessment of anatomical structures in volume-rendered images requires a proper 3D view adjustment. (*A, D*) The surgical view of the mitral valve (*white arrows*) can be defined in 2D images (multiplanar reconstructions) with two clicks only (D↑ art). The results of this view adjustment are shown in *B* and *E*. (*C, F*) The corresponding en face views of a human mitral valve. *Abbreviations:* AMVL, anterior mitral valve leaflet AoV, aortic valve; LA, left atrium; LVOT, left ventricular outflow tract; LV, left ventricle; MPR, multiplanar reconstruction; PMVL, posterior mitral valve leaflet. (*Courtesy of* N. Pandian, MD, Boston, MA.)

transverse plane (short axis view) [1] can be displayed side by side in real time.

Morphological and quantitative valve assessment

3DE greatly improved the assessment and understanding of valvular anatomy and function [6]. It can provide a detailed en face visualization of valve structures [9] like leaflet scallops, prolapses, or commissures for example for a better preoperative assessment. Fig. 2A shows a 3DE en face view from the left atrium to the mitral valve (MV), clearly depicting a prolapse. Fig. 2B shows the same MV and the prolapse in a side view.

Mitral valve assessment

The MV can be acquired in a 3DE data set with the 3DTEE or RT3DE approach. For RT3DE, a parasternal or apical window shall be used. The anterior leaflet can be visualized best from a parasternal long-axis position. As the posterior leaflet has a much smaller excursion compared with the anterior leaflet, it is sometimes more challenging to visualize. Then, an apical four-chamber position is preferable [10].

The imaging of the MV and various pathologies is feasible in most patients [6]. RT3DE gives additional information in the assessment of MV prolapse [11], flail leaflets, mitral stenosis, cleft mitral valves, and MV perforation. It helps to increase diagnostic confidence and to plan the surgical approach (MV repair or replacement) [3,9].

Based on the acquired and digitally stored 3DTEE or RT3DE data set, the MV can be assessed in a qualitative and quantitative way using dedicated MV analysis software tools like 4D MV-Assessment (TomTec Imaging Systems, Unterschleissheim, Germany). Such tools support in particular the interdisciplinary communication between cardiac surgeons and cardiologists/anesthesiologists.

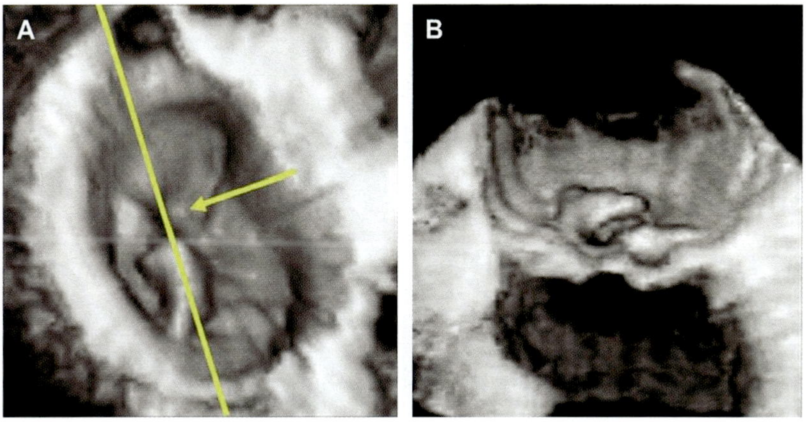

Fig. 2. Morphological assessment of mitral valve with 3D echocardiography. (*A, B*) A transesophageal 3D reconstruction of prolapsed mitral valve. The spatial location and shape of the prolapse can be assessed in the surgical (*A*) and side view (*B*). (*Courtesy of* A. Franke, MD, Aachen, Germany.)

Fig. 3A shows a 3DTEE en face view or so-called surgical view from the atrium to the MV with the aortic valve (AoV) at 12 o'clock position. The software outlines the MV annulus, which is displayed as an overlay contour (Fig. 3B). In addition it extracts the MV coaptation line from the anteriolateral to the posteriomedial commissure and is labeling the three anterior and posterior mitral leaflet segments (A1, A2, A3, P1, P2, P3). Fig. 4A shows a surgical view of a prolapsed (A2, A3) mitral valve. The white line represents the MPR shown in Fig. 4B. Leaflets can be segmented (turquoise line) in reconstructed 2D views (see Fig. 4B) and visualized together with anatomical structures in three dimensions (Fig. 4C). In Fig. 5, 3DE color flow information is displayed additionally. Here a simultaneous side-by-side display of three reconstructed cut planes (MPRs) (see Fig. 5A, C, D) and the 3D en face reconstruction (see Fig. 5B) is shown. By cropping the 3D color flow display of the regurgitant jet slightly above the level of the vena contracta, the relationship

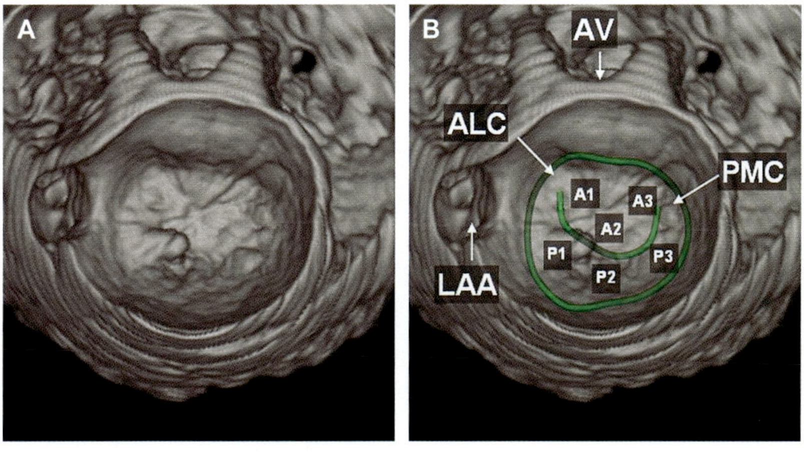

Fig. 3. (*A*) Transesophageal 3D reconstruction of a prolapsed (P1) mitral valve. (*B*) The morphological assessment can be simplified by visualizing the mitral valve annulus and the coaptation line into the volume-rendered image (TomTec 4D MV-Assessment CAP, TomTec Imaging Systems, Unterschleissheim, Germany). (*B*) The major anatomical structures can be labeled automatically if required. *Abbreviations:* ALC, anteriolateral commissure; AoV, aortic valve; LAA, left atrial appendage; PMC, posteriomedial commissure. A1-A3 and P1-P3 refer to the three scallops of the anterior (*A*) and posterior (*P*) leaflet.

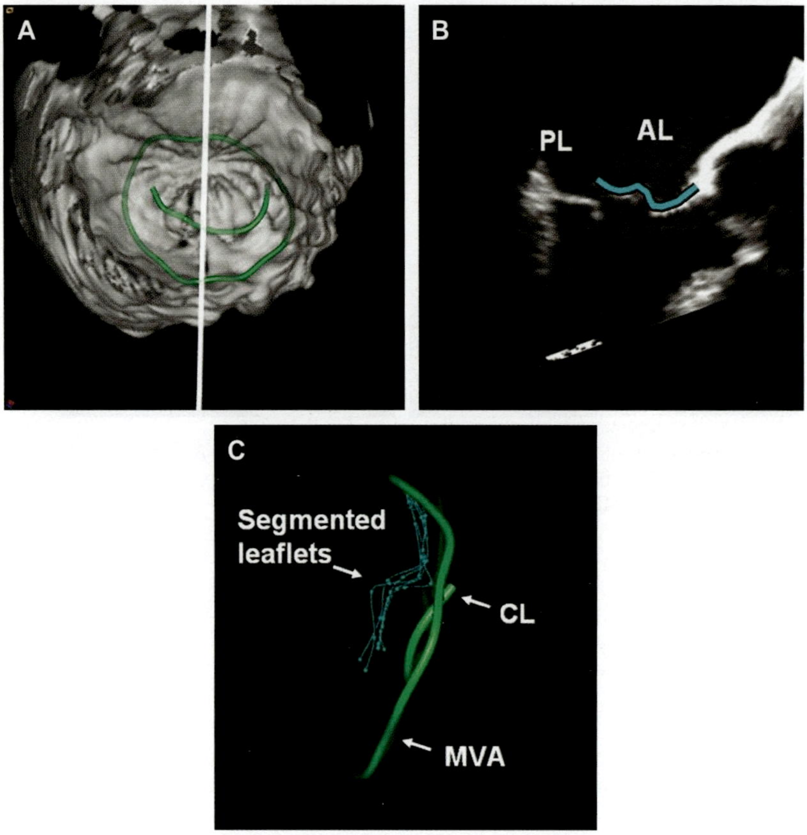

Fig. 4. (*A*) A surgical view of a prolapsed (A2, A3) mitral valve. The white line represents the multiplanar reconstruction (*B*). Leaflets can be segmented (*turquoise line*) in reconstructed 2D views (*B*) and visualized together with anatomical structures in three dimensions (*C*). *Abbreviations:* AL, anterior leaflet; CL, coaptation line; MVA, mitral valve annulus; PL, posterior leaflet (4D MV-Assessment CAP, TomTec Imaging Systems, Unterschleissheim, Germany).

of the jet origin to the valve closure line can be visualized (see Fig. 5B), and the jet origin area can be quantified. In Fig. 6A, a transesophageal 3D reconstruction of MV regurgitation is shown. The relationship between the regurgitant jet, MV annulus, and coaptation line is visualized in Fig. 6B. The jet at the level of the mitral valve is shown in Fig. 6C, allowing easy assessment of its exact spatial location. Fig. 7A shows a mitral valve regurgitation caused by P2 flail. As shown in Fig. 7B, the exact jet origin, size (turquoise line), and the prolapsed area (yellow) are measured.

Global and regional annular ring and coaptation line geometry can be calculated automatically. Fig. 8A, B shows a schematic view of global MV annulus measurements. Fig. 8C displays a selection of automatically generated MV annulus parameters.

Advanced 3D analysis technology allows such segmentation and quantification of MV annulus, leaflets, and subvalvular apparatus. Tenting area, tenting height, and papillary muscle geometry are visualized in Fig. 9A. Fig. 9B shows the aorto–mitral relationship. Fig. 10 shows the analysis of the displacement (longitudinal motion) of the MV and the valve surface area change over one heart cycle.

Mitral valve prolapse

As shown in Figs. 2–7, a MV prolapse can be visualized and quantified with 3DE [12–18]. Such preoperative assessment of the MV morphology is very important to plan the surgical approach (MV repair is preferable to MV replacement [19]). Here 3D has big advantages compared with 2D echocardiography [20] in the communication with the cardiac surgeon describing which scallops are involved or are prolapsing.

Mitral regurgitation

Accurate quantitative grading of mitral regurgitation (MR) is a powerful predictor of the

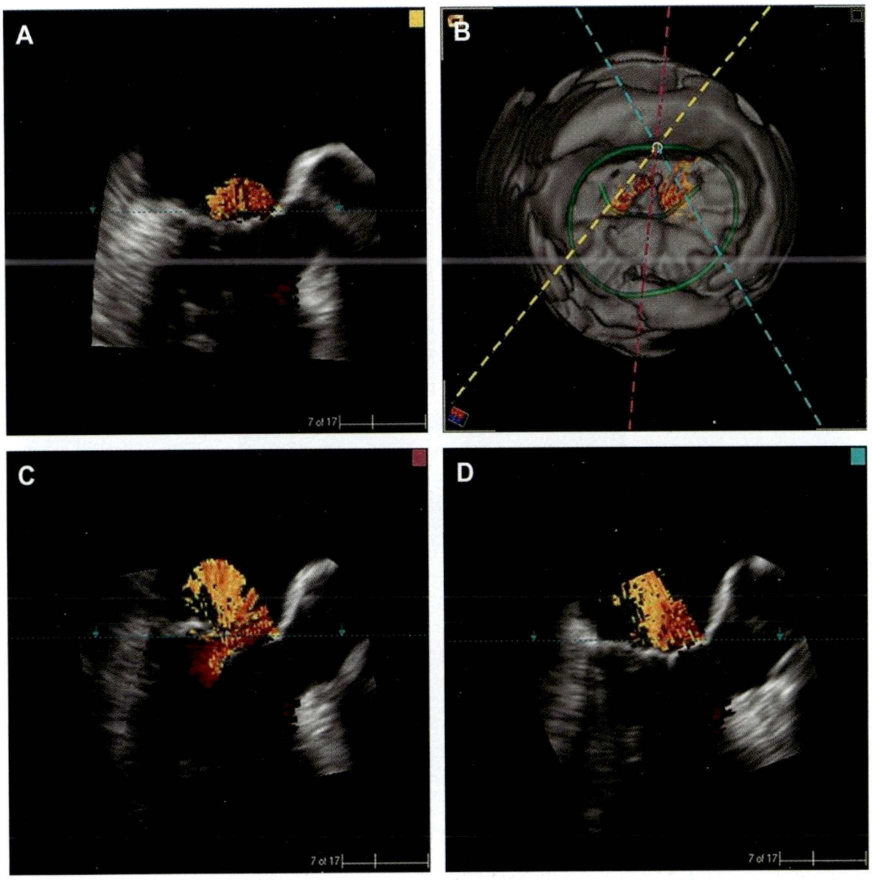

Fig. 5. The simultaneous side-by-side display of three reconstructed cut planes (multiplanar reconstructions) (*A, C, D*), and the 3D en face reconstruction (*B*) simplifies the morphological assessment of the mitral valve (TomTec 4D MV-Assessment CAP, TomTec Imaging Systems, Unterschleissheim, Germany).

clinical outcome of MR [21]. It would be desirable to precisely quantify the regurgitant flow volume per beat and the effective regurgitant orifice. This is difficult, however, using conventional color Doppler and 2D echocardiography techniques [22]. The addition of color flow to 3DE has provided improved visualization of regurgitant lesions and has the potential to play an increasing role to better quantify MR [23–25]; however, the temporal resolution of 3DE color flow still needs to be enhanced. 3DE can give new insights into the geometry of MR, which can lead to a better surgical strategy planning. It is particularly useful in patients who have multiple or eccentric jets. Fig. 11 shows a patient who had severe MR and presented with heart failure after MV repair. On 2D TEE, there is an echo density at the level of the MV annulus (see Fig. 11A), and on color flow Doppler (see Fig. 11B) there is severe MR, so that it is difficult to differentiate whether there is valvular or para-ring regurgitation. Using a TEE rotational approach (3DE TEE), a 3D reconstruction of the valve demonstrated dehiscence of the anterior portion of the MV ring (see Fig. 11C) and severe mitral valvular and para-ring regurgitation (see Fig. 11D).

In case of dilated left ventricles (LV) and ischemic cardiomyopathy, MR usually results from a dilatation of the mitral annulus and papillary muscle displacement and tethering of the mitral leaflets, leading to incomplete closure of the leaflets [1]. Here a 3DE-based analysis of the mitral annulus and its motion throughout the cardiac cycle is a promising new approach (see Fig. 10) to better understand MR mechanisms [26].

As 3DE is not based on any geometric assumptions, it can overcome the limitations of the

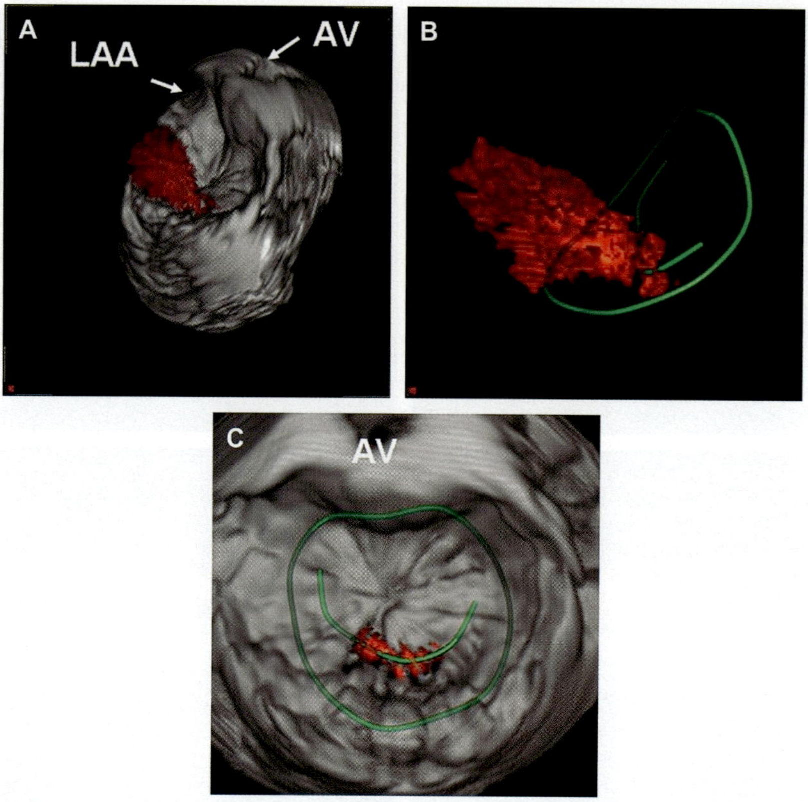

Fig. 6. (*A*) Transesophageal 3D reconstruction of mitral valve regurgitation. The relationship between regurgitant jet, mitral valve annulus, and coaptation line are visualized (*B*). The jet at the level of the mitral valve is shown (*C*), allowing easy assessment of its exact spatial location (4D MV-Assessment CAP, TomTec Imaging Systems, Unterschleissheim, Germany). *Abbreviations:* AoV, aortic valve; LAA, left atrial appendage.

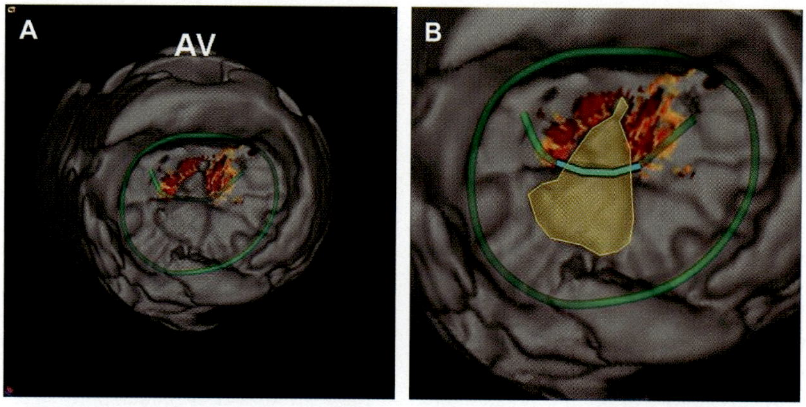

Fig. 7. (*A*) Mitral valve regurgitation caused by P2 flail. (*B*) The exact jet origin, size (*turquoise line*), and the prolapsed area (*yellow*) are measured: Jet size = 1.6 cm; Prolapsed area = 3.2 cm^2. Abbreviation: AoV, aortic valve (4D MV-Assessment CAP, TomTec Imaging Systems, Unterschleissheim, Germany).

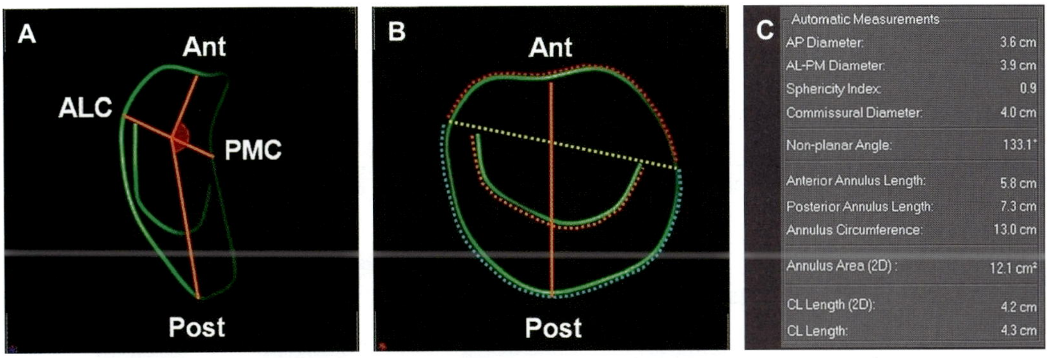

Fig. 8. Global and regional annular ring and coaptation line geometry can be calculated automatically. (*A, B*) A schematic view of global mitral valve (MV) annulus measurements. (*C*) A selection of MV annulus parameters. *Abbreviations:* ALC, anteriolateral commissure; Ant, anterior; PMC, posteriomedial commissure; Post, posterior (TomTec 4D MV-Assessment CAP, TomTec Imaging Systems, Unterschleissheim, Germany).

2D echocardiography-based proximal isovelocity surface area (PISA) method, which is assuming a perfect hemisphere for the quantification of mitral regurgitation. 3DE can address the real geometry and area of the isovelocity surface [27]. Iwakura and colleagues [28] published a comparison of the mitral orifice area measured by transthoracic 3D Doppler echocardiography versus the 2D echocardiography-based PISA method for assessing MR.

Khanna and colleagues [29] demonstrated the quantification of MR by live 3D transthoracic echocardiographic measurements of vena contracta area.

Mitral valve stenosis

Several studies have demonstrated the utility of 3DE for assessing the severity of mitral stenosis. Sugeng and colleagues [30] validated the accuracy of mitral valve area measurements in comparison with noninvasive 2DE and invasive hemodynamic methods. Zamorano and colleagues published a comparable study based on RT3DE stating that the 3D assessment of the MV area had an excellent correlation with the invasive determined area [31,32]. Fig. 12 is an example of the quantification of the MV orifice in a stenotic MV, before (see Fig. 12A) and after balloon valvuloplasty (see Fig. 12B).

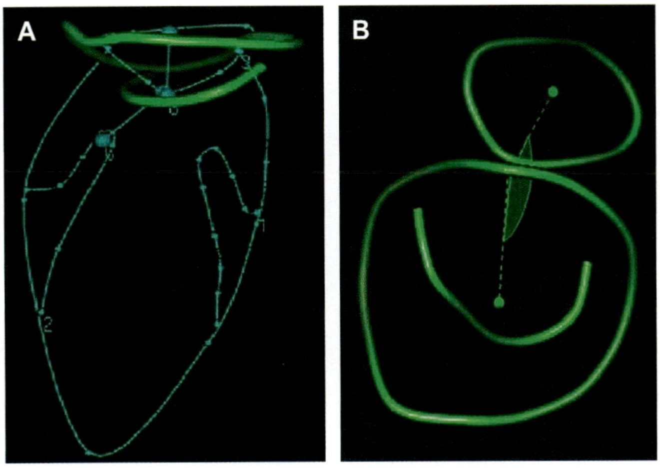

Fig. 9. Advanced 3D analysis technology allows segmentation and quantification of mitral valve annulus, leaflets, and subvalvular apparatus (TomTec 4D MV-Assessment CAP, TomTec Imaging Systems, Unterschleissheim, Germany). (*A*) Tenting area, tenting height, and papillary muscle geometry are visualized. (*B*) The aorto–mitral relationship.

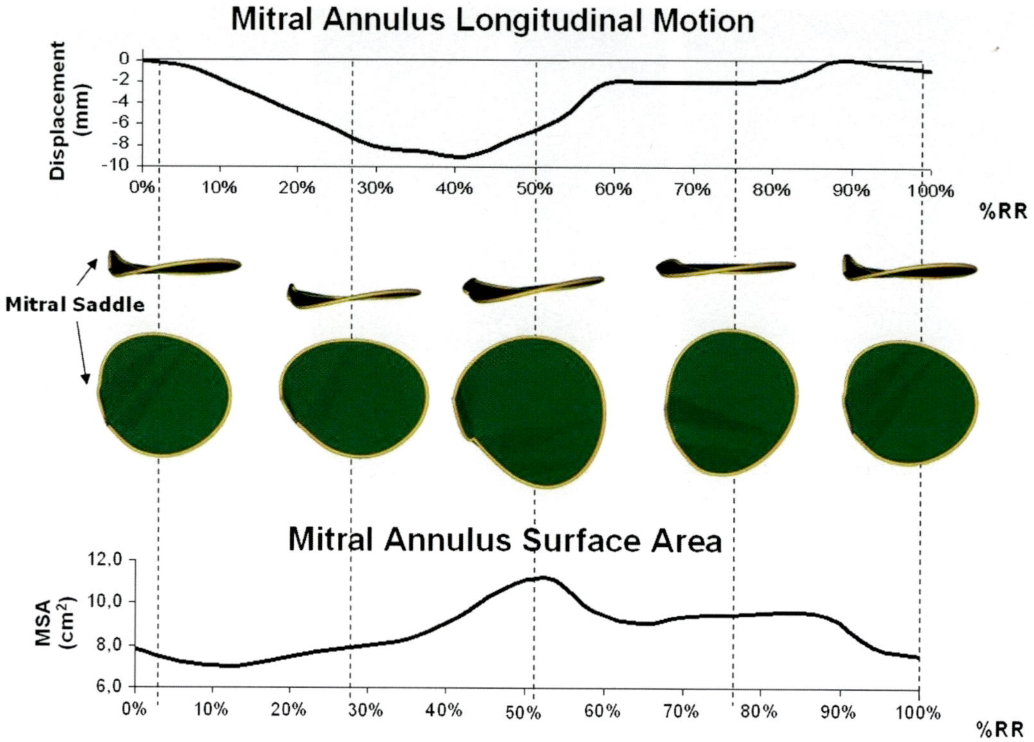

Fig. 10. Numerous parameters can be derived by dynamic annulus analysis. This image shows the dynamic changes in mitral valve longitudinal motion and annulus surface area. (*Courtesy of* L. Sugang, MD and R. Lang, MD, Chicago, IL.)

Aortic valve assessment

To examine the AoV with RT3DE, a high right or left parasternal approach gives the best results [10]. The apical window is another option but has the AoV positioned in the far field. For a complete valvular assessment, the AoV becomes more and more important. Studies have shown that 3DE improves the morphological assessment of the AoV leaflets, the quantification of the valve orifice area in aortic stenosis, and the quantification of aortic regurgitation. Fig. 13 shows a 3D long-axis view of the aortic valve. Fig. 14 shows a quadricuspid AoV from aortic perspective (see Fig. 14A) and in a 3D long-axis view (see Fig. 14B). The noncoronary cusp (NCC) is marked with a red dot. Fig. 15 shows an aortic valve sclerosis case. Fig. 15A demonstrates the aortic valve seen from an aortic perspective looking down on a sclerosed aortic valve in diastole (see Fig. 15A) and in systole (see Fig. 15B).

Limitations of 3DE for assessing the AoV are the temporal resolution of 3DE. Handke and colleagues [33] evaluated a 3DE prototype solution for a very high temporal resolution to study the mitral and aortic valve. Especially the rapid AoV opening phase could be analysed in three dimensions with such a high frame rate of more than 160 frames per second. This study could show how AoV movement is influenced by myocardial and valvular factors.

Tricuspid valve and pulmonary valve assessment

Compared with the MV and AoV, much less work has been published to study the tricuspid valve (TV) and pulmonary valve (PV) with 3DE techniques. In order to acquire a RT3DE data set of the TV, it is recommended to use more gain than normal [10] while positioning the RT3DE transducer in a modified parasternal long axis position, centering the TV in the 3D volume. From an apical four-chamber view, the TV can be visualized in relation to other intracardiac structures. Thus RT3DE allows the visualization of all three TV leaflets, their attachment in the TV annulus, and their relation with the interventricular septum [10]. 3DE also can provide an accurate visualization of the TV from a surgical viewpoint from

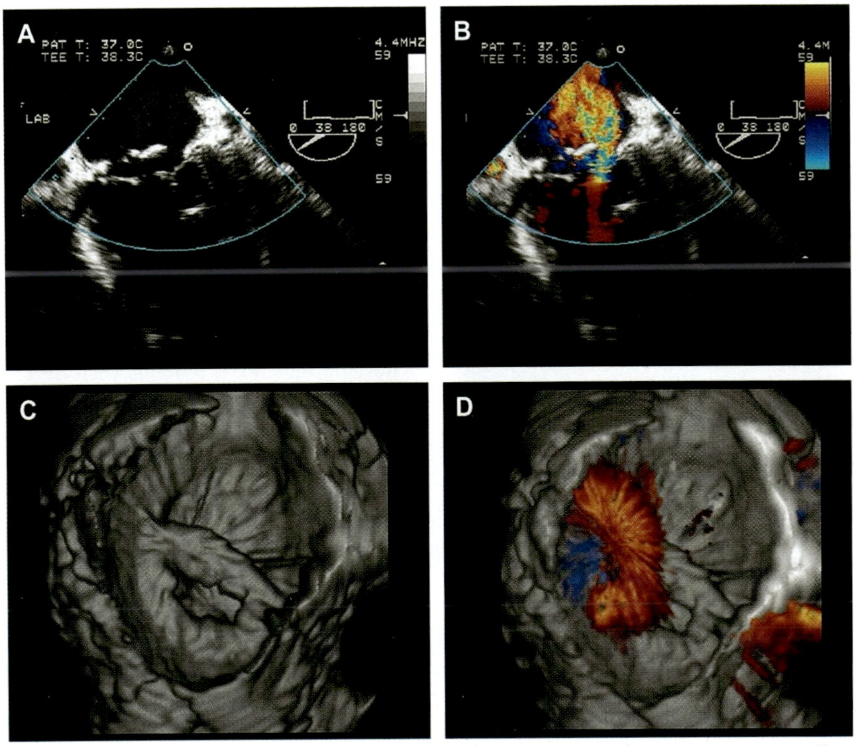

Fig. 11. Patient with severe mitral regurgitation and presented with heart failure after mitral valve repair. On transesophageal echo (TEE) there is an echo density at the level of the mitral valve annulus (*A*), and on color flow Doppler (*B*) there is severe mitral regurgitation, so that it is difficult to differentiate whether there is valvular or para-ring regurgitation. Using a TEE rotational approach, a 3D reconstruction of the valve demonstrated dehiscence of the anterior portion of the mitral valve ring (*C*), severe mitral regurgitation that is valvular, and para-ring regurgitation (*D*). (*Courtesy of* L. Sugang, MD, and R. Lang, MD, Chicago, IL.)

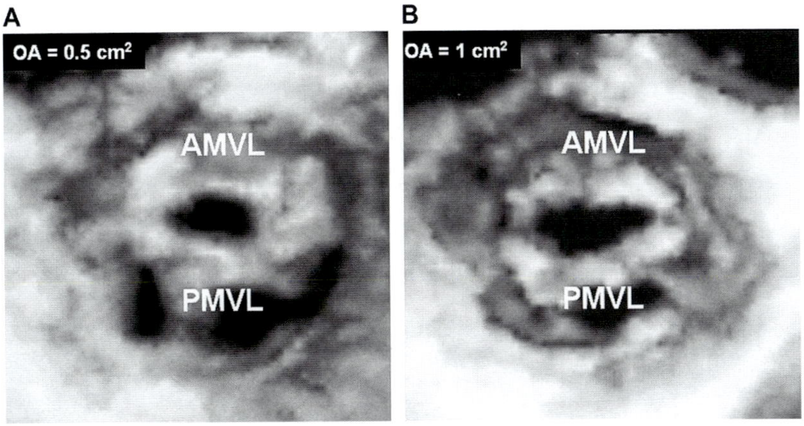

Fig. 12. Patient with mitral stenosis before (*A*) and after (*B*) balloon valvuloplasty. *Abbreviations:* AMVL, anterior mitral valve leaflet; OA, orifice area; PMVL, posterior mitral valve leaflet. (*Courtesy of* L. Sugang, MD, and R. Lang, MD, Chicago, IL.)

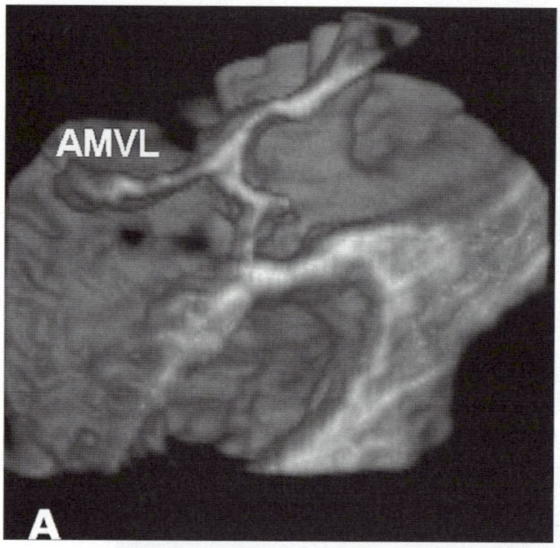

Fig. 13. (*A*) A side view (3D long-axis view) of the aortic valve. *Abbreviation:* AMVL, anterior mitral valve leaflet. (*Courtesy of* N. Nanda, MD, Birmingham, AL.)

the right atrium to help in the surgical decision-making process [4].

In a recent publication, Masaki and colleagues [34] studied the tricuspid annular function and dynamics in children who had RT3DE acquired from an apical view. The authors studied the interaction between the TV and the MV and reported the interplay between the TV annulus and its supporting tension apparatus.

The PV can be acquired and visualized from two parasternal positions, first from a modified parasternal short axis, and second from a modified parasternal long-axis view [10]. In 3DE, the visualization of PV leaflet details can be limited. A better visualization is achieved if the PV is thickened or calcified.

Future outlook

Because 3DE provides unique tools to assess valves preoperatively, it will play an important role in surgical planning in the future. Valve annulus size, shape, and dynamic changes can be determined accurately, and the patient's individual case can be considered in the treatment by developing and providing customized implants. Models of customized implants can be implanted virtually with the help of 3DE data sets to simulate the outcome of the surgery (Fig. 16B). Fig. 16A shows the coronary sinus (CS) together with mitral valve annulus and coaptation line. Future 3D color Doppler technologies may allow quantifying the regurgitation volume (Fig. 16C).

Most of the work for the assessment of valve geometry and function so far has been done for the mitral valve. 3DE enables the collection of completely new parameters describing the valve. Several parameters have been established to describe the mitral annulus geometry and its changes during the cardiac cycle (see Fig. 10). 3DE also has the potential to assess the closing pattern of the leaflets and performed measurements like tenting volume, which has been described by Watanabe and colleagues [33,35]. Because valve pathologies are extremely complex, it is necessary to address the whole valve apparatus, like for the MV, the annulus, the leaflets, the chordae length, and the positioning of the papillary muscles, being influenced by myocardial conditions. 3DE greatly

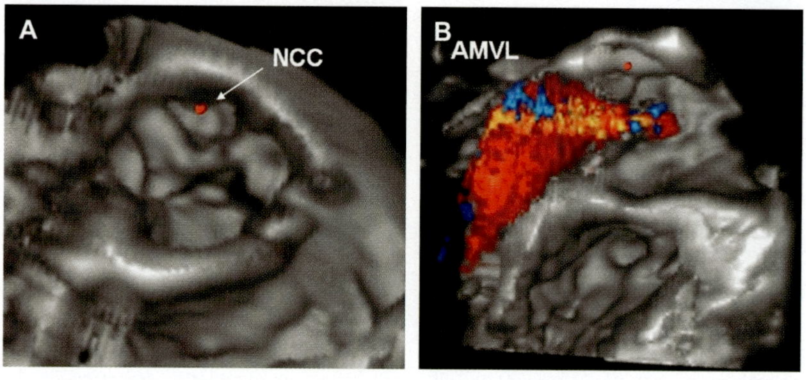

Fig. 14. The same quadricuspid aortic valve from aortic perspective (*A*) and in 3D long-axis view (*B*). The noncoronary cusp (NCC) is marked with a red dot. *Abbreviation:* AMVL, anterior mitral valve leaflet.

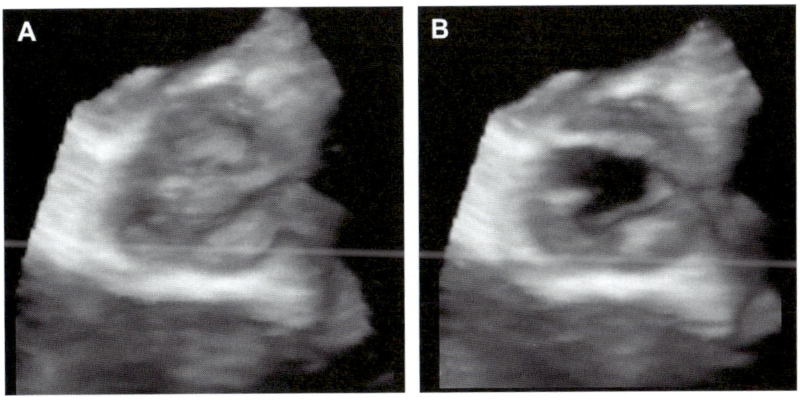

Fig. 15. Aortic valve sclerosis. The aortic valve seen from an aortic perspective looking down on a sclerosed aortic valve in diastole (*A*) and in systole (*B*). (*Courtesy of* L. Sugang, MD, and R. Lang, MD, Chicago, IL.)

improves the understanding of the interaction of those components and therefore leads to a more complete picture of the pathology and to a more profound choice of treatment.

With the improvement of spatial and temporal resolution of 3D color Doppler, the assessment of regurgitations of valves also will enter a new dimension. The current geometric

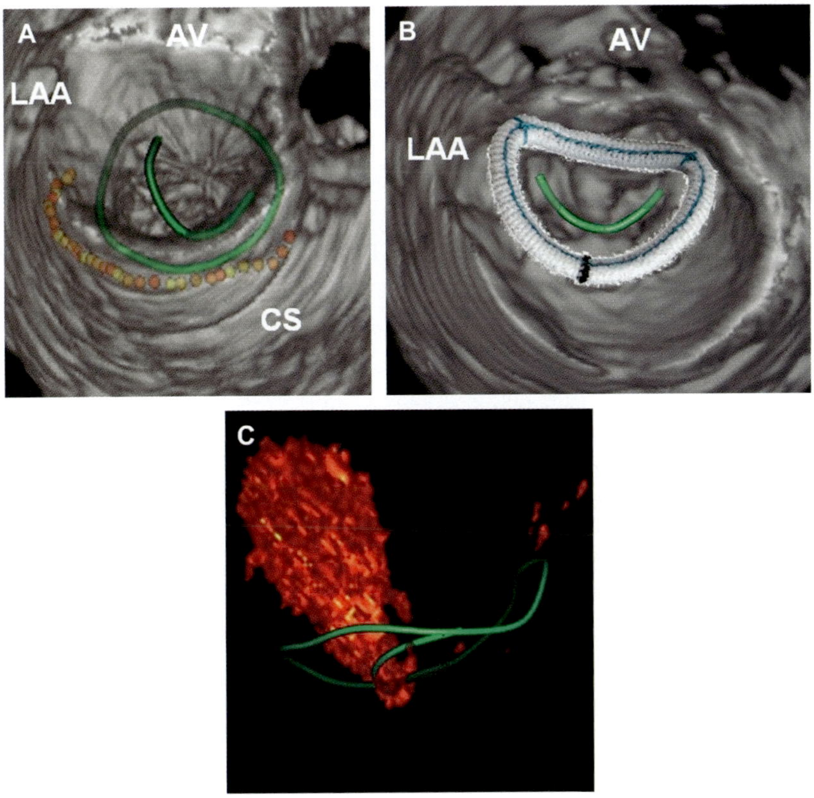

Fig. 16. (*A*) The coronary sinus (CS) together with mitral valve annulus and coaptation line (4D MV-Assessment CAP, TomTec Imaging Systems, Unterschleissheim, Germany). Visualizing the ring into the volume-rendered image (*B*) may help to assess the correct ring size preoperatively. Future 3D color Doppler technologies may allow quantifying the regurgitation volume (*C*).

assumptions for all 2D methods to quantify flow based on color Doppler like the hemispherical surface in the PISA method are not required with 3DE. In 3DE, the flow can be examined in its true dimensions, which will improve understanding and accuracy of the measurements.

Although surgical planning will be one important application of 3DE before treatment, guiding the procedure itself is becoming increasingly important. RT3DE is an ideal tool for offering visual feedback during the procedure, especially with percutaneous interventions like valvuloplasty or minimally invasive aortic valve replacements. This new way of guiding will help to reduce procedure time and will improve the efficiency, quality, and safety of the treatment.

With 3DE overcoming the current limitations of 2D echocardiography, it might change the workflow in laboratories for many applications that do not have to be performed in real time. The ability to reslice a volume offline will transfer a substantial part of the work currently done on the ultrasound system to offline review workstations. Automatic slicing algorithms will display predefined slices of the heart derived from the 3DE data set, but in doubtful cases, the physician still has the option to virtually rescan the patient and generate any 2D slice or 3D view of the structures acquired in the 3DE data volume. Also, physicians from remote places can have access to such a virtual rescan and deliver a second opinion, which makes telemedicine a more realistic scenario rather than just exchanging images and clips.

Summary

3DE is a valuable tool to be used in addition to and not instead of 2D echocardiography by providing complementary information and improved quantitative accuracy and reproducibility compared with 2D techniques [1]. More and more, ultrasound systems will be equipped with a 3DE option. By overcoming the current limitations like the lower temporal resolution, compared with 2D echocardiography, 3DE has the potential to become the standard echocardiographic examination procedure for the assessment of valvular disease.

Acknowledgment

The authors gratefully acknowledge the support of Dr. Lissa Sugeng and Dr. Roberto Lang in providing material for this manuscript.

References

[1] Hung J, Lang R, et al. 3D echocardiography: a review of the current status and future directions. J Am Soc Echocardiogr 2007;20(3):213–33.

[2] Nanda N, Sorrell V. Atlas of 3D echocardiography. Valvular heart disease. Armonk (NY): Futura Publishing; 2002. p. 49–94.

[3] Valocik G, Kamp O, Visser CA. Three-dimensional echocardiography in mitral valve disease. Eur J Echocardiogr 2005;6(6):443–54.

[4] Salehian O, Chan KL. Impact of 3D echocardiography in valvular heart disease. Curr Opin Cardiol 2005;20(2):122–6.

[5] Hoda MR, Schwarz T, Wolf I, et al. Three-dimensional echocardiography in cardiac surgery: current status and perspectives. Chirurg 2007;78(5):435–42.

[6] Sugeng L, Coon P, Weinert L, et al. Use of real-time 3-dimensional transthoracic echocardiography in the evaluation of mitral valve disease. J Am Soc Echocardiogr 2006;19(4):413–21.

[7] Sugeng L, Shernan SK, Lang R, et al. Realtime 3D transesophagel echocardiographic assessment of cardiac structures. J Am Soc Echocardiogr 2007; 20(5):570.

[8] Roelandt JRTC, Salustri A, Vletter W, et al. Precordial multiplane echocardiography for dynamic anyplane, paraplane, and 3D imaging of the heart. The Thoraxcentre J 1994;6/5:6–15.

[9] De Castro S, Salandin V, Cartoni D, et al. Qualitative and quantitative evaluation of mitral valve morphology by intraoperative volume-rendered 3D echocardiography. J Heart Valve Dis 2002;11(2): 173–80.

[10] van den Bosch A. Real-time 3D echocardiography: an extra dimension in the echographic diagnosis of congenital heart disease. Rotterdam, Netherlands; Erasmus University: 2006. p. 31–41.

[11] Goktekin O, Matsumura M, Omoto R, et al. Evaluation of mitral valve prolapse using newly developed real-time 3D echocardiographic system with real-time volume rendering. Int J Card Imaging 2003; 19(1):43–9.

[12] Chauvel C, Bogino E, Clerc P, et al. Usefulness of 3D echocardiography for the evaluation of mitral valve prolapse: an intraoperative study. J Heart Valve Dis 2000;9(3):341–9.

[13] Levine RA, Handschumacher MD, Sanfilippo AJ, et al. Three-dimensional echocardiographic reconstruction of the mitral valve, with implications for the diagnosis of mitral valve prolapse. Circulation 1989;80(3):589–98.

[14] Chung R, Pepper J, Henein M. Images in cardiology: mitral valve anterior leaflet prolapse by real- time 3D transthoracic echocardiography. Heart (British Cardiac Society) 2005;91(9):e55.

[15] Pepi M, Tamborini G, Maltagliati A, et al. Head-to-head comparison of 2- and 3D transthoracic and transesophageal echocardiography in the

localization of mitral valve prolapse. J Am Coll Cardiol 2006;48(12):2524–30.
[16] Delabays A, Jeanrenaud X, Chassot PG, et al. Localization and quantification of mitral valve prolapse using 3D echocardiography. Eur J Echocardiogr 2004;5(6):422–9.
[17] Patel V, Hsiung MC, Nanda NC, et al. Usefulness of live/real time 3D transthoracic echocardiography in the identification of individual segment/scallop prolapse of the mitral valve. Echocardiography 2006; 23(6):513–8.
[18] Müller S, Bartel T. Comparison of 3D imaging to transesophageal echocardiography for preoperative evaluation in mitral valve prolapse. Am J Cardiol 2006;98:243–8.
[19] Galloway AC, Colvin SB, Baumann FG, et al. A comparison of mitral valve reconstruction with mitral valve replacement: intermediate-term results. Ann Thorac Surg 1989;47(5):655–62.
[20] Ahmed S, Nanda NC, Miller AP, et al. Usefulness of transesophageal 3D echocardiography in the identification of individual segment/scallop prolapse of the mitral valve. Echocardiography 2003;20(2): 203–9.
[21] Enriquez-Sarano M, Avierinos J, et al. Quantitative determinants of the outcome of asymptomatic mitral regurgitation. N Engl J Med 2005;352:875–83.
[22] Khanna D, Miller AP, Nanda NC, et al. Transthoracic and transesophageal echocardiographic assessment of mitral regurgitation severity: usefulness of qualitative and semiquantitative techniques. Echocardiography 2005;22(9):748–69.
[23] Macnab A, Ray SG. Three-dimensional echocardiography is superior to multiplane transoesophageal echo in the assessment of regurgitant mitral valve morphology. Eur J Echocardiogr 2004;5(3):212–22.
[24] Macnab A, Jenkins NP, Ewington I, et al. A method for the morphological analysis of the regurgitant mitral valve using 3D echocardiography. Heart 2004; 90(7):771–6.
[25] Franke A, Kuehl HP. Regurgitant mitral valve and 3D echocardiography—meant for each other? Eur J Echocardiogr 2004;5(3):212–22.
[26] Diamon M, Gillinov M, Liddicoat JR, et al. Dynamic change in mitral annular area and motion during percutaneous mitral annuloplasty for ischemic mitral regurgitation: preliminary animal study with real-time 3-dimensional echocardiography. J Am Soc Echocardiogr 2007;20(4):381–8.
[27] Paszczuk A, Wiegers S. Quantitative assessment of mitral insufficiency: its advantages and disadvantages. Heart Fail Rev 2006;11:205–17.
[28] Iwakura K, Ito H, Kawano S, et al. Comparison of orifice area by transthoracic 3D Doppler echocardiography versus proximal isovelocity surface area (PISA) method for assessment of mitral regurgitation. Am J Cardiol 2006;97(11):1630–7.
[29] Khanna D, Vengala S, Miller AP, et al. Quantification of mitral regurgitation by live 3D transthoracic echocardiographic measurements of vena contracta area. Echocardiography 2004;21(8):737–43.
[30] Sugeng L, Weinert L, Lammertin G, et al. Accuracy of mitral valve area measurement using transthoracic rapid freehand 3-dimensional scanning: comparison with noninvasive and invasive methods. J Am Soc Echocardiogr 2003;16:1292–300.
[31] Zamorano J, Cordeiro P, Sugeng L, et al. Real-time 3D echocardiography for rheumatic mitral valve stenosis evaluation: an accurate and novel approach. J Am Coll Cardiol 2004;43(11):2091–6.
[32] Sugeng L, Weinert L, Lang RM. Accuracy of mitral valve area measurements using transthoracic rapid freehand 3-dimensional scanning: comparison with noninvasive and invasive methods. J Am Soc Echocardiogr 2003;16(12):1292–300.
[33] Handke M, Jahnke C, Heinrichs G, et al. New 3D echocardiographic system using digital radiofrequency data—visualization and quantitative analysis of aortic valve dynamics with high resolution: methods, feasibility, and initial clinical experience. Circulation 2003;107(23):2876–9.
[34] Masaki N, Guerra V, Roman KS, et al. Three-dimensional tricuspid annular function provides insight into the mechanism of tricuspid valve regurgitation in classic hypoplastic left heart syndrome. J Am Soc Echocardiogr 2006;19(4): 391–402.
[35] Watanabe N, Ogasawara Y, Yamaura Y, et al. Quantitation of mitral valve tenting in ischemic mitral regurgitation by transthoracic real-time 3D echocardiography. J Am Coll Cardiol 2005;45(5): 763–9.

ELSEVIER
SAUNDERS

Cardiol Clin 25 (2007) 297–303

CARDIOLOGY
CLINICS

Current Status of Three-Dimensional Color Flow Doppler

Lissa Sugeng, MD*, Roberto M. Lang, MD, FACC, FASE, FAHA

Section of Cardiology, Department of Medicine, University of Chicago Medical Center, MC 5084, 5841 South Maryland Avenue, Chicago, IL 60637, USA

The first effort to image intracardiac flow in three dimensions to obtain gray-scale reconstructions of jets was performed using a transthoracic sequential multiplanar–rotational gated acquisition. Acquisition of color information from 2D echocardiography images was not possible at the time, resulting in the inability to separate tissue from intracardiac flow [1]. Nevertheless, it permitted visualization of flow convergence zones that set in motion other studies to observe the effects of orifice shape, impact of the geometry of the regurgitant orifice, and enable the validation of 3D echocardiography (3DE) as a more accurate method to estimate the vena contracta area [2–5].

Method of 3D color-flow acquisition

A 3D volume of a color-flow jet was acquired from the transthoracic or transesophageal approach using a rotational gated sequential acquisition method (Fig. 1A). The transthoracic approach required a commercially available transducer to be inserted into a cylindrical device that mechanically rotated the probe. From the transesophageal approach, the image sector was rotated electronically. When using the latter approach, the regurgitant jet was positioned in the middle of the sector. Sequential 2D color-flow images were collected from a single window every 3° to 5° over a 180° rotation gated to the patient's electrocardiogram and respiration (end exhalation). Images were stored on a disc and subsequently processed on an off-line computer. These images were reformatted in time and space to produce a Cartesian volume data set. Further manipulation of this data usually was performed using special software to allow volume, surface, or wire frame display and quantitation of regurgitant volume. This technique is limited because of the multiple cardiac cycles that need to be acquired to obtain a volume data set. This introduces radial artifacts if the transesophageal echocardiography (TEE) probe moves during data acquisition because of respiration or peristaltic motion. On the other hand, this approach allowed simultaneous data collection and reconstruction of color flow data superimposed on valve leaflet and chamber structures. Another mode of acquisition used in early investigational studies of 3D color flow was a free-hand method (Fig. 1B) using a magnetic sensor and transmitter that was attached to the probe. Multiple images were obtained from a single window in a fan-like manner gated to ECG and respiration. Images were reformatted and analyzed on an off-line computer.

With the advent of a fully-sampled matrix array transducer (Fig. 1C), the number of cardiac cycles required to acquire a color-flow data set was reduced. Data collection necessitated ECG gating and a breath hold by the patient, which reduced the incidence of artifact. Although frame rates are higher using this method, the sector size is narrower along with restricted visualization of the regurgitant volume and surrounding valve leaflets.

* Corresponding author.
E-mail address: lsugeng@medicine.bsd.uchicago.edu (L. Sugeng).

doi:10.1016/j.ccl.2007.06.006

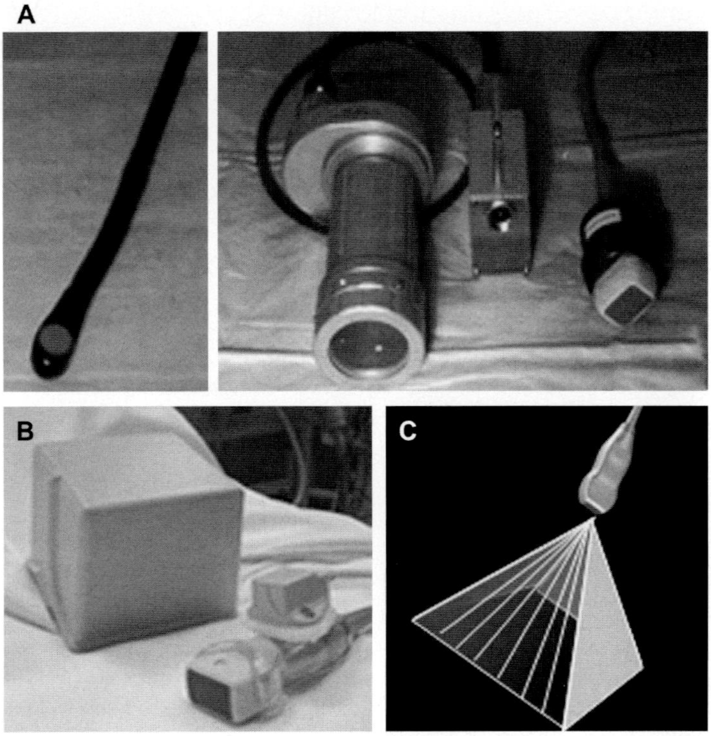

Fig. 1. Acquisition methods. (*A*) Rotational gated sequential acquisition method using a transesophageal probe or transthoracic transducer coupled in a mechanical rotational device. (*B*) Free-hand method using magnetic sensor and transmitter. (*C*) Fully-sampled matrix array transducer acquires a pyramidal volume data set consisting of seven subvolumes for color acquisition.

Regurgitant jets and shunts

Early 3D reconstructions of jets were feasible using a rotational gated sequential method of acquisition using a transthoracic probe coupled with a motorized device. These images provided in still-frame or in a dynamic format an appreciation of the shape, its relative location and size relative to the cardiac chamber, and the jet shape of the flow convergence surface over the regurgitant orifice [1]. With the ability to visualize 3D reconstructions of flow convergence, subsequent studies focused on the quantitation of regurgitant orifice areas and regurgitant volumes derived from 3DE data sets. As the regurgitant orifice shapes are noncircular along with wall-hugging jets, 2D echocardiography easily underestimates the orifice size (35% to 44%) and regurgitant flow (22% to 32%) [6]. These findings also were demonstrated in animal models of aortic regurgitation, confirming that 3DE was more accurate in the estimation of regurgitant orifice area, regurgitant volumes, and vena contracta [2,7,8]. Similarly, this approach also was applied to pulmonary regurgitant jets to estimate volumes, which agreed well with the reference standard [4]. Most of these studies demonstrating regurgitant jets and flow convergence were derived from video composite data, which have the same variability as 2D color Doppler flow mapping such as gain settings, wall filtering, and aliasing velocities. During this development period, 3D reconstruction of regurgitant jets was also in gray-scale map without velocity information. Differentiation between flow and anatomy were not possible at this time.

3D reconstruction displaying color flow first was demonstrated in patients who had mitral regurgitation (MR) (Fig. 2) [9,10]. 3D mitral regurgitant jets, acquired using a gated sequential rotational TEE approach, were processed off line using the Heidelberg ray tracing method, which enabled display of 3D color flow while simultaneously allowing quantitation of jet volumes [11]. Qualitatively, these reconstructed images of MR

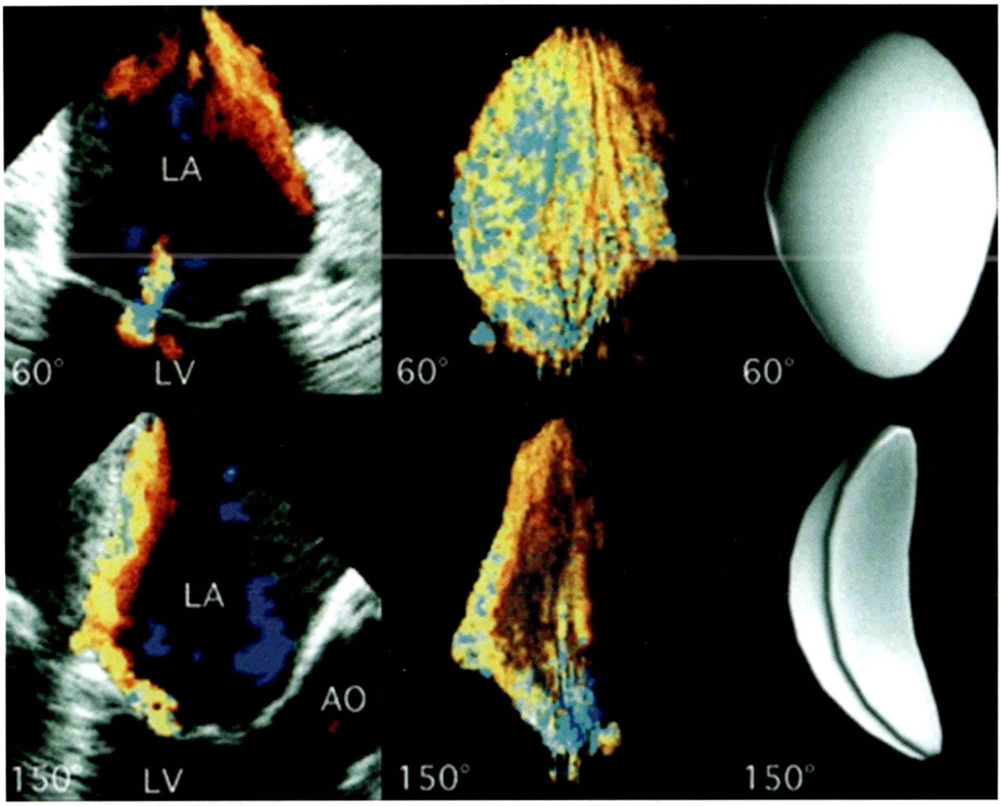

Fig. 2. Mitral regurgitation jet with a spoon pattern in a patient with anterior prolapse. Visualization of the jet in two dimensions at 600 and 1500 only demonstrates portion of the jet (left, top, and bottom panels). 3D reconstructions, using the Heidelberg Ray tracing method enables display of 3D color flow (*middle panels*) and surface-rendered images (*right, top, and bottom panels*). (*From* De Simone R, Glombitza G, Vahl CF, et al. 3D color Doppler: a clinical study in patients with mitral regurgitation. J Am Coll Cardiol 1999;33:1646–54; with permission.)

aid in demonstrating jets in three dimensions rather than with mental conceptualization using multiple 2D views. The direction of the jet, extent, and geometry were recognized using this 3DE technique. Besides having a display of jet geometry, the more significant strength of this methodology lies in its ability to quantitate. When 3D jet volumes were compared with 2D quantitative methods for MR (continuity method for regurgitant volume and fraction and jet area), 3D jet volume had a better correlation compared with 2D methods using angiography as the reference standard. In addition, 3D jet volumes of eccentric jets were significantly larger compared with calculated 2D methods. One may conclude that 3DE correctly identifies severe mitral regurgitation when 2D methods underestimate severity, particularly when using the jet area calculation, and to a lesser degree if the regurgitant volume formula is used [11,12]. Nevertheless, there are limitations to the previous 3D methods that are not real-time; the jet size is dependent on gain settings, velocity scale, frame rate, and filters, and a transesophageal approach was required in a controlled setting (under general anesthesia). Moreover, comparison of 2D jet volumes with more current 2D quantitative method such as flow convergence was not used and angiography, as the gold standard has its own set of limitations for assessing MR. The absence of gray-scale information such as the valve morphology and left atrial chamber also provided an incomplete demonstration of the relation of the jet to cardiac anatomy.

The ability to incorporate both color-flow data and gray-scale information has enabled the quantitation of MR severity using 3DE by visualizing the vena contracta, measuring the proximal isovelocity surface area (PISA) radius, or estimating tricuspid or mitral regurgitant volume relative to the atrial chambers. In an in vitro setting, 3D quantitation of flow-convergent zones are more accurate (2.6% underestimation) compared with 2D or M-mode methods, which underestimate regurgitant volumes (44.2% and 32.1%, respectively) [13]. Recent development of a fully sampled matrix array probe allows color-flow Doppler and gray-scale information to be acquired simultaneously over seven cardiac cycles (Fig. 3A, B). When comparing 3D derived vena contracta (Fig. 3C) measurements for tricuspid regurgitation (TR) jets, the minimum diameter measurements were similar to 2D measurements but in an orthogonal view. The maximum diameters were larger in three dimensions compared with two dimensions. Whereas for mitral regurgitant flow, 3D derived maximum and minimum vena contracta measurements were significantly larger than 2D measurements but more circular/oval than TR vena contractas, which appear more elliptical in shape [14]. Similarly, a comparison of 3D derived vena contracta area to MR angiography demonstrated a better agreement for quantitative assessment of MR than 2D derived vena contracta width and jet/left atrial (LA) area ratio to estimate the severity of MR. When comparing 3D MR jet/LA volume ratios and TR jet/right atrial volume rations with 2D MR jet/LA area and 2D TR jet/right atrial area ratios, 3D ratios were significantly smaller than 2D ratios (Fig. 4D). This could be explained by the larger atria volumes, low frame rates in 3D imaging, poor delineation of the jet, and averaging of high velocity flow lending to smaller 3D jet volumes [15].

Assessment of function

Measurements of stroke volume (SV) and cardiac output (CO) using the Thermodilution method are useful for serial hemodynamic monitoring. This methodology requires an invasive procedure that may result in complications while

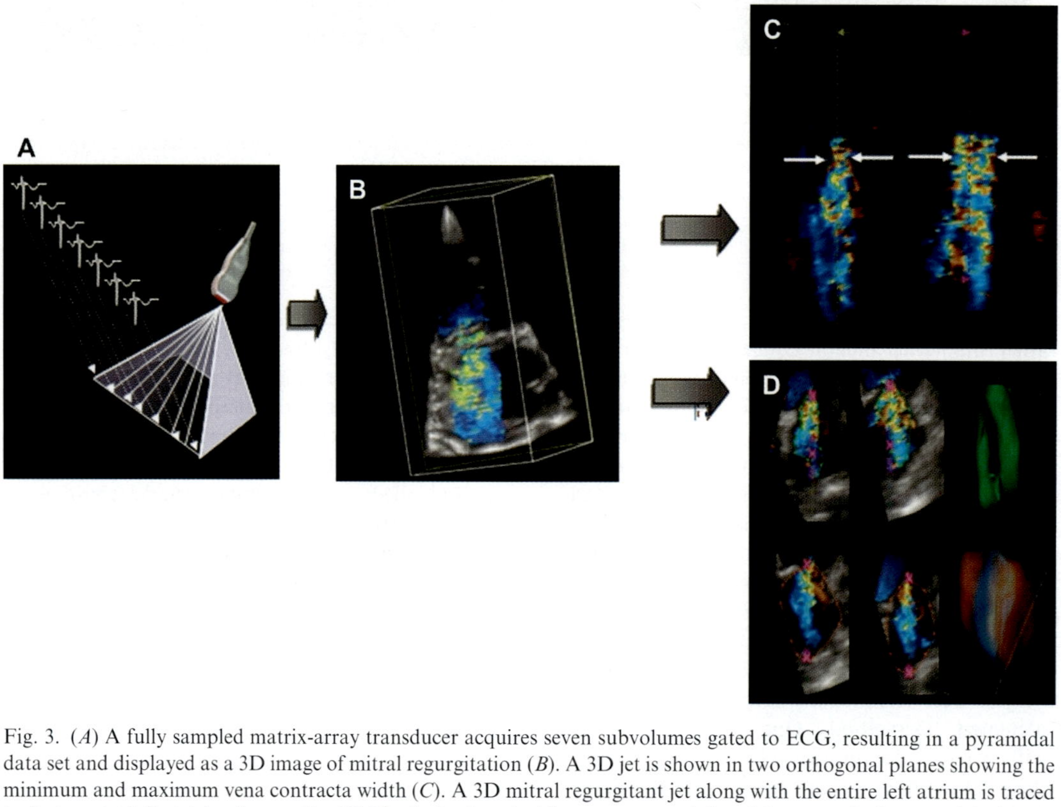

Fig. 3. (*A*) A fully sampled matrix-array transducer acquires seven subvolumes gated to ECG, resulting in a pyramidal data set and displayed as a 3D image of mitral regurgitation (*B*). A 3D jet is shown in two orthogonal planes showing the minimum and maximum vena contracta width (*C*). A 3D mitral regurgitant jet along with the entire left atrium is traced to derive a jet/left atrial volume ratio. (*D*) The jet is viewed with a transparent left atrial cast on the bottom right image.

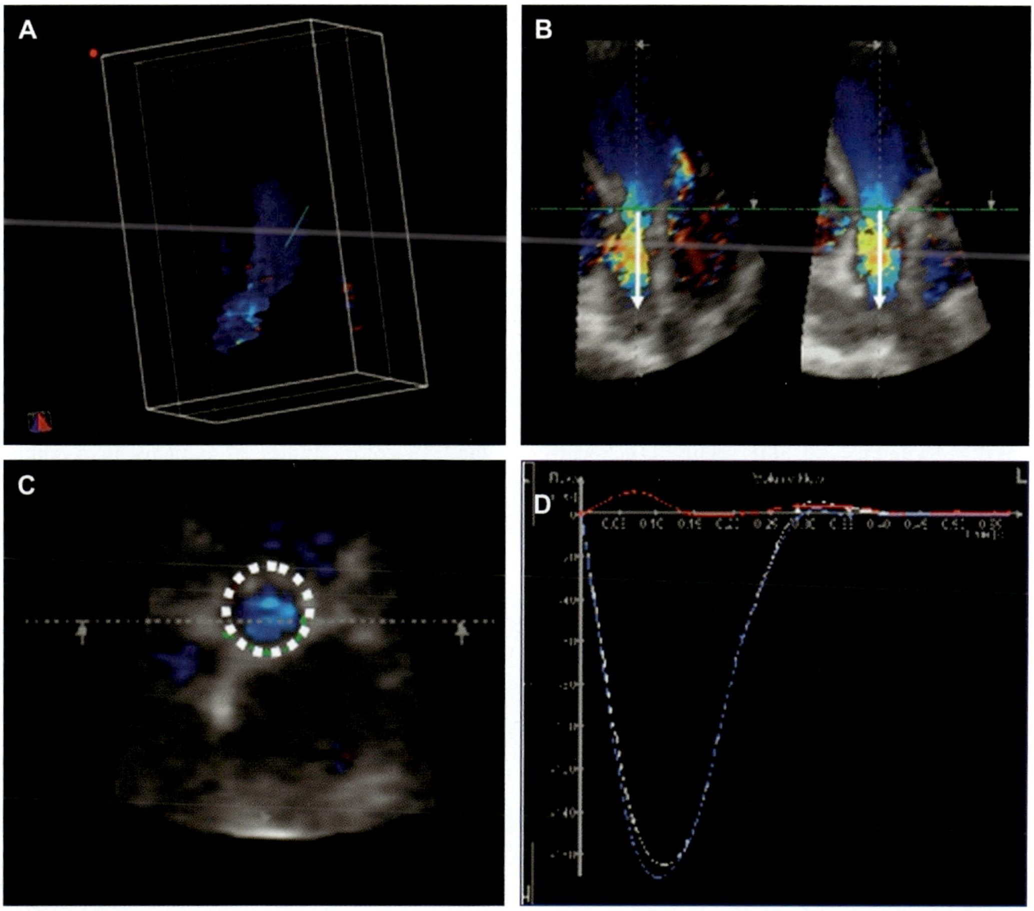

Fig. 4. Cardiac output estimation using off-line analysis software to quantitate flow rate (TomTec Imaging Systems, Unterscheissheim, Germany). A 3D color Doppler volume data set (*A*) subsequently is displayed in two orthogonal planes (*B*). Arrows (*white*) indicate the direction of flow, which automatically is aligned perpendicularly along a curved surface. In a third multiplanar view, a circular region of interest is drawn to calculate flow rate (*C and D*).

being prone to inaccuracies. Noninvasive methods such as 2D echocardiography and pulsed wave Doppler measurements of cardiac output provide an estimate of these measurements but are also fraught with limitations because of geometric assumptions of the left ventricular outflow tract (LVOT), alignment of Doppler flow, and inaccuracies with the LVOT velocity profile. Real-time 3DE data contain Doppler and gray-scale volume information that are obtained initially using an optimized 2D echocardiography image acquired in a biplane view. Subsequently, a region of interest is placed surrounding the LVOT and aortic valve to calculate aortic flow. Gated to ECG and using a breath hold, a 3D volume is acquired over seven cardiac cycles. Thus, the final volume consists of seven subvolumes with smaller color subvolumes contained within the region of interest. 3D color Doppler may overcome these limitations by using a semiautomated method of integrating flow traversing the LVOT to derive SV and CO calculations. The foundation of this method was established in-vitro and later in vivo in animal studies that determined the feasibility and accuracy of 3DE [16–21]. Of note, calculation of stroke volume from real-time 3DE data performed in an in vitro study depends on the depth of imaging. Stroke volumes are less accurate with depths greater than 13 cm, particularly with higher SV caused by decreased resolution and reduced frame rates [22].

Human studies have yielded similar correlations against gold standards, such as thermodilution and 2DE [23,24]. Both studies used real-time

3DE color volume data set and off-line analysis (TomTec Imaging Systems, Unterscheissheim, Munich, Germany) to quantitate flow volumes based on Gaussian control surface theory. Direction of flow automatically is aligned perpendicularly along a curved surface; thus the flow rate is equal to the sum of all vectors [25]. Placement of this curved surface is defined in two orthogonal views. Subsequently, in a third multiplanar view a circular region of interest is drawn to calculate flow rate (Fig. 4 A–D). Using this methodology, stroke volumes derived using 3DE correlate well with 2D echocardiography, but when 2D echocardiography and 3DE calculations were compared against thermodilution, 3DE had better correlations ($r = .94$ and $r = .75$, 3DE versus 2D echocardiography, respectively) with smaller biases and narrower limits of agreement (1.84 ± 16.8 versus -8.6 ± 36.2 mol). When this methodology was applied to mitral inflow in children, it also compared well against phase velocity MRI at the ascending aorta and left volumetric MRI measurements [26]. Similarly, mitral valve inflow using 3DE compared better than 2D echocardiography ($r = .93$ and $r = .75$, respectively) [23].

Limitations

Real-time 3DE acquisition using a fully sampled matrix array probe has improved and overcome significantly many of the limitations encountered with previous methods of data collection. This technology allows shorter data collection and concurrent color Doppler information and gray scale. Shortcomings of this technology still exist, however. The 3D volume data set consists of seven subvolumes that are acquired over 7 to 14 cardiac cycles during a breath hold. This introduces the possibility of stitch artifact, seen as misalignment between subvolumes, caused by either movement of the probe, inability to maintain a breath hold, or arrhythmias during acquisition. Another drawback is that the sector sizes for both color Doppler and gray scale are too narrow to compensate for low frame rates, particularly if one wants to image the extent of the jet contained within an atrial chamber. If the region of interest is either the flow convergence or the outflow tract, this latter drawback is not as problematic. As technology advances, a single-volume acquisition would be preferable with high frame rates, depending on the density of the 3D volume.

Another major impediment of using 3D Color Doppler clinically is that data analysis must be performed off line. Other challenges are the continued presence of aliasing and color bleeding. Although current software enables the operator to adjust for aliasing by shifting Doppler baseline during off-line analysis, overt baseline shifting results in overestimation of cardiac output. Color bleeding may be adjusted by changing write priority (parameter or threshold that balances between 3D color and gray scale), but this also may confound the results.

Though much has been learned about the potential advantages of 3D color Doppler over 2D echocardiography, the feasibility of performing 3D color studies in patients in a clinical practice is challenging. Reasons for these continued obstacles are poor acoustic windows, inadequate color gain settings, and respiratory artifacts [23].

Summary

3D color Doppler has provided new physiologic insight into regurgitant jets, an alternative method for quantitation, and more accurate estimates of regurgitant volume, vena contracta, and effective regurgitant orifice areas. It is a relatively new noninvasive tool that also enables quantitation of cardiac output, stroke volume, pulmonary outflow, and shunt calculations. With further advances in computer and ultrasound technology, this modality will become a viable tool in clinical practice.

References

[1] Delabays A, Sugeng L, Pandian NG, et al. Dynamic three-dimensional echocardiographic assessment of intracardiac blood flow jets. Am J Cardiol 1995; 76(14):1053–8.

[2] Shiota T, Jones M, Delabays A, et al. Direct measurement of three-dimensionally reconstructed flow convergence surface area and regurgitant flow in aortic regurgitation: in vitro and chronic animal model studies. Circulation 1997;96(10):3687–95.

[3] Shiota T, Jones M, Aida S, et al. Calculation of aortic regurgitant volume by a new digital Doppler color-flow mapping method: an animal study with quantified chronic aortic regurgitation. J Am Coll Cardiol 1997;30(3):834–42.

[4] Mori Y, Rusk RA, Jones M, et al. A new dynamic three-dimensional digital color Doppler method for quantification of pulmonary regurgitation:

validation study in an animal model. J Am Coll Cardiol 2002;40(6):1179–85.
[5] Guo Z, Boughner DR, Dietrich JM, et al. Quantitative assessment of in vitro jets based on three-dimensional color Doppler reconstruction. Ultrasound Med Biol 2001;27(2):235–43.
[6] Shiota T, Sinclair B, Ishii M, et al. Three-dimensional reconstruction of color Doppler flow convergence regions and regurgitant jets: an in vitro quantitative study. J Am Coll Cardiol 1996;27(6):1511–8.
[7] Mori Y, Shiota T, Jones M, et al. Three-dimensional reconstruction of the color Doppler-imaged vena contracta for quantifying aortic regurgitation: studies in a chronic animal model. Circulation 1999; 99(12):1611–7.
[8] Acar P, Jones M, Shiota T, et al. Quantitative assessment of chronic aortic regurgitation with 3-dimensional echocardiographic reconstruction: comparison with electromagnetic flow meter measurements. J Am Soc Echocardiogr 1999;12(2): 138–48.
[9] De Simone R, Glombitza G, Vahl CF, et al. Assessment of mitral regurgitant jets by three-dimensional color Doppler. Ann Thorac Surg 1999;67(2):494–9.
[10] De Simone R, Glombitza G, Vahl CF, et al. Three-dimensional Doppler. Techniques and clinical applications. Eur Heart J 1999;20(8):619–27.
[11] De Simone R, Glombitza G, Vahl CF, et al. Three-dimensional color Doppler: a clinical study in patients with mitral regurgitation. J Am Coll Cardiol 1999;33(6):1646–54.
[12] De Simone R, Glombitza G, Vahl CF, et al. Three-dimensional color Doppler: a new approach for quantitative assessment of mitral regurgitant jets. J Am Soc Echocardiogr 1999;12(3):173–85.
[13] Coisne D, Erwan D, Christiaens L, et al. Quantitative assessment of regurgitant flow with total digital three-dimensional reconstruction of color Doppler flow in the convergent region: in vitro validation. J Am Soc Echocardiogr 2002;15(3):233–40.
[14] Sugeng L, Weinert L, Lang RM. Real-time 3-dimensional color Doppler flow of mitral and tricuspid regurgitation: feasibility and initial quantitative comparison with 2-dimensional methods. J Am Soc Echocardiogr, in press.
[15] Khanna D, Vengala S, Miller AP, et al. Quantification of mitral regurgitation by live three-dimensional transthoracic echocardiographic measurements of vena contracta area. Echocardiography 2004;21(8): 737–43.
[16] Berg S, Torp H, Haugen BO, et al. Volumetric blood flow measurement with the use of dynamic 3-dimensional ultrasound color flow imaging. J Am Soc Echocardiogr 2000;13(5):393–402.
[17] Irvine T, Li XN, Mori Y, et al. A digital 3-dimensional method for computing great artery flows: in vitro validation studies. J Am Soc Echocardiogr 2000;13(9):841–8.
[18] Li J, Li X, Mori Y, et al. Quantification of flow volume with a new digital three-dimensional color Doppler flow approach: an in vitro study. J Ultrasound Med 2001;20(12):1303–11.
[19] Li XN, Sahn DJ. Quantifying cardiac flow with freehand 3D scan. Eur J Echocardiogr 2000;1(3): 152–3.
[20] Pemberton J, Li X, Karamlou T, et al. The use of live three-dimensional Doppler echocardiography in the measurement of cardiac output: an in vivo animal study. J Am Coll Cardiol 2005;45(3):433–8.
[21] Rusk RA, Li XN, Irvine T, et al. Surface integration of velocity vectors from 3D digital colour Doppler: an angle-independent method for laminar flow measurements. Eur J Echocardiogr 2002;3(3):177–84.
[22] Pemberton J, Hui L, Young M, et al. Accuracy of 3-dimensional color Doppler-derived flow volumes with increasing image depth. J Ultrasound Med 2005;24(8):1109–15.
[23] Lodato JA, Weinert L, Baumann R, et al. Use of 3-dimensional color Doppler echocardiography to measure stroke volume in human beings: comparison with thermodilution. J Am Soc Echocardiogr 2007;20(2):103–12.
[24] Pemberton J, Li X, Kenny A, et al. Real-time 3-dimensional Doppler echocardiography for the assessment of stroke volume: an in vivo human study compared with standard 2-dimensional echocardiography. J Am Soc Echocardiogr 2005;18(10): 1030–6.
[25] Pemberton J, Ge S, Thiele K, et al. Real-time three-dimensional color Doppler echocardiography overcomes the inaccuracies of spectral Doppler for stroke volume calculation. J Am Soc Echocardiogr 2006;19(11):1403–10.
[26] Ge S, Bu L, Zhang H, et al. A real-time 3-dimensional digital Doppler method for measurement of flow rate and volume through mitral valve in children: a validation study compared with magnetic resonance imaging. J Am Soc Echocardiogr 2005; 18(1):1–7.

ELSEVIER
SAUNDERS

Cardiol Clin 25 (2007) 305–309

CARDIOLOGY
CLINICS

Three-Dimensional Echocardiography: An Alternative Imaging Choice for Evaluation of Tricuspid Valve Disorders

Alicia A. Ahlgrim, BS, RDCS, RDMS[a],
Navin C. Nanda, MD, FACC, FAHA, FSOC, FISCU[b],
Elenise Berther, RDCS[a], Edward A. Gill, MD, FACC, FASE, FACP[c,*]

[a]*Harborview Medical Center, 325 Ninth Avenue, Box 359748, Seattle, WA 98104, USA*
[b]*University of Alabama at Birmingham, Heart Station SW/S102, 619 19th Street South, Birmingham, AL 35249, USA*
[c]*Division of Cardiology, Harborview Medical Center, University of Washington School of Medicine, 325 Ninth Avenue, Box 359748, Seattle, WA 98104, USA*

Historically, precise echocardiographic depiction of the tricuspid valve anatomy has proven to be illusive. Simultaneous visualization of all leaflets has not been achieved routinely from standard two-dimensional echo (2DE) imaging views, especially the posterior leaflet [1]. Therefore, 2DE evaluates the valvular structure and function with only two leaflets represented within the imaging plane. The result is that determination of individual tricuspid leaflet involvement is challenging when pathologic processes are present, and is perhaps accomplished best by acquiring a multiple cardiac cycle capture with an anterior to posterior sweep.

Conversely, the left-sided valves are visualized easily en face from parasternal short axis view. The aortic valve is of course particularly well visualized en face, and very frequently all three leaflets are visualized easily. Imaging for the bileaflet mitral valve is also often quite pleasing by 2D imaging in the parasternal short axis view.

Real-time three-dimensional (RT3D) imaging previously has been used to aid quantification of tricuspid regurgitation using color flow [2]. In addition, a series of 29 patients has been presented with various tricuspid pathologies. In this series, the main advantage of the RT3D was the ability to see all three leaflets. The authors particularly re-emphasized that the posterior leaflet is particularly difficult to visualize by 2DE [3]. This article presents an approach to RT3D imaging the tricuspid valve from three different views. This is followed by some representative cases that illustrate these views and some unique tricuspid valve abnormalities, including one case of corrected transposition.

Approaches to 3D imaging of the tricuspid valve

Like 2DE, there are three main views for use with RT3D imaging: parasternal, apical, and subcostal. In RT3D imaging, however, there is also the truly real-time acquisition, and then there is the four cardiac cycle full volume. Both of these approaches are useful for tricuspid valve imaging, particularly from the apical and parasternal views. A major advantage that RT3D imaging offers in terms of physical imaging is the ability to steer the 3D beam without actually moving the transducer. Here, in addition to basic RT3D imaging, the authors provide some tips for using the beam steering and some examples.

Parasternal views

From the parasternal long axis view, sweeping to the right will yield the tricuspid valve. With the 3D matrix probe, again, the beam can be steered

* Corresponding author.
E-mail address: eagill@u.washington.edu (E.A. Gill).

doi:10.1016/j.ccl.2007.06.001

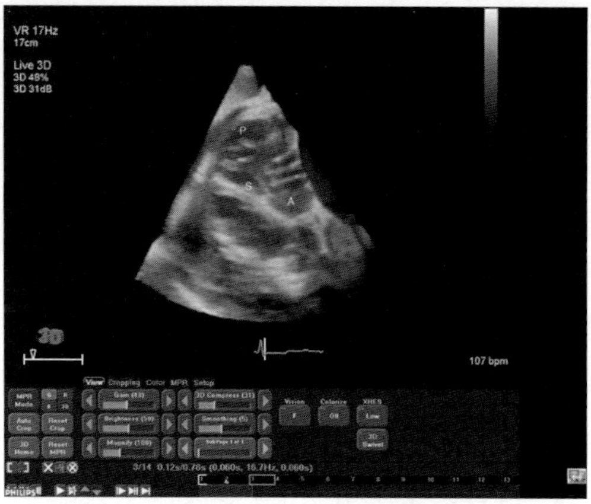

Fig. 1. Subcostal view of the tricuspid valve showing all three leaflets (case 1). In this case, the tricuspid valve is viewed from the right ventricle and looking toward the right atrium. The individual valve leaflets are depicted as A, anterior, P, posterior, and S, septal.

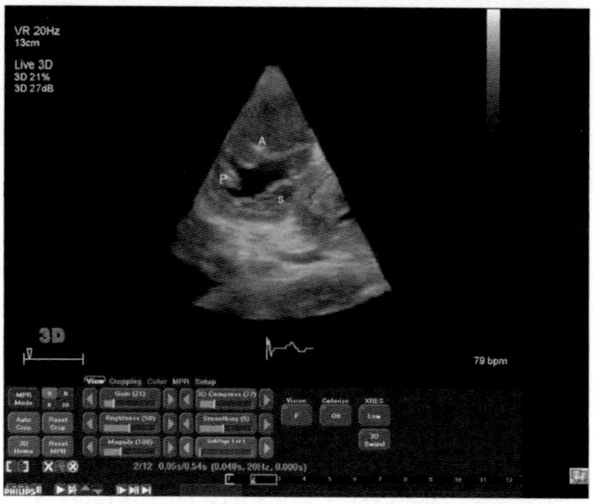

Fig. 3. The tricuspid valve obtained from the parasternal short axis view with tilting toward the right. Electronic beam steering was employed to optimize the image (case 3).

electronically, a major advantage for this particular purpose. That is because viewing the tricuspid valve from this vantage often requires a very acute angle between the transducer and the skin. The combination of the acute angle to the skin and the need to fit between a rib interspace to discover an optimal ultrasound window do indeed welcome the electronic steering. Often initial 2D scanning is used to identify the tricuspid valve, and then switching to real-time 3D imaging (RT3D) will yield the tricuspid valve in an enface view, although often slight manipulation of the transducer either manually or with electronic steering is necessary to optimize the image to simultaneously view all three leaflets. Examples are provided in cases 3,4,5, and 6.

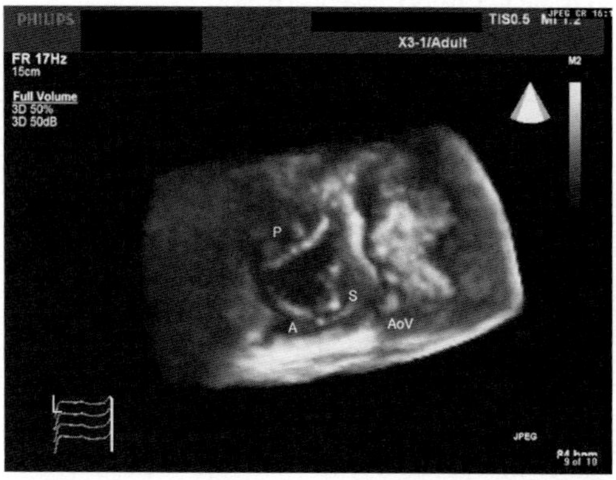

Fig. 2. Apical 4 chamber view. Full volume obtained from the apical view shows the tricuspid valve en face. The image has been cropped from apex to base, showing the tricuspid valve looking from the right ventricle toward the RA (case 2). Note the interventricular septum. Valve leaflet designation same. AoV depicts aortic valve. The aortic valve and left ventricular outflow tract are not imaged optimally.

Apical imaging

From the apex, the tricuspid valve can be imaged in a similar plane as would be used for 2D imaging. Optimization for the right heart structures of course is required. In addition,

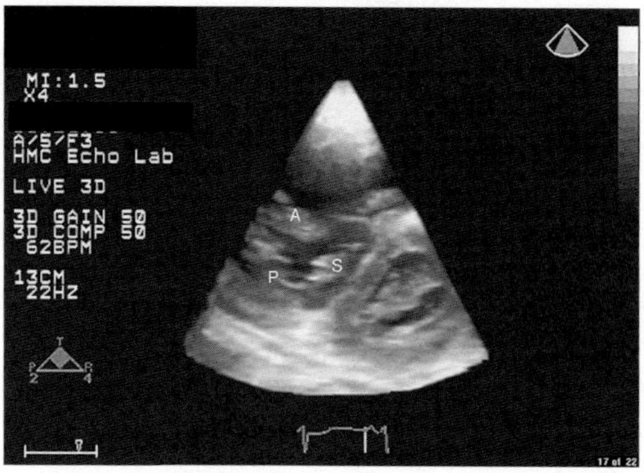

Fig. 4. Parasternal short axis view with the right ventricle cropped in order to view the tricuspid valve from the right ventricle side. Right ventricular volume overload is noted with compression of the interventricular septum in diastole (case 4).

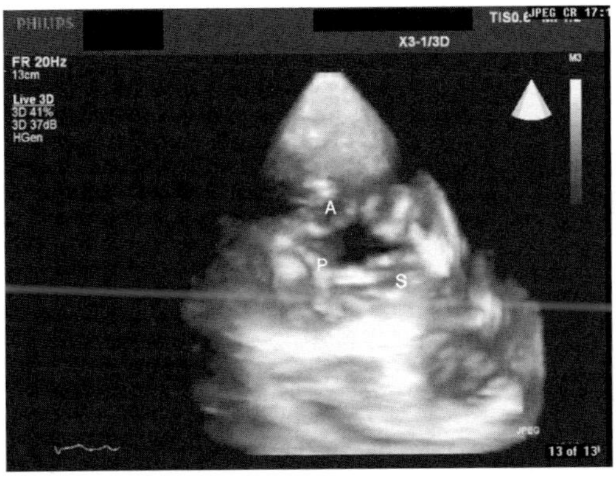

Fig. 5. Parasternal long axis FV. Full-volume acquisition is shown obtained from the parasternal long axis view. The view is seen looking into the right atrium from the parasternal long axis and was obtained by angling toward the right heart and cropping from the right ventricle apex toward the tricuspid valve to show this trileaflet tricuspid valve. The view is looking into the right atrium (case 5).

acquisition of a full-volume data set (a stitching together of four cardiac volumes) will allow the widest field of visualization for the tricuspid valve from this view. Once the full-volume data set has been acquired, cropping from either the apex toward the base or from base to apex frequently will yield side-by-side views of the tricuspid and mitral valves, and both can be viewed from either the apical or basilar side. And of course the main advantage is visualization of all three leaflets of the tricuspid valve with the ability to distinguish the anterior leaflet from the posterior leaflet. Cases 2 and 7 provide examples.

Subcostal imaging

In some patients, the subcostal view is also useful for obtaining similar views for the tricuspid valve. Beam steering again can be advantageous for this view given the acute angle to the skin that often is required to place the probe adjacent to the liver and under the costochondral junction. Case 1 is an example.

Cases

The authors describe seven cases involving eight patients who had particularly outstanding views of the tricuspid valve that were all obtained en face from various imaging planes/angles. They further describe in detail as much as possible how the images were obtained. Note that there are still frames as well as movie (avi) clips for all of these cases.

Case 1. This patient had underlying mitral stenosis leading to an enlarged right heart. The trileaflet tricuspid valve was imaged from a subcostal short axis at the base of the heart. This demonstrates that various imaging windows may yield an optimal RT3D image of the valve en face (See Fig. 1).

Case 2. A 37-year-old woman who had mild pulmonary hypertension and a mildly enlarged right ventricle presented with dyspnea. A full 3D volume acquired from an apical four-chamber view allows for simultaneous visualization of the

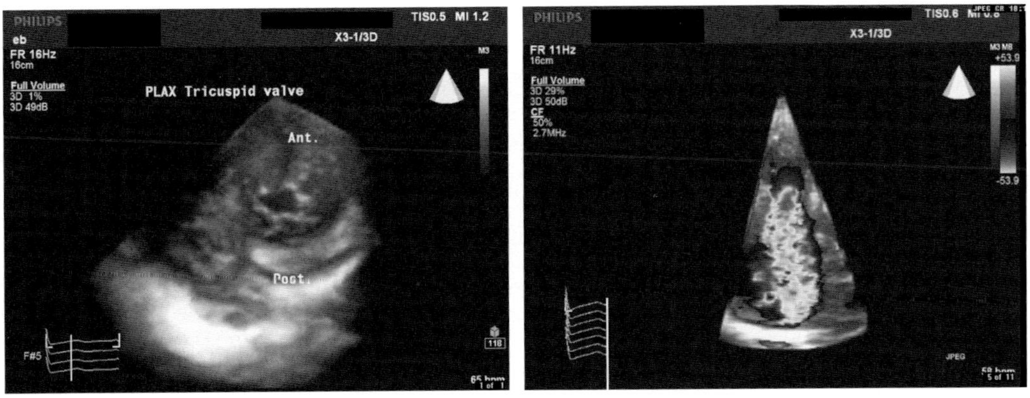

Fig. 6. Parasternal long axis view. (*A*) In this patient status post endocarditis of the tricuspid valve. It was clear from 2D imaging that there was lack of coaptation between two of the tricuspid valve leaflets. Which two leaflets failed to coapt was much less clear. The view that the authors obtained from the parasternal long axis view showed unequivocally that the septal leaflet was normal, and it was lack of coaptation between the anterior and posterior leaflets that resulted in the severe tricuspid regurgitation. (*B*) The severe tricuspid regurgitation 3D color jet (case 6).

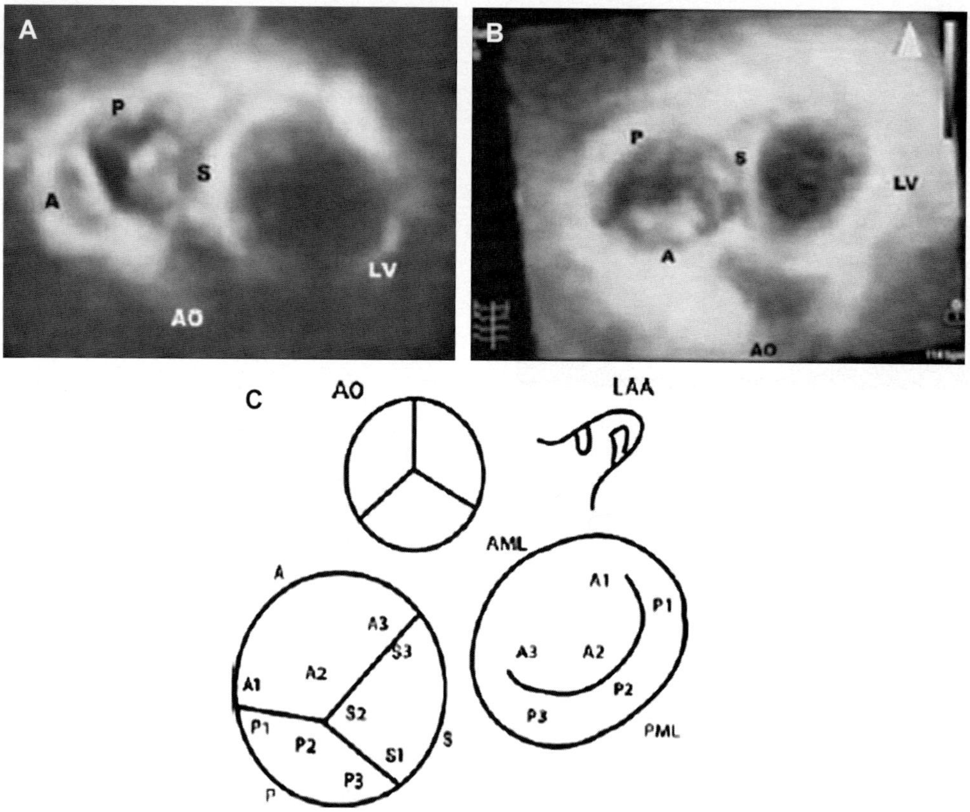

Fig. 7. Apical 4 chamber view full volume. Two patients with tricuspid valve prolapse are shown in this full-volume data set obtained from the apical view. (*A*) En face view from the atrial side showing prolapse of S1, S2, A2, A3, P1, and P2 tricuspid valve segments. (*B*) Another en face view in a patient with prominent systolic prolapse of A1, A2, A3, S2, and S3 tricuspid valve segments. Also present is mild prolapse of the P2 segment. (*C*) Schematic of a proposal for divisions of the segment for the tricuspid valve. *Abbreviations:* AML, anterior mitral leaflet; LAA, left atrial appendage; PML, posterior mitral leaflet. (*Reproduced from* Pothineni KR, et al. Live/real-time 3D transthoracic echocardiographic assessment of tricuspid valve pathology: incremental value over the 2D technique. Echocardiography 2007;24:541–52; with permission.)

leaflets. Cropping the full volume from the RV apex toward the base will reveal the TV en face as demonstrated here. 3D cropping is important to understand when trying to maintain proper orientation and identification of the anatomy (See Fig. 2).

Case 3. This image was obtained from a 95-year-old woman who sustained chest trauma and suffered from atrial fibrillation. A trileaflet tricuspid valve can be imaged from the parasternal window both from the long and short axis. This TV was imaged from a parasternal short axis (PSAX) window with image optimization focused on the right heart. The leaflets are seen from the right ventricular side of the valve. Medial and anterior angulations may be necessary to obtain visualization of all leaflets. The 3D matrix probe's electronic beam steering was used for this case (See Fig. 3).

Case 4. A 45-year-old man who had severe pulmonary hypertension presented with dyspnea. His right ventricle was dilated severely with severely reduced systolic function. This image was obtained from a PSAX with the RV apex cropped to view the valve from the ventricular side (See Fig. 4).

Case 5. A 51-year-old woman with end-stage renal failure and severe pulmonary hypertension presented with an arterio-venous fistula infection. The right ventricle was dilated moderately, and systolic function was reduced severely. A full volume from the parasternal long axis was obtained by angling toward the right heart and cropping from the RV apex toward the TV to show this trileaflet TV. The view is looking into the right atrium (See Fig. 5).

Case 6. This patient had a history of endocarditis leading to noncoaptation of the valve leaflets. The question was which leaflets. The view that the authors obtained from the parasternal long axis view showed unequivocally that the septal leaflet was normal, and it was coaptation between the anterior and posterior leaflets that resulted in the severe tricuspid regurgitation (See Fig. 6).

Case 7. Two patients with tricuspid valve prolapse are shown. Both images are obtained from the apical view with cropping from the atrial side. In both cases, the prolapsed sections are coming into the plane of view (See Fig. 7).

Access Videos in online version of this article at: http://www.CardiologyClinics.TheClinics.com.

Discussion

Imaging of the tricuspid valve by 2DE is limited severely by the inability to view all three leaflets simultaneously. For years, this limitation has been overcome partially by using an anterior/posterior sweep to see both the anterior and posterior leaflets in the apical four-chamber view or the subcostal view. The echocardiographer then interpolates the results of the sweep into his or her own imagined 3D image of the entire valve. The advent of RT3D imaging largely eliminates for this exercise when all three leaflets are viewed en face. The can be accomplished in three ways:

1. Parasternal short axis imaging with beam steering
2. Apical imaging with full-volume acquisition and subsequent cropping
3. Subcostal views, again with either short-axis orientation, sometimes optimized with beam steering, or with full-volume acquisition and cropping

It should be pointed out that full-volume acquisition is of course not truly real-time, as typically four cardiac cycles are stitched together. In situations where full-volume acquistion is suboptimal, such as patient movement or irregular heart rhythm, beam steering can be a particularly useful feature of RT3D, because imaging planes not possible with transducer movement only are made imminently approachable just by steering the ultrasound beam electronically.

Summary

In 2DE imaging, the tricuspid valve presents a challenge for pinpointing individual leaflets, because it is rare to see all three in one two-dimensional imagine plane. RT3DE circumvents this problem, with the additional plane of elevation such that all three leaflets are seen.

References

[1] Feigenbaum H, Armstrong WF, Ryan T. In: Echocardiography. 6th edition. Philadelphia (PA): Lippincott, Williams and Wilkins; 2005. p. 361–2.
[2] Velayudhan DE, Brown TM, Nanda NC, et al. Quantification of tricuspid regurgitation by live three-dimensional transthoracic echocardiographic measurements of vena contracta area. Echocardiography 2006;23:793–800.
[3] Pothineni KR, Duncan K, Yelamanchili P, et al. Live/real-time three-dimensional transthoracic echocardiographic assessment of tricuspid valve pathology: incremental value over the two-dimensional technique. Echocardiography 2007;24:541–52.

ELSEVIER
SAUNDERS

Cardiol Clin 25 (2007) 311–318

CARDIOLOGY
CLINICS

The Use of Three-Dimensional Echocardiography for the Evaluation of and Treatment of Mitral Stenosis

Jose A. de Agustin, MD[a],
Navin C. Nanda, MD, FACC, FAHA, FSOC, FISCU[c],
Edward A. Gill, MD, FACC, FASE, FACP[b],
Leopoldo Pérez de Isla, MD, PhD[a], Jose L. Zamorano, MD[a,*]

[a]*CV Imaging Unit, University Clinic San Carlos, Madrid, Spain*
[b]*Harborview Medical Center, University of Washington, Seattle, WA, USA*
[c]*University of Alabama Birmingham, Birmingham, AL, USA*

Rheumatic mitral stenosis remains an important public health concern in both developing and developed countries, the latter because of immigration from the former. Percutaneous mitral valvuloplasty (PMV) has developed into the treatment of choice for selected patients who have favorable mitral valve anatomy [1]. Choosing the subset of patients with mitral stenosis who are the most favorable for PMV requires precise evaluation of valve and particularly commissural anatomy. More specifically, echocardiography is used to define the valve area, the degree of calcification, valve mobility and thickening, the degree of mitral regurgitation, and finally, degree of commissural fusion.

Dating back to the 1950s, the catheter-based Gorlin's equation has been considered the standard for estimation of the mitral valve area. Gorlin's equation, however, uses hemodynamics obtained from fluid-filled catheters. It is invasive, uses numerous assumptions, and clearly can result in complications and has numerous limitations. Most notably, it is inaccurate when significant valvular regurgitation is present. In clinical practice, two-dimensional echocardiography (2DE), coupled with Doppler evaluation of mitral valve gradient and pulmonary artery pressure, has become the mainstay for evaluating mitral valve disease and more particularly mitral valve area (MVA). MVA is assessed indirectly by the PHT method or directly by planimetry. There are advantages and limitations to both methods. PHT-derived MVA can be obtained easily, but may be influenced by hemodynamic factors (heart rate, cardiac index, cardiac rhythm, left ventricular systolic and diastolic dysfunction, left ventricular and atrial compliance, left ventricular hypertrophy, and concomitant valvular disease [2,3]. These hemodynamic factors change rapidly during the immediate post-PMV period, which may explain the significant discrepancies observed in earlier studies between the PHT-derived MVA and the Gorlin's-derived MVA. In addition, there is the issue of the presence of an atrial septal defect (ASD) formed during the procedure during transseptal puncture. This is another cause for inaccuracy of the Gorlin formula [4].

Planimetry of the valve orifice has the advantage of being relatively hemodynamically independent, although one might imagine that the orifice could be truly larger when left atrial pressure is high. Until the recent development of 3D techniques, planimetry of the valve orifice was performed by 2DE, a technique that has multiple limitations (Fig. 1). The greatest limitation is that measurements of the mitral valve orifice area are made in the short axis view with no

* Corresponding author.
E-mail address: jlzamorano@vodafone.es
(J.L. Zamorano).

doi:10.1016/j.ccl.2007.06.008

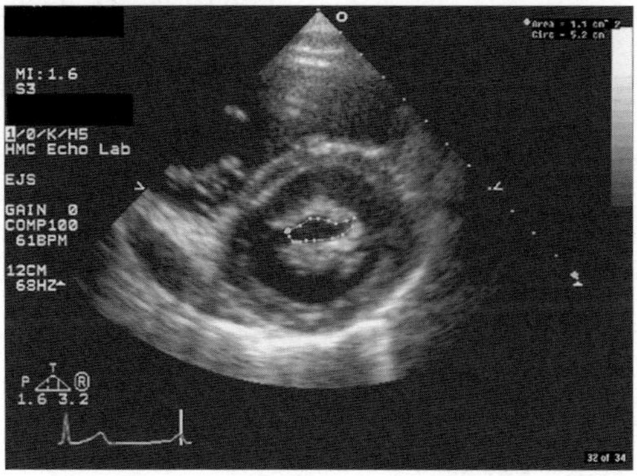

Fig. 1. Example of planimetry of a stenotic mitral valve using standard 2D imaging. Note that the extreme medial and lateral edges of the mitral orifice have dropped out of the grey scale, making accurate assessment of the area difficult. Also, there is no verification from an orthogonal plane that the measurement is at the mitral leaflet tips.

simultaneous independent imaging to verify that the imaging plane corresponds to the smallest and most perpendicular view of the mitral orifice. Because of this disadvantage, the 2D method requires significant experience and operator skill to obtain the correct imaging plane that displays the true mitral valve orifice. This limitation is amplified the more diseased the valve is and after PMV. As the disease process progresses, the border of the valve orifice becomes more calcified and irregular, making the tracing of the orifice more challenging. Likewise, after PMV, the commissural fusion can split in an asymmetric fashion, again making the tracing of the orifice less reproducible between observers. Many, but not all of these limitations are overcome with the use of 3D echo (3DE).

Advantages of 3D echocardiography

One of the most significant developments of the last decade, particularly in the field of cardiac imaging, has been real-time 3DE (RT3DE). Even before that time, other methods of 3DE were used to evaluate the mitral valve, but the required reconstructive process made them much less practical. 3DE provides unique orientations of the cardiac structures not obtainable by standard 2DE. 3DE has evolved from a research tool to having practical utility, one of them being the accurate planimetry of the MVA in rheumatic mitral stenosis. 3DE can provide not only adequate imaging of the anatomic structure of the mitral valve orifice (commissural splitting and leaflet tears) [5], but also information on the optimal plane of the smallest mitral valve orifice area (Figs. 2–4). In addition, planimetry using 3DE is not limited to the parasternal window as 2DE is, but rather it also can be performed from the apical window. This imaging view has been slower to be adopted in routine clinical practice, because it requires postprocessing, specifically cropping the acquired image, which can be time-consuming and tedious. The combination of the dense array [6] matrix transducer and the newest cropping software, however, has streamlined this process considerably.

3D echocardiography performed with transesophageal echo

3DE acquired with TEE and subsequent 3D reconstruction had shown promise for evaluating patients with mitral stenosis before the advent of RT3DE. Before rotational 3D TEE even developed by commercial vendors, the group from the Thorax center had developed its own system and studied 15 patients with it, showing good correlation between MVA by this methodology and pressure halftime [7]. In 1998, TEE acquired 3DE was shown to predict response to PMV based on commissural fusion. The visualization of commissural splitting after PMV also correlated with larger valve area [5]. Later, in a series of more than 40 mitral stenosis patients, three-dimensional reconstructions were performed from 2D TEE acquisitions. MVA correlated closely with traditional methods, and visualization of the commissures was superior to what was seen by 2DE [8]. Similar results were obtained by others [9].

Real-time 3D echocardiography compared with classic methods for the assessment of the mitral valve area

In 2003, a series of five patients with mitral stenosis was studied with RT3DE and showed favorable results compared with the traditional methods of Gorlin's equation and pressure halftime. It was suggested that RT3DE was more accurate, particularly compared with 2DE, because it was more reproducible and correlated better with the Gorlin's equation valve area. Also, in one of the cases, postprocedure mitral

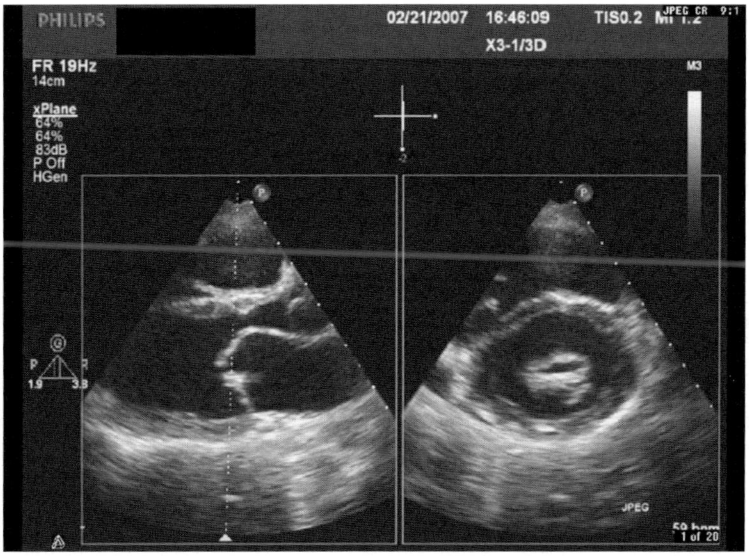

Fig. 2. Example of a view of a stenotic mitral valve using biplane 2D imaging. The 3D transducer allows simultaneous display of more than one 2D view. The advantage of this is the ability to confirm that the parasternal short axis view of the mitral orifice is in fact at the tip of the mitral leaflets.

regurgitation developed, and RT3DE detected an area of systolic noncoaptation between the mitral leaflets that was not seen by 2DE and correlated with the mitral regurgitation [10]. In a series of 48 patients, RT3D (in a subset of the group) and 3D TEE were used to evaluate mitral valve area and response to PMV. Valve area correlated well with Gorlin and pressure half time valve areas. The clear visualization of commissural fusion by 3DE was the most reliable predictor of a positive response to PMV, more so than the Wilkins valvuloplasty score [11].

Then, in a larger group of 80 patients, the accuracy of current 2DE methods (2D planimetry, PHT, and proximal isovelocity surface area method (PISA) was compared with RT3DE for the assessment of MVA in patients who had rheumatic mitral valve disease. RT3DE was compared to the standard of the invasively determined Gorlin's equation [12]. RT3DE was performed en face at the ideal cross section of the mitral valve orifice during its maximum diastolic opening. The ideal cross section was defined as the most perpendicular view in the plane with the smallest mitral valve orifice (Fig. 3). This plane also should be parallel to the flow through the most limiting part of the mitral orifice.

The PMV Wilkins score was determined by both 2DE and RT3DE. RT3DE planimetry and mitral score were measured by two independent observers and then repeated by one of them. Intermethods agreement was evaluated by means of the intraclass correlation coefficient. The analysis demonstrated a superior agreement when comparing the invasively determined MVA with RT3DE MVA than when comparing it with the current 2DE methods (Table 1) [13]. Further, the interobserver variability was nearly twice as good with RT3DE than with 2DE for the PMV Wilkins score (Table 2) [13]. Finally, RT3DE measurements had excellent inter- and intraobserver variability and the best interobserver agreement for morphologic evaluation. This study showed that RT3DE was the most accurate echocardiography parameter for measuring MVA. Similar results have been reported by others [14–16].

Real-time 3D echocardiography compared with classic methods for the assessment of mitral valve area after a mitral valvuloplasty

As previously stated, traditional methods of MVA measurement have even more limitations immediately after PMV; therefore, MVA was evaluated by RT3DE following PMV [17]. Many studies have demonstrated considerable discrepancies after PMV between MVA measurements obtained using the PHT method and invasive hemodynamic evaluation using Gorlin's equation

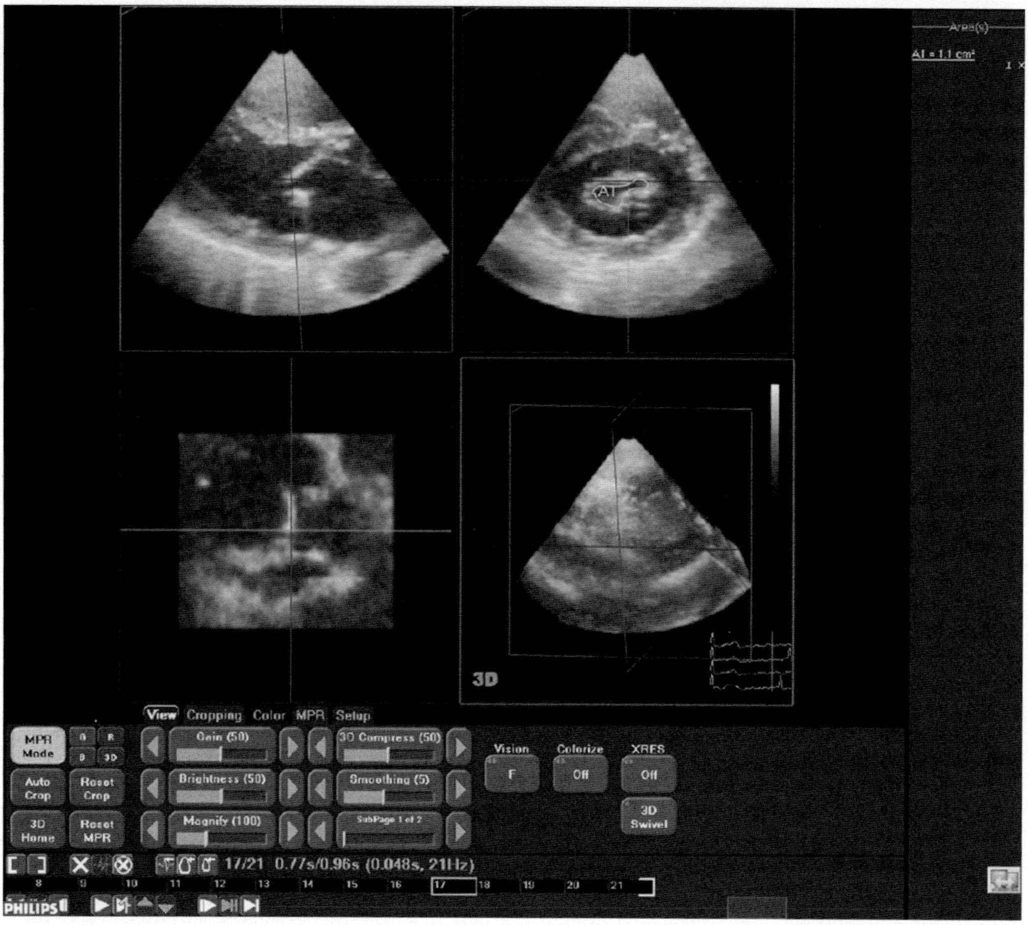

Fig. 3. A full-volume acquisition obtained from parasternal view. The data set has been cropped such that the smallest mitral valve orifice can be measured. The upper left image shows the mitral valve in parasternal long orientation, while the upper right image shows the mitral valve in parasternal short orientation. The bottom right image is a compilation of the entire volume data set. The upper left image has been used to place the cursor at the very tip of the mitral leaflets, so that the corresponding mitral valve area shown on the right is the smallest possible. See corresponding measurement.

[4,18–23]. There are several reasons for this inaccuracy. Perhaps the most obvious, especially as it adversely affects the PHT method, is the development of an atrial septal defect as an unavoidable side effect of the transseptal puncture [4,22]. Also, the PHT method assumes stability of left atrial and left ventricular compliance, an assumption that is not valid in the immediate post-PMV period [24,25]. 2D planimetry of MVA is not as dependent on hemodynamic variables [26–31], and theoretically it should be more accurate than PHT after PMV. It is not exempt of inaccuracies, however, because following PMV, the mitral orifice becomes irregular and is technically difficult to trace, particularly if significant calcification is present. Because of the variable geometry of the stenotic mitral valve orifice, correct plane orientation frequently becomes difficult, and hence minor changes in depth and angle of the ultrasound beam lead to an overestimation of the MVA that ranges between 63% to 88% [14].

RT3DE allows a unique and superior evaluation of the mitral valve apparatus, enhancing the ability to obtain an accurate measurement of the MVA. To evaluate RT3DE-based planimetry after a PMV, 29 consecutive patients who had rheumatic mitral valve disease were enrolled and underwent PMV. MVA was calculated before and after PMV using the PHT method, 2DE planimetry, RT3DE planimetry and the invasive

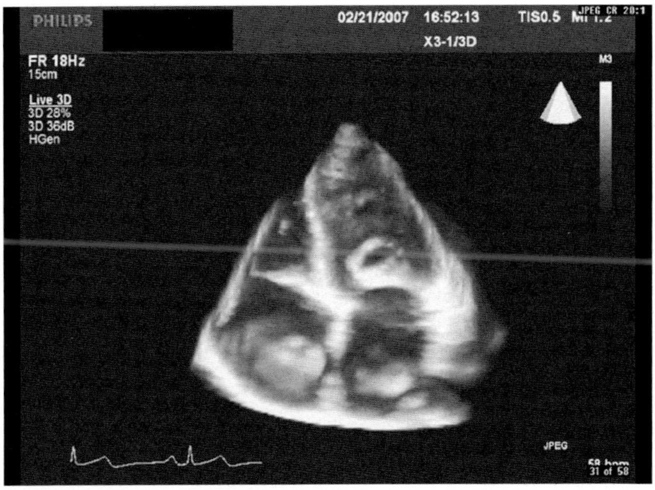

Fig. 4. Similar to Fig. 3, but obtained from an apical view, a full-volume data set is shown cropped to show the mitral orifice.

determination using the Gorlin's equation. The Gorlin's equation was considered the standard. The main findings were that RT3DE was the most accurate ultrasound technique for measuring MVA, with a superior pre- and postprocedural agreement with the Gorlin's derived MVA (see Table 2) [16]. After PMV, the agreement with the Gorlin's-derived MVA was better than two-dimensional planimetry and pressure halftime-derived MVA (Fig. 5, Table 3, Video 1).

Access video on Mitral Stenosis post cracked commissures of this article at: http://www.cardiology.TheClinics.com

Mitral valve shown with 3D rendering after having undergone percutaneous mitral valvuloplasty. In this video, the medial commissure is particularly well shown, having undergone splitting resulting in a larger orifice area.

In this study, the interobserver variability of Wilkins score [32] by using 2DE and RT3DE also was evaluated. Leaflet mobility, calcification, and subvalvular involvement were assessed using 2DE and RT3DE by two independent observers. As previously noted, the RT3DE assessment showed the best interobserver agreement for the morphologic evaluation of the rheumatic mitral valve.

In conclusion, real-time 3DE is also a very suitable technique for monitoring the efficacy of the PMV, with better accuracy compared with

Table 1
Intraclass correlation coefficient between the different echocardiographic methods and invasive estimated mitral valve area (Gorlin method)

Method	ICC (95% confidence interval)
Gorlin	
RT3DE	0.83 (0.74–0.89)
PHT	0.6 (0.39–0.75)
2D planimetry	0.57 (0.38–0.72)
PISA	0.48 (0.24–0.66)

Abbreviations: ICC, intraclass correlation coefficient; PHT, half pressure time; PISA, proximal isovelocity surface area; RT3DE, real-time 3D echocardiography.

Table 2
Intraclass correlation coefficient between the different echocardiographic methods and invasive estimated mitral valve area before and after percutaneous mitral valvuloplasty

Method	Intraclass correlation coefficient
Pre-PMV Gorlin	
Pre-PMV RT3DE	0.79
Pre-PMV 2D planimetry	0.6
Pre-PMV PHT	0.49
Post-PMV Gorlin	
Post-PMV RT3DE	0.64
Post-PMV 2D planimetry	0.5
Post-PMV PHT	0.2

Abbreviations: PHT, half pressure time PMV, percutaneous mitral valvuloplasty; RT3DE, real-time 3D echocardiography.

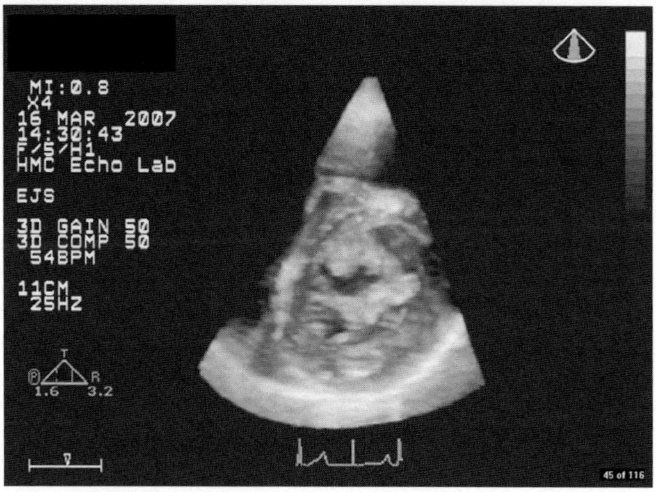

Fig. 5. The mitral valve is shown with 3D rendering after having undergone percutaneous mitral valvuloplasty. The commissures have been split, optimizing the mitral orifice.

2D planimetry and pressure halftime-derived MVA.

Real-time 3D echocardiography. The new standard for the mitral valvular area quantification?

RT3DE offers the possibility of accurately measuring the mitral valve orifice area because of its ability to crop the volume data set in any position in space, and therefore, select the en face view that includes the smallest mitral valve area. In a study by Zamorano and colleagues [33], the MV orifice area was imaged further using RT3DE. In this investigation, the gold standard was different, because it was composed of a median mitral valve orifice area calculated from the three classical 2DE methods: 2D planimetry, pressure halftime, and PISA method. This composite value was compared with MV orifice areas obtained with RT3DE planimetry and the Gorlin's method. Intraclass correlation coefficient was used to compare the different methods. Analysis showed that the accuracy of RT3DE planimetry is superior to the accuracy of the invasive Gorlin's method for assessing MVA in rheumatic mitral valve stenosis when the median (or composite data set) was used as the standard.

Summary

RT3D is a major advance in cardiac imaging, because it allows visualization of the entire mitral valve apparatus and the optimal plane to measure the smallest mitral valve orifice area. Currently, it can be argued that sufficient evidence has been compiled to prove that 3D imaging is superior to

Table 3
Advantages and limitations of the different methods to evaluate the mitral valve area

Method	Influence of hemodynamic conditions	Acoustic window needed	Useful after percutaneous mitral valvuloplasty	Invasive technique
2D planimetry	−	++	+	−
PHT	++	++	−	−
PISA	+	++	+	−
RT3DE	−	++	++	−
GORLIN	++	−	++	++

Abbreviations: PHT, half pressure time; PISA, proximal isovelocity surface area; RT3DE, real-time 3D echocardiography.

traditional 2D techniques and should be used routinely to quantify the MVA in mitral stenosis, particularly in the immediate postpercutaneous mitral valvuloplasty period, where other methods have be proven to be inaccurate [16,33–35]. RT3D is also useful to obtain accurate Wilkins score. RT3DE should be integrated into the routine echocardiographic examination, and perhaps, in the near future should replace Gorlin's method as the reference method to quantify the MVA in rheumatic mitral valve stenosis.

References

[1] Bonow RO, Carabello B, de Leon AC Jr. ACC/AHA Guidelines for the management of patients with valvular heart disease. J Am Coll Cardiol 1998;32:1486–692.

[2] Hatle L, Angelsen B, Tromsdal A. Noninvasive assessment of atrioventricular pressure half-time by Doppler ultrasound. Circulation 1979;60:1096–104.

[3] Rodriguez L, Thomas JD, Monterroso V, et al. Validation of the proximal flow convergence method: calculation of orifice area in patients with mitral stenosis. Circulation 1993;88:1157–65.

[4] Manga P, Singh S, Brandis S, et al. Mitral valve area calculations immediately after percutaneous balloon mitral valvuloplasty: effect of the atrial septal defect. J Am Coll Cardiol 1993;21:1568–73.

[5] Applebaum RM, Kasliwal RR, Kanojia A, et al. Utility of three-dimensional echocardiography during balloon mitral valvuloplasty. J Am Coll Cardiol 1998;32(5):1405–9.

[6] Houck RC, Cooke JE, Gill EA. Live three-dimensional echo—an entire replacement for traditional two-dimensional echo? Am J Roentgenol 2006; 187(4):1092–106.

[7] Chen Q, Hosir YF, Vletter WB, et al. Accurate assessment of MVA in patients with mitral stenosis by three-dimensional echocardiography. J Am Soc Echocardiogr 1997;10:133–40.

[8] Gill E, Bhola R, Carroll J, et al. Three-dimensional echocardiography predictors of percutaneous balloon mitral valvuloplasty success. Eur J Echocardiogr 2000;1:S32.

[9] Hozumi T, Yoshikawa J. Three dimensional echocardiography using a multiplane TEE probe: the clinical applications. Echocardiography 2000;17:757–64.

[10] Singh V, Nanda NC, Agrawal G, et al. Live three-dimensional echocardiographic assessment of mitral stenosis. Echocardiography 2003;20:743–50.

[11] Gill E, Bhola R, Carroll JD, et al. Live 3D echo and biplane evaluation of mitral stenosis for prediction of mitral valvuloplasty success. J Am Soc Echocardiogr 2004;17:499.

[12] Gorlin R, Gorlin SG. Hydraulic formula for calculation of the stenotic mitral valve, other cardiac valves, and central circulatory shunts. Am Heart J 1951;41: 1–12.

[13] Zamorano J, Cordeiro P, Sugeng L, et al. Real-time three-dimensional echocardiography for rheumatic mitral valve stenosis evaluation. J Am Coll Cardiol 2004;43(11):2091–6.

[14] Binder TM, Rosenhek R, Porenta G, et al. Improved assessment of mitral valve stenosis by volumetric real-time three-dimensional echocardiography. J Am Coll Cardiol 2000;36(4):1355–61.

[15] Xie MX, Wang XF, Cheng TO, et al. Comparison of accuracy of mitral valve area in mitral stenosis by real-time, three-dimensional echocardiography versus two-dimensional echocardiography versus Doppler pressure half-time. Am J Cardiol 2005; 95(12):1496–9.

[16] Sebag IA, Morgan JG, Handschumacher MD, et al. Usefulness of three-dimensionally guided assessment of mitral stenosis using matrix array ultrasound. Am J Cardiol 2005;96(8):1151–6.

[17] Zamorano J, Pérez de Isla L, Sugeng L, et al. Noninvasive assessment of mitral valve area during percutaneous balloon mitral valvuloplasty: role of real-time 3D echocardiography. Eur Heart J 2004; 25(23):2086–91.

[18] Reid CL, Rahimtoola SH. The role of echocardiography/Doppler in catheter balloon treatment of adults with aortic and mitral stenosis. Circulation 1991;84(Suppl I):240–9.

[19] Vahanian A, Michel PL, Cormier B, et al. Results of percutaneous mitral commissurotomy in 200 patients. Am J Cardiol 1989;63:847–52.

[20] Abascal VM, Wilkins GT, Choong CY, et al. Echocardiographic evaluation of mitral valve structure and function in patients followed for at least 6 months after percutaneous balloon mitral valvuloplasty. J Am Cardiol 1988;12:606–15.

[21] Nakatani S, Nagata S, Beppu S, et al. Acute reduction of mitral valve area after percutaneous balloon mitral valvuloplasty: assessment with Doppler continuity equation method. Am Heart J 1991;121:770–5.

[22] Chen CG, Wang YP, Guo BL, et al. Reliability of the Doppler pressure half-time method for assessing effects of percutaneous mitral balloon valvuloplasty. J Am Coll Cardiol 1989;13:1309–13.

[23] Pitsavos CE, Stefanadis CI, Stratos CG, et al. Assessment of accuracy of the Doppler pressure half-time method in the estimation of the mitral valve area immediately after balloon mitral valvuloplasty. Eur Heart J 1997;18:455–63.

[24] Otto CM, Davis KB, Holmes DR, et al. Methodologic issues in clinical evaluation of stenosis severity in adults undergoing aortic or mitral balloon valvuloplasty. Am J Cardiol 1992;69:1607–16.

[25] Thomas JD, Wilkins GT, Choong CY, et al. Inaccuracy of mitral pressure half-time immediately after percutaneous mitral valvotomy: dependence on mitral gradient and left atrial and ventricular compliance. Circulation 1988;78:980–93.

[26] Smith MD, Wisenbaugh T, Grayburn PA, et al. Value and limitations of Doppler pressure half-time in quantifying mitral stenosis: a comparison with micromanometer catheter recordings. Am Heart J 1991;121:480–8.
[27] Nakatani S, Masuyama T, Kodama K, et al. Value and limitations of Doppler echocardiography in the quantification of stenotic mitral valve area: comparison of the pressure half-time and the continuity equation methods. Circulation 1988;77:78–85.
[28] Karp K, Teien D, Bjerle P, et al. Reassessment of valve area determinations in mitral stenosis by the pressure half-time method: impact of left ventricular stiffness and peak diastolic pressure difference. J Am Coll Cardiol 1989;13:594–9.
[29] Fredman CS, Pearson AC, Labovitz AJ, et al. Comparison of hemodynamic pressure half-time method and Gorlin formula with Doppler and echocardiographic determinations of mitral valve area in patients with combined stenosis and regurgitation. Am Heart J 1990;119:121–9.
[30] Rifkin RD, Harper K, Tighe D. Comparison of proximal isovelocity surface area method with pressure half-time and planimetry in evaluation of mitral stenosis. J Am Coll Cardiol 1995;26:458–65.
[31] Faletra F, Pezzano A Jr, Fusco R, et al. Measurement of mitral valve area in mitral stenosis: four echocardiographic methods compared with direct measurement of anatomic orifices. J Am Coll Cardiol 1996;28:1190–7.
[32] Wilkins GT, Weyman AE, Abascal VM, et al. Percutaneous balloon dilatation of the mitral valve: an analysis of echocardiographic variables related to outcome and the mechanism of dilatation. Br Heart J 1988;60:299–308.
[33] Perez de Isla Casanova L, Almeria C, et al. Which method should be the reference method to evaluate the severity of rheumatic mitral stenosis? Gorlin's method versus 3D echo. Eur J Echocardiogr, in press.
[34] Herman FJ, Mannaerts, Otto Kamp, Cees A Visser. Should mitral valve area assessment in patients with mitral stenosis be based on anatomical or on functional evaluation? A plea for 3D echocardiography as the new clinical standard. Eur Heart J 2004;25:2073–4.
[35] Sugeng L, Weinert L, Lammertin G, et al. Accuracy of mitral valve area measurements using transthoracic rapid freehand 3-dimensional scanning: comparison with noninvasive and invasive methods. J Am Soc Echocardiogr 2003;16:1292–300.

ELSEVIER
SAUNDERS

Cardiol Clin 25 (2007) 319–325

CARDIOLOGY
CLINICS

Live/Real-Time Three-Dimensional Transthoracic Assessment of Mitral Regurgitation and Mitral Valve Prolapse

Andrew P. Miller, MD,
Navin C. Nanda, MD, FACC, FAHA, FSOC, FISCU*

Division of Cardiovascular Diseases, University of Alabama at Birmingham, Heart Station SWB/S102, 619 19th Street South, Birmingham, AL 35249, USA

Evaluation of the mitral valve requires appreciation of its complex geometry. In vertical space, the mitral annulus takes the shape of a saddle or ski slope, with the anteroseptal portion being more cephalad [1,2]. In pathologic conditions, this geometry is perturbed (eg, the annulus flattens when stretched in conditions such as dilated cardiomyopathies) [3]. When viewed en face, the mitral valve is composed of an anterior leaflet that can be divided into three segments:

A1, anterolateral
A2, middle
A3, posteromedial

and a posterior leaflet composed of three scallops:

P1, anterolateral
P2, middle
P3, posteromedial (Fig. 1) [4]

To accurately guide surgical interventions and describe pathology, familiarity with this nomenclature and orientation of the valve in 3D space is necessary. For this reason, 3D transthoracic echocardiography (TTE) is an immense improvement over the cumbersome mental reconstruction required by 2D TTE.

* Corresponding author. University of Alabama at Birmingham, Heart Station SW/S102, 619 South 19th Street, Birmingham, AL 35249.

E-mail address: nanda@uab.edu (N.C. Nanda).

Mitral regurgitation

Accurate grading of mitral regurgitation (MR) severity using qualitative and quantitative color Doppler 2D TTE techniques has been challenging [5]. The most commonly employed measure is the ratio of the regurgitant jet area to left atrial area (RJA/LAA), but this is really a semiquantitative or qualitative technique. Techniques using volumetric approaches or the proximal flow convergence provide quantitative assessment but are limited by being time-consuming and involve calculations based upon assumptions that introduce inaccuracies [6,7]. Measurement of vena contracta width (VCW) by 2D TTE has been validated against regurgitant fraction and angiography [8,9]; however, grading criteria assume a circular or elliptical shape that may not represent the true geometric appearance of the vena contracta [10]. For these reasons, the authors evaluated 3D TTE measurements of vena contracta area (VCA), with comparisons to 2D TTE measures of RJA/LAA and VCW and to angiographic grading by left ventriculography [11]. As demonstrated by the authors and others, quantification of MR by 3D TTE is superior to 2D TTE measures, which especially are hampered when the assumed geometry is not realized in practice [11–13].

Using a Philips Sonos 7500 (Andover, Massachusetts) ultrasound system equipped with a 4 × matrix transducer, B mode, and color Doppler, 3D data sets were acquired from the apical and parasternal long axis views. Color Doppler gain was set at 70%, and the Nyquist limit was set between 43 and 69 cm/sex, because VCA

0733-8651/07/$ - see front matter
doi:10.1016/j.ccl.2007.06.003

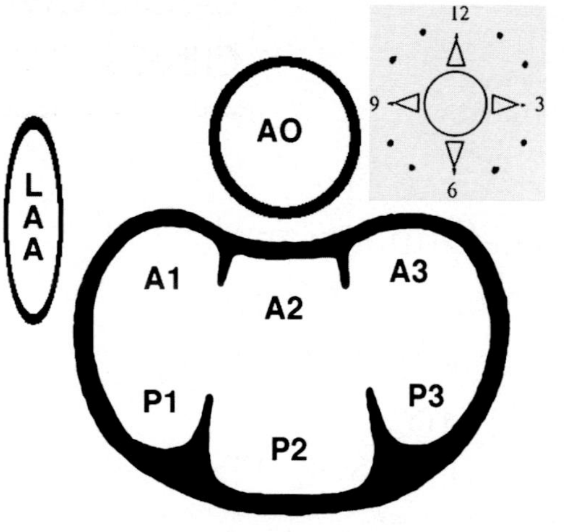

Fig. 1. Schematic diagram of the segmental classification used to describe the prolapse of mitral valve, as viewed by the surgeon. *Abbreviations:* A1, A2, and A3, anterolateral, middle, and posteromedial segments of anterior mitral valve leaflet; AO, aorta; LAA, left atrial appendage; P1, P2, and P3, anterolateral, middle, and posteromedial scallops of posterior mitral valve leaflet. (*Reproduced from* Ahmed S, Nanda NC, Miller AP, et al. Usefulness of transesophageal 3D echocardiography in the identification of individual segment/scallop prolapse of the mitral valve. Echocardiography 2003;20: 203–9; with permission.)

measurements remained relatively constant in this range. Most cropping was performed from the apical views as demonstrated in Fig. 2. First, the best vena contracta image was obtained in long axis by anterior-to-posterior cropping (see Fig. 2A). Second, by cropping from the top of the data set, an imaging plane was placed at the level of the vena contracta, at or just below the mitral valve leaflet tips in a plane that was parallel to the orifice (see Fig. 2B). The image then was rotated, to view the vena contracta en face (see Fig. 2C), and the previously cropped anterior portion was added back to obtain the maximum VCA (see Fig. 2D). This procedure was recorded in its entirety on a VHS tape. Measurements of VCA were obtained by:

- Direct video planimetry (using the VCR function on the ultrasound system to play back the recorded cropping, the depth markers viewable in the initial image, Fig. 2A, were used for calibration, and then the VCA was traced)
- Off-line (using a Tom Tec Cardio view-RT, Munich, Germany)

The authors' subsequent experience with the Q laboratory software suggests that measurements with this software package may slightly underestimate those performed in their original publication.

Using this technique, the authors assessed MR by measurements of VCA with 3D TTE and other standard 2D TTE measurements in 44 patients who underwent left ventriculography [11]. Results revealed close agreement for 3D TTE VCA measurements and angiographic grading, with discernment between angiographic grades using the following diagnostic criteria: <0.2 cm^2 for mild (grade I), 0.2 to 0.4 cm^2 for moderate (grade II), and greater than 0.4 cm^2 for severe (grade III) MR (Fig. 3). Direct video planimetry and off-line computer analysis agreed well, and interobserver variability and intraobserver variability were very low (sum of residuals $r^2 = .99$ and 0.97, respectively) for this parameter. 3D TTE measurements of VCA were superior when compared with the angiographic standard as opposed to the traditional 2D TTE measurements of RJA/LAA, RJA, VCW, and calculated VCA. A subsequent study by Iwakura and colleagues [12] yielded similar incremental value for 3D TTE measures of regurgitant orifice area over 2D TTE quantification of proximal isovelocity surface area (PISA), especially in patients who had elliptical orifice shapes. In clinical practice, the authors have found this technique robust as a clinical tool for diagnosing and following patients with MR, because 3D TTE VCA offers a quantifiable indirect measure of the hole in the mitral valve that is not load-dependent and that appreciates the complex geometry of the mitral valve and its regurgitant orifice.

In addition to quantifying MR, the three-dimensional TTE data set is useful in assessing anatomy responsible for valvar insufficiency. Leaflet geometry can be assessed with available software packages, and this may be useful in surgical decision making [14,15]. Chordae rupture and flail leaflets can be seen, improving diagnostic confidence in patients who have acute MR and often obviating the need for a transesophageal echocardiography (TEE) exam. In addition, the authors have found 3D TTE particularly useful in evaluating patients with endocarditis. En face views permit correct characterization of valvar perforations, and systematic cropping is useful in excluding abscess formation. The 3D dataset can be cropped to accurately describe and measure vegetations, which may provide a prognostic

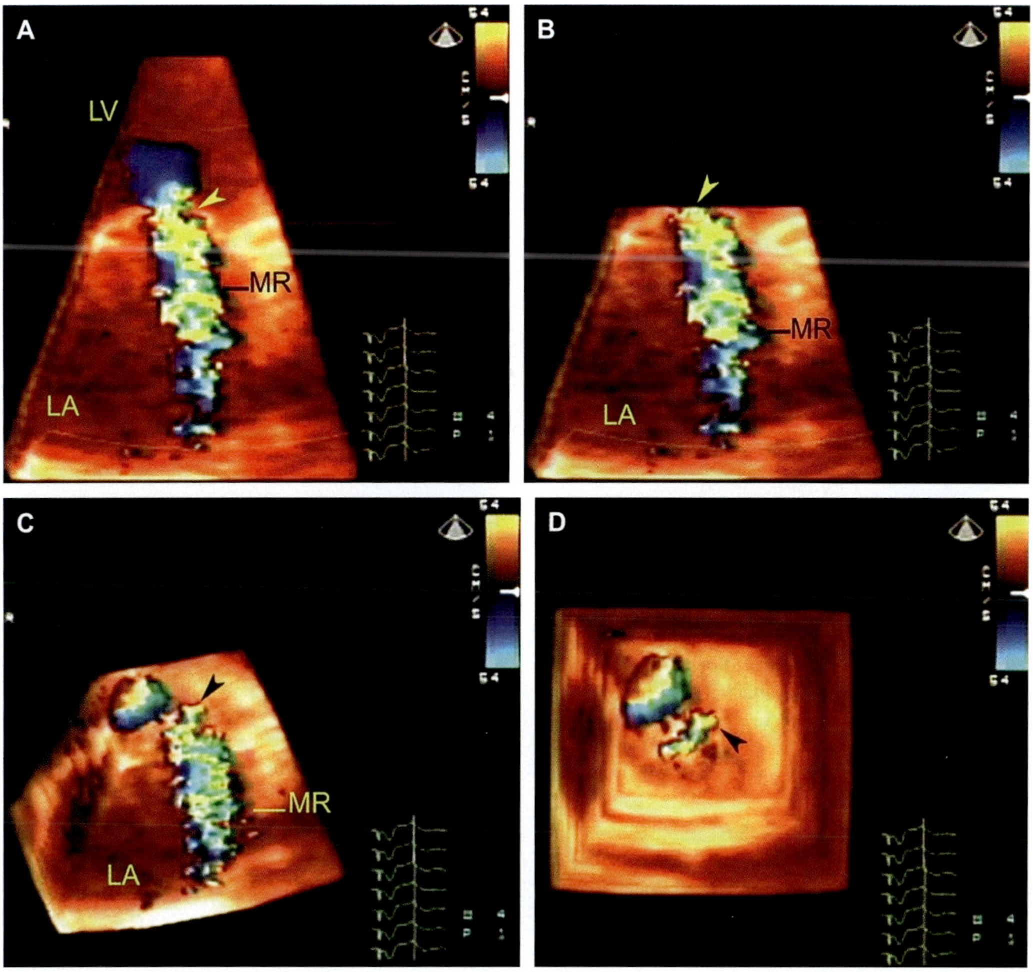

Fig. 2. Live 3D color Doppler transthoracic echocardiographic technique for assessment of vena contracta area. 3D color Doppler data set showing mitral regurgitation (MR, *A*) is cropped from top to the level of the vena contracta (*arrowhead, B*) and tilted to view it en face (*C, D*). The vena contracta then is planimetered by copying onto a videotape. *Abbreviations:* LA, left atrium; LV, left ventricle. (*Reproduced from* Khanna D, Vengala S, Miller AP, et al. Quantification of mitral regurgitation by live 3D transthoracic echocardiographic measurements of vena contracta area. Echocardiography 2004;21:737–43; with permission.)

index for embolization [16,17]. Because the 3D dataset contains the entire mitral valve apparatus, comprehensive evaluation with 3D TTE is possible in a time-efficient manner.

Mitral valve prolapse

Because mitral valve repair is always preferable to replacement for mitral valve prolapse (MVP) [18–20], preoperative evaluation of the mitral valve for suitability for repair and precise identification of the prolapsing segment/scallop (see Fig. 1) is necessary [21]. 2D TTE and TEE have been used primarily to delineate and localize MVP, and to evaluate chordae integrity, the subvalvular apparatus, annular calcification, and left ventricular size and function. Determining which segment/scallop is prolapsing is difficult by 2D echocardiography, however, and the authors and others have found utility in 3D assessment [4,22–31].

The authors evaluated 34 patients in whom surgical intervention was undertaken for severe

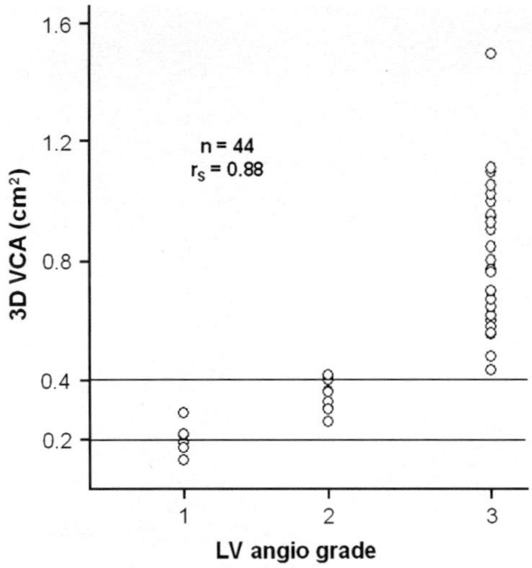

Fig. 3. Mitral regurgitation vena contracta area by live 3D color Doppler transthoracic echocardiography (3D VCA) correlated with left ventricular angiographic assessment. (*Reproduced from* Khanna D, Vengala S, Miller AP, et al. Quantification of mitral regurgitation by live 3D transthoracic echocardiographic measurements of vena contracta area. Echocardiography 2004;21:737–43; with permission.)

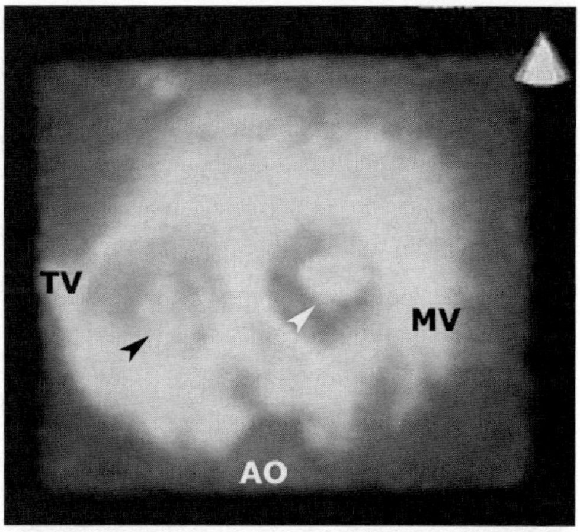

Fig. 4. Live/real-time 3D transthoracic echocardiography in the assessment of mitral valve prolapse. Apically acquired four-chamber data set was cropped from bottom to the level of mitral valve and tilted to view mitral (MV) and tricuspid (TV) valves en face. Yellow arrowhead shows prominent and echogenic prolapse of P2 scallop. Black arrowhead points to prolapse of the middle segment of septal TV leaflet. *Abbreviation:* AO, aorta. (*Reproduced from* Patel V, Hsiung MC, Nanda NC, et al. Usefulness of live/real-time 3D transthoracic echocardiography in the identification of individual segment/scallop prolapse of the mitral valve. Echocardiography 2006;23:513–8; with permission.)

mitral insufficiency caused by MVP [22]. Parasternal and apically acquired 3D datasets were analyzed using the Q laboratory 4.1 software package. By cropping from the left atrial side to just above the mitral annulus, a short axis view was obtained. Individual prolapsing parts of segments or scallops were identified by their increased echogenicity from this view. To view all parts of the saddle shaped mitral valve, two or three oblique planes were used. This procedure was performed using the apically acquired dataset (Fig. 4) and the dataset from the parasternal window (Fig. 5). Segments/scallops were identified based upon their anterior (closer to the aorta) or posterior (deeper in the left atrium) and medial (closer to the ventricular septum), middle, or lateral positions as: A3 and P3, A2 and P2, A1 and P1 for posteromedial, middle, and anterolateral segments/scallops of the mitral valve, respectively (see Fig. 1). In this report, the authors accurately determined MVP location when compared with surgical findings with 95% sensitivity and 87% specificity, and with low inter- and intraobserver variability. The authors now routinely perform 3D TTE exams on all patients the day before surgery to help guide, and hopefully improve likelihood of mitral valve repair.

Summary

Taken together, assessment of MR may play the leading role in the current echocardiography laboratory as an indication for a 3D TTE examination. In this role, 3D TTE offers incremental value over 2D techniques by providing a quantifiable measure of MR for accurate diagnostic grading and for reproducible longitudinal follow-up. Additionally, the ability to prospectively locate and quantify pathological changes provides guidance for surgical interventions, making preferable valve repair more likely. Because these direct measurements of valve anatomy and insufficiency are load-independent, time-efficient, and do not involve calculations based on assumptions, 3D TTE assessment of the mitral

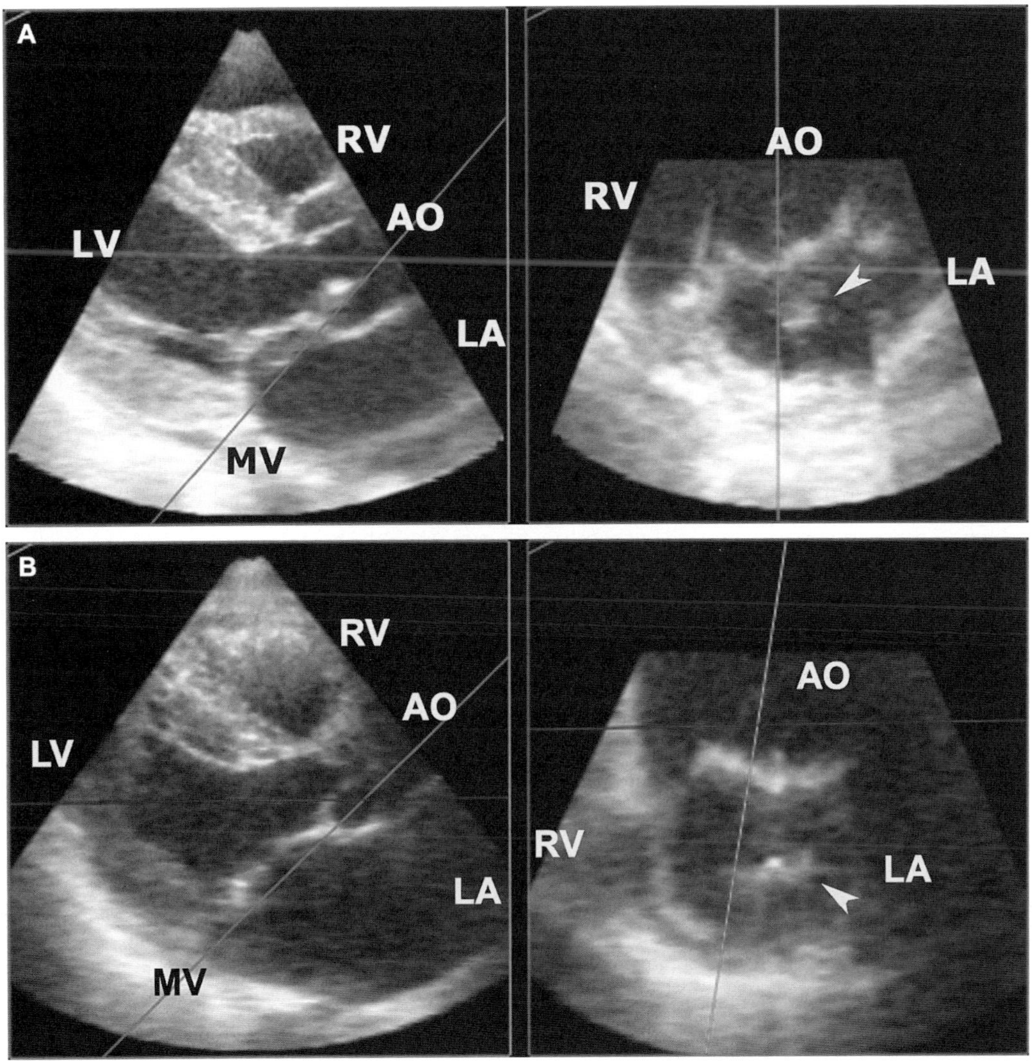

Fig. 5. Live/real-time 3D transthoracic echocardiography in the assessment of mitral valve prolapse using parasternally acquired data sets and offline Q laboratory 4.1 software. (*A, B*) The cropping plane (*red*) was placed at the level of mitral valve annulus in parasternal long axis view (*left panels*) and the prolapsing segment identified in the corresponding short axis view (*right panels*). The position of aorta (AO) and the right ventricle (RV) was used for anatomical orientation. Anterior mitral valve (MV) leaflet prolapse will appear in the left atrium anteriorly (adjacent to aorta), while posterior leaflet prolapse will be located more posteriorly. Depending on whether prolapsing MV leaflet tissue is located medially toward the ventricular septum, in the middle, or laterally, posteromedial (A3/P3), middle (A2/P2), and anterolateral (A1/P1) segment/scallop prolapse can be identified. Arrowheads show A2 prolapse in A and P2 prolapse in B. *Abbreviation:* LA, left atrium. (*Reproduced from* Patel V, Hsiung MC, Nanda NC, et al. Usefulness of live/real-time 3D transthoracic echocardiography in the identification of individual segment/scallop prolapse of the mitral valve. Echocardiography 2006;23:513–8; with permission.)

valve is an important addition to the echocardiography armamentarium.

References

[1] Pai RG, Tanimoto M, Jintapakorn W, et al. Volume-rendered three-dimensional dynamic anatomy of the mitral annulus using a transesophageal echocardiographic technique. J Heart Valve Dis 1995;4(6):623–7.

[2] Flachskampf FA, Chandra S, Gaddipatti A, et al. Analysis of shape and motion of the mitral annulus in subjects with and without cardiomyopathy by echocardiographic 3-dimensional reconstruction. J Am Soc Echocardiogr 2000;13(4):277–87.

[3] Kwan J, Qin JX, Popovic ZB, et al. Geometric changes of mitral annulus assessed by real-time 3-dimensional echocardiography: becoming enlarged and less nonplanar in the anteroposterior direction during systole in proportion to global left ventricular systolic function. J Am Soc Echocardiogr 2004; 17(11):1179–84.

[4] Ahmed S, Nanda NC, Miller AP, et al. Usefulness of transesophageal three-dimensional echocardiography in the identification of individual segment/scallop prolapse of the mitral valve. Echocardiography 2003;20(2):203–9.

[5] Khanna D, Miller AP, Nanda NC, et al. Transthoracic and transesophageal echocardiographic assessment of mitral regurgitation severity: usefulness of qualitative and semiquantitative techniques. Echocardiography 2005;22(9):748–69.

[6] Grossmann G, Giesler M, Stein M, et al. Quantification of mitral and tricuspid regurgitation by the proximal flow convergence method using two-dimensional colour Doppler and colour Doppler M mode: influence of the mechanism of regurgitation. Int J Cardiol 1998;66(3):299–307.

[7] Enriquez-Sarano M, Bailey KR, Seward JB, et al. Quantitative Doppler assessment of valvular regurgitation. Circulation 1993;87(3):841–8.

[8] Fehske W, Omran H, Manz M, et al. Color-coded Doppler imaging of the vena contracta as a basis for quantification of pure mitral regurgitation. Am J Cardiol 1994;73(4):268–74.

[9] Hall SA, Brickner ME, Willett DL, et al. Assessment of mitral regurgitation severity by Doppler color flow mapping of the vena contracta. Circulation 1997;95(3):636–42.

[10] Velayudhan DE, Brown TM, Nanda NC, et al. Quantification of tricuspid regurgitation by live three-dimensional transthoracic echocardiographic measurements of vena contracta area. Echocardiography 2006;23(9):793–800.

[11] Khanna D, Vengala S, Miller AP, et al. Quantification of mitral regurgitation by live three-dimensional transthoracic echocardiographic measurements of vena contracta area. Echocardiography 2004;21(8): 737–43.

[12] Iwakura K, Ito H, Kawano S, et al. Comparison of orifice area by transthoracic three-dimensional Doppler echocardiography versus proximal isovelocity surface area (PISA) method for assessment of mitral regurgitation. Am J Cardiol 2006;97(11): 1630–7.

[13] Buck T, Plicht B, Hunold P, et al. Broad-beam spectral Doppler sonification of the vena contracta using matrix-array technology: a new solution for semiautomated quantification of mitral regurgitant flow volume and orifice area. J Am Coll Cardiol 2005; 45:770–9.

[14] Watanabe N, Ogasawara Y, Yamaura Y, et al. Geometric differences of the mitral valve tenting between anterior and inferior myocardial infarction with significant ischemic mitral regurgitation: quantitation by novel software system with transthoracic real-time three-dimensional echocardiography. J Am Soc Echocardiogr 2006;19(1): 71–5.

[15] Watanabe N, Ogasawara Y, Yamaura Y, et al. Quantitation of mitral valve tenting in ischemic mitral regurgitation by transthoracic real-time three-dimensional echocardiography. J Am Coll Cardiol 2005;45(5):763–9.

[16] Vilacosta I, Graupner C, San Roman JA, et al. Risk of embolization after institution of antibiotic therapy for infective endocarditis. J Am Coll Cardiol 2002;39(9):1489–95.

[17] Tischler MD, Vaitkus PT. The ability of vegetation size on echocardiography to predict clinical complications: a meta-analysis. J Am Soc Echocardiogr 1997;10(5):562–8.

[18] Carpentier A, Chauvaud S, Fabiani JN, et al. Reconstructive surgery of mitral valve incompetence: ten-year appraisal. J Thorac Cardiovasc Surg 1980; 79(3):338–48.

[19] Galloway AC, Colvin SB, Baumann FG, et al. A comparison of mitral valve reconstruction with mitral valve replacement: intermediate-term results. Ann Thorac Surg 1989;47(5):655–62.

[20] Sand ME, Naftel DC, Blackstone EH, et al. A comparison of repair and replacement for mitral valve incompetence. J Thorac Cardiovasc Surg 1987; 94(2):208–19.

[21] Hellemans IM, Pieper EG, Ravelli AC, et al. Prediction of surgical strategy in mitral valve regurgitation based on echocardiography. Interuniversity Cardiology Institute of The Netherlands. Am J Cardiol 1997;79(3):334–8.

[22] Patel V, Hsiung MC, Nanda NC, et al. Usefulness of live/real-time three-dimensional transthoracic echocardiography in the identification of individual segment/scallop prolapse of the mitral valve. Echocardiography 2006;23(6):513–8.

[23] Fabricius AM, Walther T, Falk V, et al. Three-dimensional echocardiography for planning of mitral valve surgery: current applicability? Ann Thorac Surg 2004;78(2):575–8.

[24] Delabays A, Jeanrenaud X, Chassot PG, et al. Localization and quantification of mitral valve prolapse using three-dimensional echocardiography. Eur J Echocardiogr 2004;5(6):422–9.

[25] Hozumi T, Yoshikawa J, Yoshida K, et al. Assessment of flail mitral leaflets by dynamic three-dimensional echocardiographic imaging. Am J Cardiol 1997;79(2):223–5.

[26] De Castro S, Salandin V, Cartoni D, et al. Qualitative and quantitative evaluation of mitral valve morphology by intraoperative volume-rendered three-dimensional echocardiography. J Heart Valve Dis 2002;11(2):173–80.

[27] Chauvel C, Bogino E, Clerc P, et al. Usefulness of three-dimensional echocardiography for the evaluation of mitral valve prolapse: an intraoperative study. J Heart Valve Dis 2000;9(3):341–9.

[28] Levine RA, Handschumacher MD, Sanfilippo AJ, et al. Three-dimensional echocardiographic reconstruction of the mitral valve, with implications for the diagnosis of mitral valve prolapse. Circulation 1989;80(3):589–98.

[29] Chung R, Pepper J, Henein M. Images in cardiology: mitral valve anterior leaflet prolapse by real-time three-dimensional transthoracic echocardiography. Heart 2005;91(9):e55.

[30] Sugeng L, Coon P, Weinert L, et al. Use of real-time 3-dimensional transthoracic echocardiography in the evaluation of mitral valve disease. J Am Soc Echocardiogr 2006;19(4):413–21.

[31] Pepi M, Tamborini G, Maltagliati A, et al. Head-to-head comparison of two- and three-dimensional transthoracic and transesophageal echocardiography in the localization of mitral valve prolapse. J Am Coll Cardiol 2006;48(12):2524–30.

ELSEVIER
SAUNDERS

Cardiol Clin 25 (2007) 327–334

CARDIOLOGY
CLINICS

Three-Dimensional Transthoracic Echocardiographic Assessment of Aortic Stenosis and Regurgitation

Ravi K. Mallavarapu, MD,
Navin C. Nanda, MD, FACC, FAHA, FSOC, FISCU*

Division of Cardiovascular Diseases, University of Alabama at Birmingham, Heart Station, SWB/S102, 619 19th Street South, Birmingham, AL 35249, USA

Noninvasive echocardiographic methods have revolutionized the assessment of patients who have valvular heart disease. Transthoracic 2D echocardiography (2DTTE) with color Doppler is the standard modality for the initial evaluation of the patient who has aortic valvular disease to help with the diagnosis and quantification of the severity of the condition. Color-guided continuous-wave Doppler, however, has important limitations in the assessment of aortic stenosis (AS) and aortic regurgitation (AR). This article outlines the limitations of conventional echocardiographic methods and describes the 3D echocardiographic assessment of AS and AR.

Aortic stenosis

Limitations of transthoracic 2D echocardiography/color Doppler

2DTTE/color Doppler has several limitations in the assessment of AS. Errors in the measurement of the left ventricular outflow tract (LVOT) diameter may occur because of calcification at the junction of the aortic root and the outflow tract. LVOT velocity also may be erroneous depending on how close or far from the aortic valve (AV) it is estimated. The AS jet has a 3D configuration and consists of a central core of high-velocity flow and an outer region of relatively low-velocity flow. Thus, even if it appears that the cursor lies parallel by color Doppler, it may not be in the central core (Fig. 1) [1,2]. Occasionally, an eccentric stenotic jet escapes accurate recording despite meticulous technique, possibly leading to underestimation of the true gradient. In a significant number of patients, Doppler may overestimate AS severity because of various reasons. These include erroneous identification of a jet (the high velocity jet of mitral regurgitation can be mistaken for aortic regurgitation), contamination of the AS jet by the jet of mitral regurgitation, downstream pressure recovery, possible detection of localized high-velocity gradients [3] around the AV that do not represent the true gradient across the valve itself, nonrepresentative jet selection (for eg, a postextrasystolic beat), and coexisting stenotic lesions present in tandem [4,5]. The pressure recovery phenomenon (caused by the change of kinetic to potential energy downstream of the stenosed aortic valve) results in the overestimation of AS severity, especially in the presence of tubular rather than discrete AS, domed bicuspid or tricuspid aortic valves, a small ascending aorta (<3 cm width just beyond sinotubular junction), and a narrow LVOT diameter (≤ 2 cm) [6,7].

Incremental value of 3D transthoracic echocardiography

Live, real-time 3D transthoracic echocardiography (3DTTE) has the potential to become a new noninvasive modality that complements conventional techniques in the assessment of AS [5,8–12]. 3DTTE can be used for assessing the aortic valve and root morphology and also to calculate the valve area in aortic stenosis. First, a parasternal long-axis or apical five-chamber view of the AV

* Corresponding author.
E-mail address: nanda@uab.edu (N.C. Nanda).

doi:10.1016/j.ccl.2007.06.005

cardiology.theclinics.com

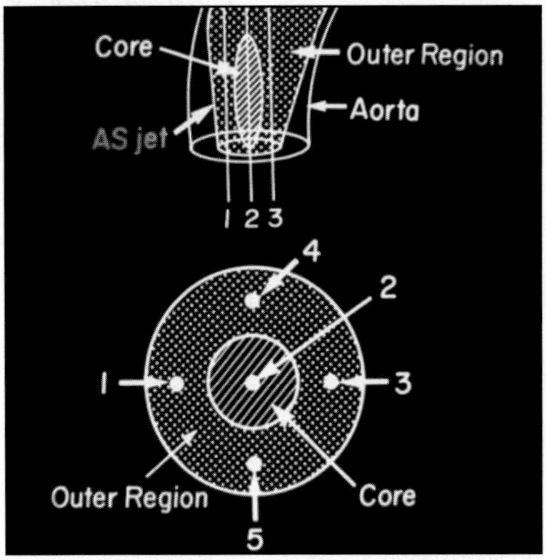

Fig. 1. Because a stenotic jet consists of a small central region or core of high velocity and a larger outer region of lower velocity, the continuous wave Doppler cursor must be positioned in the jet core in addition to being aligned parallel to the jet direction to measure the maximum jet velocity. The 3D structure of the jet may cause the continuous wave cursor to appear to be positioned correctly in the jet while, in reality, the cursor may not be placed properly in the jet core. Therefore, after the initial alignment of the continuous wave cursor in the visualized jet, minimal transducer angulations still are required to interrogate the jet core, which may be in the azimuthal plane. Failure to interrogate the core results in an underestimation of the peak transvalvular velocity and thus the severity of the stenotic lesion. In this illustration, the aortic stenosis (AS) jet is shown to consist of a central core, which has the highest velocity, and this central core is surrounded by an outer region of lower velocity flows. The highest velocity thus is obtained if the continuous wave Doppler cursor is aligned parallel to the core of the jet (cursor 2), while lower velocities are recorded if the cursor is positioned outside the core (cursors 1, 3, 4, 5). (*Reproduced from* Nanda NC (editor). Atlas of Color Doppler Echocardiography. Philadelphia: Lea & Febiger; 1989:112; with permission.)

is obtained in a standard manner using the 3D transducer. The patient then typically is asked to hold his or her breath for a few seconds to acquire and store several electrocardiogram-triggered subvolumes. These subvolumes are then time-aligned to render a full-volume 3D color data set. From the 3D pyramidal data set, a cropping plane aligned exactly parallel to the flow-limiting AV orifice (AVO), viewed in long axis, is used to obtain a short-axis 3D image of the AVO. The AVO area then can be measured accurately by direct planimetry, because the face of any 3D structure is a 2D image. More conveniently, AVO orifice can be planimetered using an online software system provided by the manufacturer [5].

Direct imaging of the 3D contoured anatomy allows an excellent appreciation of spatial anatomy. 3DTTE also affords the opportunity to obtain 2D cut planes using the 3D data set, allowing imaging at any plane desired by the interpreter [13]. This is especially useful in assessing domed AVs and angulated orifices, as the cropping plane in the 3D data set can be aligned perfectly parallel to the flow-limiting tip of the stenosed AV orifice, allowing for accurate visualization of the aortic orifice, the area of which can be obtained by planimetry (Fig. 2). Another advantage of 3DTTE is the ability to estimate the AV orifice area in patients who have combined AS and other stenotic lesions in tandem like supravalvular stenosis and discrete subaortic stenosis. These lesions can be studied in detail also [14]. In addition, measurements like LVOT width and LVOT/AV velocity that can introduce significant errors in calculating the AV orifice area using the continuity equation are not required with 3DTTE. On occasion, reliable identification of the aortic orifice may be practically impossible by 3DTTE in patients who have severe calcific AS caused by immobility of the valve leaflets. In this situation, color Doppler 3DTTE may be used to detect the initial appearance of flow at the onset of systole. These color Doppler signals can be cropped at the valve level using a parallel plane to estimate the orifice area.

Limitations of 2D transesophageal echocardiography

2D transesophageal echocardiography (2DTEE) has the advantage of allowing for direct estimation of the aortic valve area and superior quality imaging as compared with 2DTTE. It is especially useful when there is a poor acoustic window that prevents a satisfactory 2D examination. Careful advancement of the transesophageal probe from the supravalvular area until it first encounters the tip of the aortic orifice is required, and it is dependent on operator skill. This is because overshooting the tip and measuring the area or near the base will underestimate the severity of stenosis. Depending upon the anatomic relation of the esophagus to the aortic valve, the 2D echocardiographic plane may not be aligned parallel to the flow-limiting tip of the aortic valve,

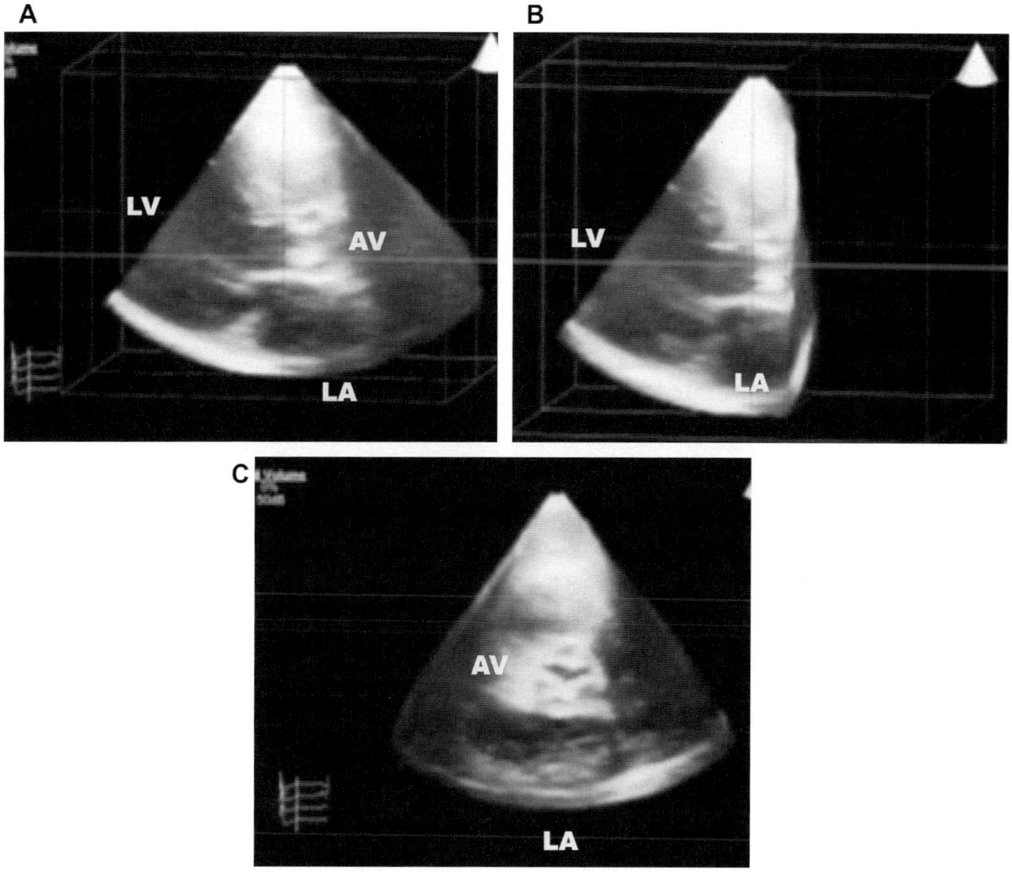

Fig. 2. Live, real time 3D echocardiography in aortic stenosis. (*A*) The aortic valve (AV) is viewed in the parasternal long-axis view showing calcified leaflets. The data set then was cropped from right to the level of the flow-limiting tip of the AV leaflets (*B*) and rotated en face to view the very narrow aortic orifice in short axis consistent with severe stenosis (*C*). The patient has the so-called acquired bicuspid aortic valve because of fusion of two of the three cusps. *Abbreviations:* LA, left atrium; LV, left ventricle.

leading to inaccurate estimation of the orifice. Other limitations include the semi-invasive nature of the procedure, associated patient discomfort, and the accompanying risks including laryngospasm, arrhythmias, aspiration and very rarely, esophageal rupture.

Incremental value of 3D transesophageal echocardiography

3DTEE accurately assesses the severity of AS and provides additional complementary information about valvular morphology as compared with 2DTTE. The TEE probe is inserted in the usual manner and 3D echocardiographic data acquisition is performed by transducer rotation at 3° to 5° increments over a span of 180° using a predetermined heart rate window [15]. It must be noted that slightest motion on part of the patient or examiner interferes with proper data acquisition, and the process has to be repeated. 3D images subsequently are reconstructed, allowing clear delineation of the aortic orifice, allowing direct and accurate planimetry [15,16]. The direct measurements obtained from 3DTEE would be expected to be more accurate than 2DTTE/TEE and cardiac catheterization. In addition, leaflet morphology, severity, and extent of valvular thickening and calcification can be demonstrated graphically (Fig. 3). 3DTEE is limited by the fact that 3D reconstruction of 2D transesophageal images is difficult and full of artifacts when there is patient

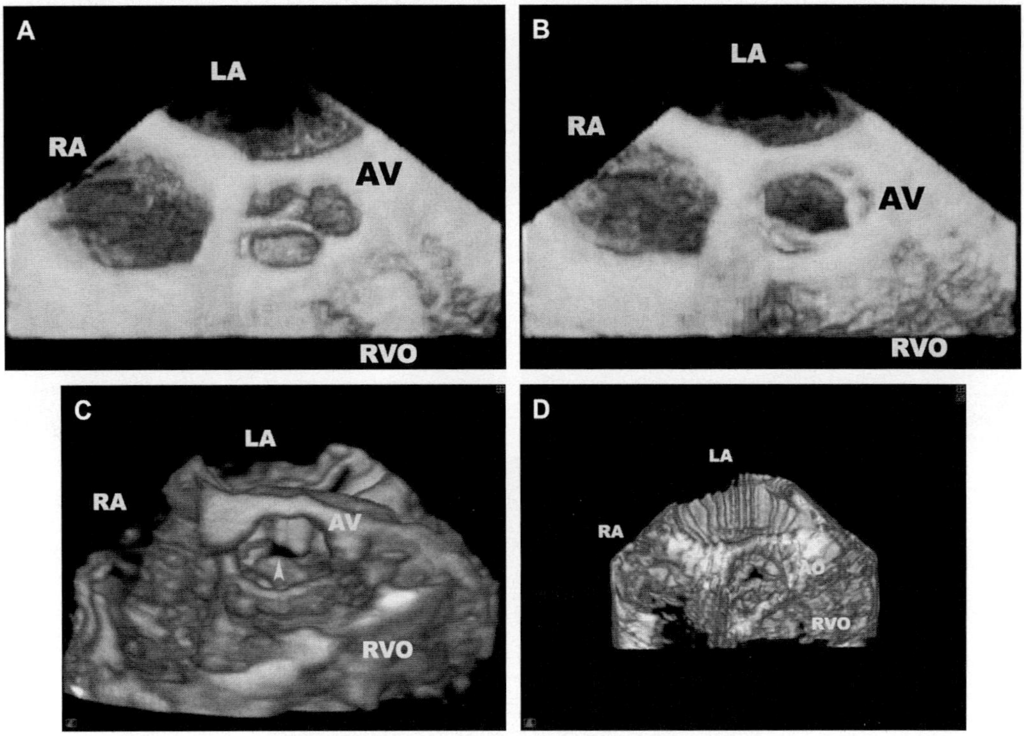

Fig. 3. 3D transesophageal echocardiographic reconstruction in aortic valve stenosis. Thickened bicuspid aortic valve without significant stenosis, shown in the closed (*A*) and open (*B*) positions. (*C*) Severe, calcified bicuspid aortic valve stenosis. Note the transversely oriented very small aortic orifice (*arrowhead*). (*D*) Another patient with calcific severe stenosis. Note that despite severe calcification, the tricuspid morphology of the valve is evident. *Abbreviations:* AO, aorta; RA, right atrium; RVO, right ventricular outflow tract. (*Reproduced from* Dod HS, Nanda NC, Baweja G, et al. Three-dimensional transesophageal echocardiographic assessment of aortic valve pathology. Am J Geriatric Cardiology 2003:12:209–13; with permission.)

motion and in scenarios like atrial fibrillation because of variation in RR intervals with consequent increased time for acquisition of cardiac cycles [12]. This would also be a problem in hemodynamically unstable patients who have wide variations in heart rate and respirations. 3DTEE is not commercially available as a live or real time modality so far.

Aortic regurgitation

Limitations of 2D transesophageal echocardiography/color Doppler

Conventional echocardiographic methods have several limitations in the assessment of AR just as in AS. The reliable and accurate quantification of the severity of AR using various qualitative and quantitative 2DTTE/color Doppler techniques continues to be a challenge. This is primarily because they use a 2D plane to describe and quantify a 3D object. Quantitative methods of assessment like the volumetric approach and proximal flow convergence are limited, because they require assumptions that are mostly inaccurate [17]. Assessing the deceleration slope and pressure halftime of the continuous-wave Doppler spectrum is limited by the fact that the flow velocity profile is dependent on systemic vascular resistance and left ventricular compliance [18,19]. Measurement of the regurgitant fraction and volume by pulsed-wave Doppler determination of aortic forward flow combined with left ventricular volume by 2DTTE cannot be used in the presence of mitral regurgitation, and it requires assumptions of the left ventricular shape and of the aortic flow profile [20,21]. Although color Doppler allows measurements of different components of the jet by allowing visualization of velocity flow maps in real time, there are important limitations. The proximal flow-convergence method for determining regurgitant volume is limited by geometric assumptions and also requires, in many instances, angle correction for AR [22,23]. The proximal jet width or height taken on the ventricular aspect of the aortic valve essentially represents the vena contracta (the size of the regurgitant jet within the leaflets and extending for a variable extent downstream into the LVOT) [24]. The regurgitant volume may be calculated by multiplying the vena contracta area (VCA) with the velocity time integral (VTI) of the continuous-wave Doppler waveform of the AR jet. Only one dimension of the AR jet is visualized in the two-dimensional parasternal long-axis or apical five-chamber views, however, and hence the VCA cannot be measured unless one makes the assumption that its shape is circular or elliptical, which is mostly incorrect [25]. Capturing the complex geometry of the vena contracta by obtaining a short-axis view of the aortic valve is limited when using two-dimensional echocardiography because of cardiac motion, making it difficult to ascertain whether one is measuring the jet width at the level of the aortic valve or at a level further downstream, where it tends to be larger [26]. In addition, it is difficult to ascertain that the 2DTTE short-axis plane is aligned exactly parallel to the AR jet imaged in short axis. This is especially important in patients who have eccentric AR. Studies have shown that the AR jet in short axis does not correlate with the aortographic criteria of AR severity as reliably as the proximal jet width divided by LVOT width [24,27].

Incremental value of 3D transthoracic echocardiography

3DTTE has demonstrated feasibility and accuracy in quantifying aortic regurgitation [25,28,29]. After completion of the standard 2DTTE, live and real time 3DTTE images can be obtained in the apical and parasternal views. Vena contracta width can be measured as the smallest neck of flow at the level of the aortic valve interposed between the area of flow acceleration and the jet [28,30]. Systematic cropping of the acquired 3DTTE data set can be used to measure VCA. The first step is obtaining the best AR jet in long axis from a parasternal long axis view or from an apical view (when the parasternal window is poor) by posterior-to-anterior cropping of the 3DTTE data set. Then the 3DTTE color Doppler data set can be cropped from the aortic or left ventricular side to the level of the vena contracta, at or just below the aortic valve leaflets, in a plane exactly perpendicular to the AR jet viewed in long axis. The image now is tilted en face, and the cropped portion of the data set is added back to obtain the maximum area of vena contracta viewed in short axis in systole (Fig. 4). In patients who have more than one AR jet, the VCW may be taken as the sum of all individual vena contracta widths. Measurements of VCA can be obtained by direct planimetry or by using an online or offline software system like the Q-Lab (Phillips, Bothell, Washington) [28]. There are several advantages to using 3DTTE for assessing AR by the method described. The VCA can be multiplied with the velocity time integral obtained by color Doppler-directed continuous wave Doppler to accurately estimate the regurgitant volume. In addition, 3DTTE has the advantage of being fairly simple and more accurate, and it obviates the need to make mostly incorrect assumptions that the vena contracta is circular or elliptical in shape, which is done when using 2DTTE/Doppler [25].

A more confident estimation of the VCA is possible, because the entirety of the vena contracta can be appreciated and planimetered by using imaging planes exactly perpendicular to the AR jet in long axis. The 3DTTE-measured VCA essentially signifies the actual regurgitant hole in the aortic orifice in diastole [31,32].

Summary

3D echocardiography is a safe, noninvasive imaging modality that has the potential to be complementary to 2D imaging in the assessment of both AS and AR. 3DTTE can be used to increase the confidence level of assessment of AS and AR, especially when there is discordance between 2D echocardiographic and clinical findings. Unlike cardiac catheterization and 2DTTE/Doppler, which are indirect methods of assessment, 3DTTE allows direct visualization of the aortic valve orifice in aortic stenosis and therefore can be expected to be more reliable. En face delineation of aortic valve stenosis allows direct planimetry and thus accurate estimation of severity. In the assessment of AR, aortography has been the time-honored gold standard for assessing severity but is limited by factors such as different background densities between two orthogonal

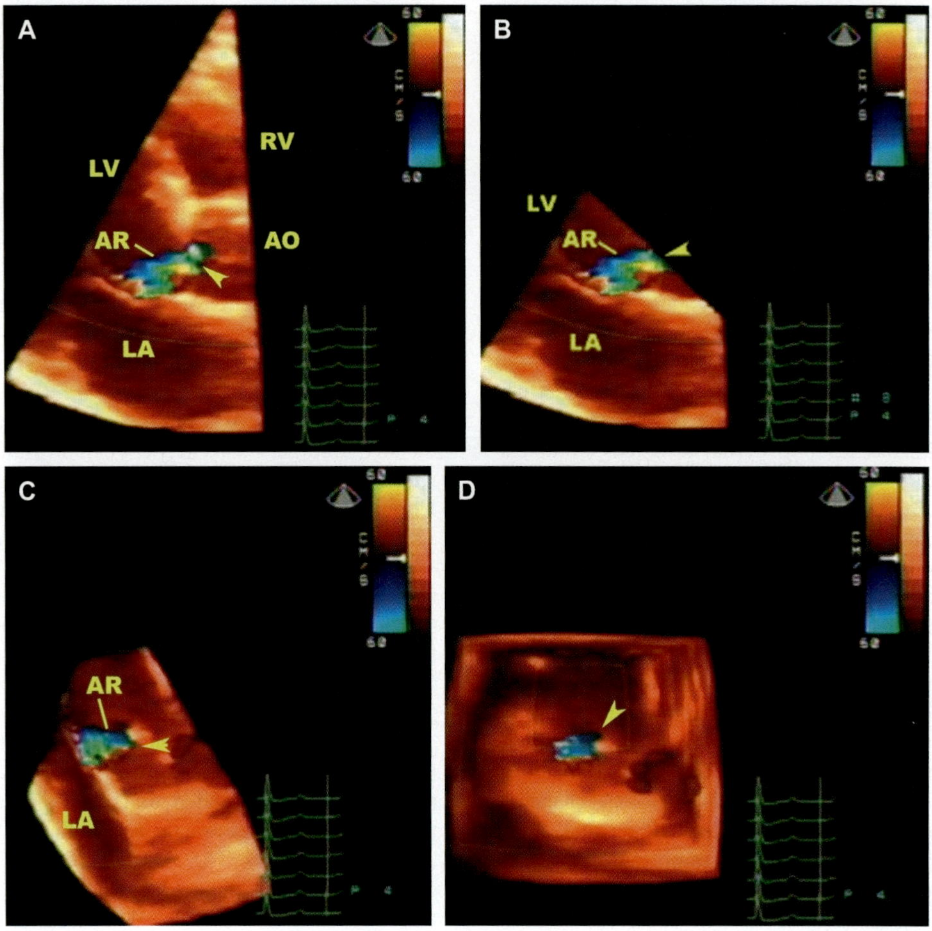

Fig. 4. Live 3D color Doppler transthoracic echocardiographic technique for assessment of aortic regurgitation (AR) vena contracta. The 3D color Doppler data set showing AR (*A*) is cropped using an oblique plane to the level of the vena contracta (*arrowhead, B*) and tilted to view it en face (*C, D*). The vena contracta then is planimetered. *Abbreviations:* AO, aorta; LA, left atrium; LV, left ventricle; RV, right ventricle. (*Reproduced from* Fang L, et al. Assessment of aortic regurgitation by live 3D transthoracic echocardiography measurements of vena contracta area: usefulness and validation. Echocardiography 2005;22:775–81; with permission.)

projections and the presence of dysrhythmias. Additionally, it is especially variable in patients who have enlarged ventricles [33]. Similarly, 2DTTE/color Doppler has several limitations as described previously. Because it is frequently eccentric in shape, the AR jet cannot be appreciated easily in its totality by 2DTTE. The ability of 3DTTE to dissect the complex geometry of a regurgitant jet makes it a more accurate method to appreciate the true geometry and spatial extent of jet flow, enabling accurate quantification of the severity of AR. Future improvements in technology and further research will continue to expand the role of 3DTTE for evaluating both AS and AR.

References

[1] Kececioglu-Draelos Z, Goldberg SJ, Areias J, et al. Verification and clinical demonstration of the echo Doppler series effect and vortex shed distance. Circulation 1981;63:1422–8.

[2] Peronneau P, Diebold JP, Guglielmi O, et al. Structure and performance of mono and bidimensional pulsed Doppler systems. In: Roelandt J, editor. Color Doppler imaging and other advances in Doppler echocardiography. Boston: Martinus Nijhoff Publishers, Inc; 1986. p. 3–18.

[3] Baumgartner H, Khan S, DeRobertis M, et al. Discrepancies between Doppler and catheter gradients in aortic prosthetic valves in vitro. A manifestation of localized gradients and pressure recovery. Circulation 1990;82:1467–75.

[4] Nanda NC. Textbook of color Doppler echocardiography. Philadelphia: Lea and Febiger, Inc; 1989. p. 178–90.
[5] Vengala S, Nanda NC, Dod SH, et al. Images in geriatric cardiology. Usefulness of live three-dimensional transthoracic echocardiography in aortic valve stenosis evaluation. Am J Geriatr Cardiol 2004;13:279–84.
[6] Baumgartner H, Stefenelli T, Niederberger J, et al. Overestimation of catheter gradients by Doppler ultrasound in patients with aortic stenosis: a predictable manifestation of pressure recovery. J Am Coll Cardiol 1999;33:1655–61.
[7] Laskey WK, Kussmaul WG. Pressure recovery in aortic valve stenosis. Circulation 1994;89:116–21.
[8] Ge S, Warner JG Jr, Abraham TP, et al. Three-dimensional surface area of the aortic valve orifice by three-dimensional echocardiography: clinical validation of a novel index for assessment of aortic stenosis. Am Heart J 1998;136:1042–50.
[9] Handke M, Jahnke C, Heinrichs G, et al. New three-dimensional echocardiographic system using digital radiofrequency data: visualization and quantitative analysis of aortic valve dynamics with high resolution: methods, feasibility, and initial clinical experience. Circulation 2003;107: 2876–9.
[10] Kasprzak JD, Nosir YF, Dall'Agata A, et al. Quantification of the aortic valve area in three-dimensional echocardiographic data sets: analysis of orifice overestimation resulting from suboptimal cut-plane selection. Am Heart J 1998;135: 995–1003.
[11] Menzel T, Mohr-Kahaly S, Kolsch B, et al. Quantitative assessment of aortic stenosis by three-dimensional echocardiography. J Am Soc Echocardiogr 1997;10:215–23.
[12] Nanda NC, Roychoudhury D, Chung SM, et al. Quantitative assessment of normal and stenotic aortic valve using transesophageal three-dimensional echocardiography. Echocardiography 1994;11: 617–25.
[13] Nanda NC, Sorrell VL. Atlas of three-dimensional echocardiography. Armonk (NY): Futura Publishing Co., Inc; 2002. p. 49–94.
[14] Rajdev S, Nanda NC, Patel V, et al. Live, real time three-dimensional transthoracic echocardiographic assessment of combined valvar and supravalvular aortic stenosis. Am J Geriatr Cardiol 2006;15: 188 90.
[15] Dod HS, Nanda NC, Agrawal GG, et al. Three-dimensional transesophageal echocardiographic assessment of aortic valve pathology. Am J Geriatr Cardiol 2003;12:209–13.
[16] Pandian NG, Nanda NC, Schwartz SL, et al. Three-dimensional and 4-dimensional transesophageal echocardiographic imaging of the heart and aorta in human using a computed tomographic probe. Echocardiography 1992;9:677–87.
[17] Tribouilloy CM, Enriquez-Sarano M, Fett SL, et al. Application of the proximal flow convergence method to calculate the effective regurgitant orifice area in aortic regurgitation. J Am Coll Cardiol 1998;32:1032–103.
[18] Teague SM, Heinsimer J, Anderson JL, et al. Quantification of aortic regurgitation utilizing continuous wave Doppler ultrasound. J Am Coll Cardiol 1986; 8:592–9.
[19] Labovitz AJ, Ferrara RP, Kern MJ, et al. Quantitative evaluation of aortic insufficiency by continuous-wave Doppler echocardiography. J Am Coll Cardiol 1986;8:1341–7.
[20] Enriquez-Sarano M, Bailey KR, Seward JB, et al. Quantitative Doppler assessment of valvular regurgitation. Circulation 1993;87:841–8.
[21] Rokey R, Sterling LL, Zoghbi WA, et al. Determination of regurgitant fraction in isolated mitral or aortic regurgitation by pulsed Doppler 2-dimensional echocardiography. J Am Coll Cardiol 1986; 7:1026–36.
[22] Recusani F, Bargiggia GS, Yoganathan AP, et al. A new method for quantification of regurgitant flow rate using color Doppler flow imaging of the flow convergence region proximal to a discrete orifice: an in vitro study. Circulation 1991;83:594–604.
[23] Cape EG, Thomas JD, Weyman AE, et al. Three-dimensional surface geometry correction is required for calculating flow by the proximal isovelocity surface area technique. J Am Soc Echocardiogr 1995;8: 585–94.
[24] Perry GJ, Helmcke F, Nanda NC, et al. Evaluation of aortic insufficiency by Doppler color flow mapping. J Am Coll Cardiol 1987;9:952–9.
[25] Shiota T, Jones M, Tsujino H, et al. Quantitative analysis of aortic regurgitation: real-time 3-dimensional and 2-dimensional color Doppler echocardiographic method: a clinical and a chronic animal study. J Am Soc Echocardiogr 2002;15:966–71.
[26] Cape EG, Kim YH, Heinrich RS, et al. Cardiac motion can alter proximal isovelocity surface area calculations of regurgitant flow. J Am Coll Cardiol 1993;22:1730–7.
[27] Byard CE, Perry GJ, Roitman DI, et al. Quantitative assessment of aortic regurgitation by color Doppler [abstract]. Circulation 1985;72:III-146.
[28] Fang L, Hsiung MC, Miller AP, et al. Assessment of aortic regurgitation by live three-dimensional transthoracic echocardiographic measurements of vena contracta area: usefulness and validation. Echocardiography 2005;22:775–81.
[29] Acar P, Jones M, Shiota T, et al. Quantitative assessment of chronic aortic regurgitation with 3-dimensional echocardiographic reconstruction: comparison with electromagnetic flow meter measurements. J Am Soc Echocardiogr 1999;12:138–48.
[30] Tribouilloy CM, Enriquez-Sarano M, Bailey KR, et al. Assessment of severity of aortic regurgitation using the width of the vena contracta: a clinical color

Doppler imaging study. Circulation 2000;102: 558–64.
[31] Nanda NC, Miller AP. Real-time three-dimensional echocardiography: specific indications and incremental value over traditional echocardiography. J Cardiol 2007;48:291–303.
[32] Dod HS, Nanda NC, Baweja G, et al. Online three-dimensional transesophageal echocardiography reconstruction. Am J Geriatr Cardiol 2003;12:328–32.
[33] Hunt D, Baxley WA, Kennedy JW, et al. Quantitative evaluation of cineaortography in the assessment of aortic regurgitation. Am J Cardiol 1973;31:696–700.

ELSEVIER
SAUNDERS

Cardiol Clin 25 (2007) 335–340

CARDIOLOGY
CLINICS

Interventional Three-Dimensional Echocardiography: Using Real-Time Three-Dimensional Echocardiography to Guide and Evaluate Intracardiac Therapies

Edward A. Gill, MD, FACC, FASE, FACP[a],
David H. Liang, MD, PhD[b,*]

[a]*Department of Medicine, Division of Cardiology, University of Washington School of Medicine, Harborview Medical Center, 325 Ninth Avenue, Box 359748, Seattle, WA 98104, USA*
[b]*Division of Cardiovascular Medicine, Stanford University School of Medicine, Stanford, CA, USA*

The growing movement toward less invasive therapies for disease creates a need for improved imaging guidance as more complicated procedures are contemplated. Echocardiography, with its ability to provide real-time imaging and resolve soft tissue structures without using ionizing radiation or very special environments required by other imaging modalities such as CT and MRI, holds promise in addressing those needs. A major limitation of 2D echocardiography is its ability to image only in a thin 2D slice, making it distinctly unusual to see a device's relative position to its surrounding environment. To obtain an understanding of the 3D position of a device, the echocardiographer must acquire several views and then integrate them into a mental 3D model to determine the actual spatial location of the device. This interpreter-based approach has proven to be effective for many years as echocardiographers have applied it to the understanding of complex objects such as the mitral valve. Relying upon the operator to assemble a series of images in his or her head, however, is not feasible during an intervention, because the devices are moving constantly. Real-time 3D echocardiography (RT3DE) has the potential to address this limitation of echocardiography.

* Corresponding author.
E-mail address: dliang@cvmed.stanford.edu (D.H. Liang).

The use of RT3DE for this purpose is in its infancy. 3D echocardiography can visualize intracardiac tools such as bioptomes, pacemaker wires, and ablation catheters along most of their course by the addition of depth or the elevation dimension, whereas typically with 2D echocardiography, only short segments are seen where they cross the imaging plane. The third dimension has proven to be helpful locating the right ventricular (RV) bioptome used during endomyocardial biopsy [1–3]. Others have reported viewing pacemakers by means of 3D echocardiography. Finally, a few other anecdotal cases illustrate the use of the technology for general catheter location, potentially aiding movement of the catheter through the heart and detecting masses on the catheters. Early experiments also have been undertaken to examine the feasibility of 3D echocardiography to guide more complex intracardiac procedures.

Visualization of right ventricular bioptome by 3D echocardiography

Like catheters, the RV bioptome, used to perform right RV endomyocardial biopsies frequently can be visualized along its entire course by RT3DE as opposed to only part of the device by 2D echocardiography (Figs. 1 and 2). There have been three studies that have evaluated the use of RT3DE for guiding a bioptome while performing RV biopsy. Most recently, in a study by Amitai and

0733-8651/07/$ - see front matter
doi:10.1016/j.ccl.2007.06.004

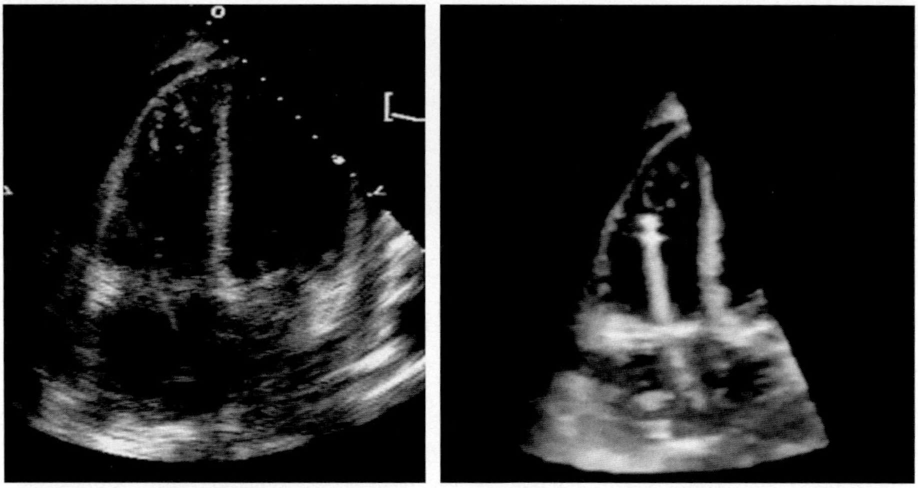

Fig. 1. Example of 2D (*left*) and 3D (*right*) echocardiography of a right ventricular bioptome for performing endomyocardial biopsy. Note that as opposed to the 2D image, which shows only a partial view of the bioptome and poor visualization of the tip, the 3D image shows the complete bioptome and tip. (*Courtesy of* D. Liang, MD, PhD, Stanford, CA.)

colleagues, 38 consecutive endomyocardial biopsies performed under fluoroscopic guidance in 26 patients were monitored using 2D echocardiography and RT3DE alternately [1]. It is important to emphasize that the operators of the bioptome were using fluoroscopy for their primary guidance and were blinded to the echocardiography images. A total of 243 biopsy attempts were made during the 38 endomyocardial biopsy procedures. The location of the biopsy could be determined in 74% of the biopsies by RT3DE compared with only 43% located by 2D echocardiography ($P < .0001$). With regard to specific location of the bioptome tip, RT3DE was superior to 2D echocardiography in 23 of 38 biopsies, compared with 1 of 38 for 2D echocardiography. In 14 of the 38 biopsies, there was no difference between 2D echocardiography and RT3DE. Arguably the most important finding of this study, despite it not being emphasized in the statistical evaluations, is that more than half the time when the biopsy site could be identified by echocardiography, it was suboptimal and potentially unsafe. It was noted in this study that no cooperation was needed between the biopsy operators and the echocardiographers to obtain diagnostic 3D images; this is in contrast to 2D imaging when there often has to be interaction between the two to capture the tip of the bioptome and the site of biopsy.

In a study by Scheurer and colleagues [3], RT3DE was performed in 28 consecutive children, aged 18 months to 16 years, who were undergoing endomyocardial biopsy. This group also found that RT3DE was a reliable method to properly

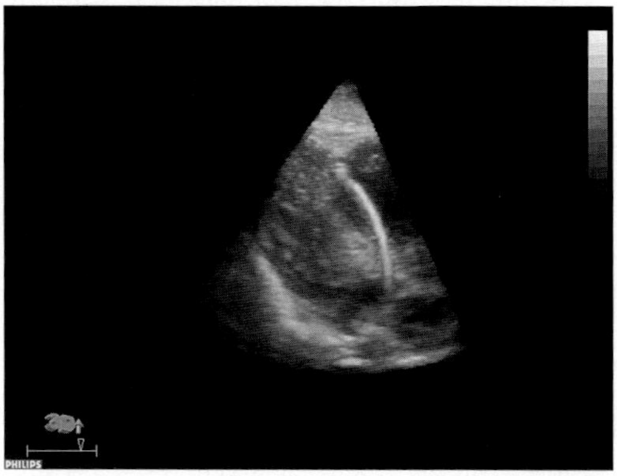

Fig. 2. Real-time 3D echocardiography shows the tip of the bioptome as it pulls away a piece of endocardium resulting in actual eversion of the right ventricular apex (in fact apical free wall, in fact a dangerous area for biopsy because of risk of rupture, nicely demonstrated by RT3D). (See video. Access video in the online version of this article at: http://www.cardiology.theclinics.com.) The still image shows the bioptome everting the right ventricular apex moments before extracting some myocardial tissue. (*Courtesy of* L. Ward, RCS, RVT, Bothell, WA, and G. Shirali, MD, Charleston, SC.)

direct the bioptome. Over time, the need for fluoroscopic guidance was less. There was no comparison done in their study to 2D echocardiography. Also, the operators were not blinded to the echocardiography results, and in fact over time, learned how to use the echocardiography results to minimize fluoroscopy time. This approach was particularly taken in children because of the issue with radiation in young children. It is interesting that of the nine patients who underwent biopsy with 3D guidance, one was a patient with intact pericardium done for evaluation of cardiomyopathy. Although this study was more a report of the operators' experience with RT3DE, there were no complications while guiding biopsy with RT3DE, particularly no new tricuspid valve flail leaflet or pericardial effusion.

In 2001, McCreery and colleagues [2] also reported the use of RT3D for endomyocardial biopsy. The early system used in this study did not produce a volume rendering of the volume containing the heart and the bioptome. Instead a series of 2D slices encompassing the region of interest was produced in real time. Despite the limitations of such a system, the position of the biopsy was identified. They reported that with fluoroscopic guidance, the bioptome was placed against the RV free wall, a suboptimal and potentially dangerous location, in 19% of patients. Further, 1% of patients had the bioptome in the coronary sinus.

In all three of these studies, the value of 3D echocardiography in tracking bioptomes in the heart through its more complete coverage of heart has been demonstrated.

Evaluation of pacemaker leads by real-time 3D echocardiography

The use of RT3DE for evaluation of pacing leads is reported sparsely currently and hence essentially is limited to a few case reports. Despite this, anecdotally, both authors have had experience with using 3D echocardiography for this purpose. Particularly, they have used RT3DE to evaluate the relationship between the RV pacing lead and the tricuspid valve leaflets and subvalvular apparatus in patients who have severe tricuspid regurgitation. The relationship between the pacing RV pacing lead and all three pacing leaflets often can be discerned (Fig. 3). Often in this situation the pacing lead is causing the tricuspid regurgitation by one of the following mechanisms:

Perforation of a tricuspid leaflet
Pinning one of the leaflet against the ventricular wall resulting in lack of coaptation

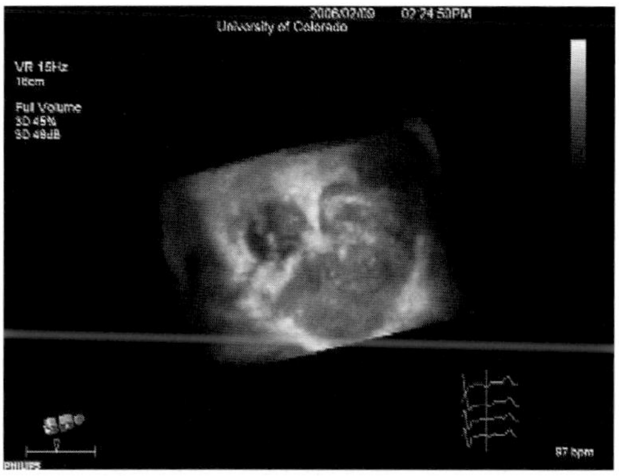

Fig. 3. Short axis of tricuspid valve with pacing wire passing through the tricuspid valve. In this case, the pacing wire can be seen in an optimal position between all three leaflets. (*Courtesy of* S. Popylisen, RDCS, Denver, CO, and L. Ward, RCS, RVT, Bothell, WA.)

Contributing to endocarditis of the lead/valve
A combination of one or some of the previous three

RT3D can help with all of these diagnoses.

RT3DE has been used to visualize the pacemaker lead in a patient with the wire perforating the interventricular septum (Fig. 4). The patient presented after a syncopal episode and had a chest radiograph, 2D echocardiogram, and CT scan, none of which were conclusive for malposition of the pacemaker. Interrogation of the pacemaker showed episodes of ventricular noncapture and

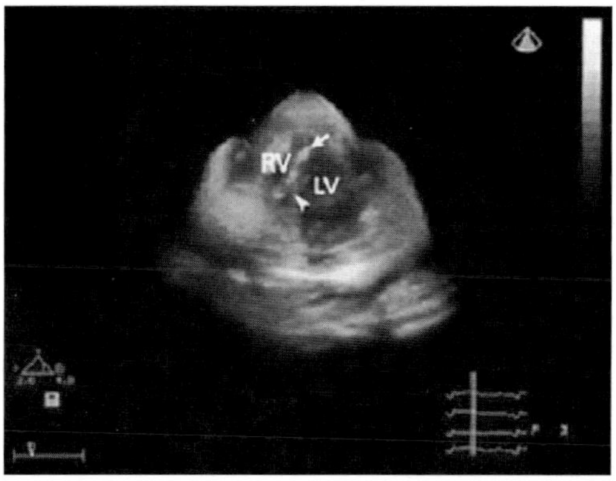

Fig. 4. Real-time 3D full-volume data set showing pacemaker present in the left ventricle, implying that it has perforated the interventricular septum. (*From* Daher IN, Saeed M, Schwarz ER, et al. Live 3D echocardiography in diagnosis of interventricular septal perforation by pacemaker lead. Echocardiography 2006;23(5):428–9; with permission.)

ventricular oversensing, suggestive of lead malfunction. A full-volume RT3D data set was acquired and conclusively showed the pacer wire in the left ventricle, diagnostic of interventricular septal perforation [4].

Masses, vegetations on pacer wires, catheters

RT3D has detected vegetations successfully on a pacemaker/defibrillator lead when other imaging technologies could not. The patient was a 71-year-old man who had history of cardiomyopathy with ejection fraction of 20% and nonsustained ventricular tachycardia. The patient had been treated with a biventricular pacer/defibrillator. The patient had had a transesophageal echocardiogram and a transthoracic 2D echocardiogram, and no definitive diagnosis had been made, but there was suspicion for vegetation, and the blood cultures were positive for methicillin-resistant *Staphylococcus aureus*. A full-volume RT3D echocardiography data set was acquired and cropped revealing a clear mass on the pacer wire (Fig. 5). The pacer wire subsequently was extracted. The diagnosis was confirmed and the patient did well [5].

Complex intracardiac procedures

The groundwork also has been laid in animal models for more complex intracardiac procedures guided by 3D echocardiography. Early work by Downing and colleagues demonstrated that even with a sparse array system adequate resolution was achieved for visualizing tools and anatomy needed to repair atrial septal defects [6]. Following these studies, Suematsu and colleagues, beginning in 2003, undertook a series of studies to develop the use of 3D echocardiography for guiding atrial septal defect repairs. Initial studies were based upon a mechanically scanned 2D echocardiography probe [7]; however frame rate limitations led to subsequent studies being performed with 2D matrix transducers [8–10]. In these studies, 3D echocardiography demonstrated accurate suture placement (deviation 1.7 plus or minus 0.7 mm from desired target) and a 21% improvement in speed over 2D guided suture placement in an in vitro experiment [8]. The value of 3D echocardiography subsequently has been verified further in in vivo experiments [10]. Limited visualization of small details by RT3D echocardiography, however, have led to subsequent experiments combining videocardioscopic guidance with RT3DE [11].

RT3D echocardiography also has been shown to be a potential guidance tool for mitral valve repairs using an edge-to-edge technique [8].

Precise catheter placement also has been shown to benefit from RT3D echocardiography guidance. Cannulation of the coronary sinus has been shown to be improved significantly with epicardial RT3D echocardiography [12]. Intramyocardial injections, such as those that may be required for delivery of pharmacologic and biologic treatments, also have been shown to guided accurately by RT3D [13].

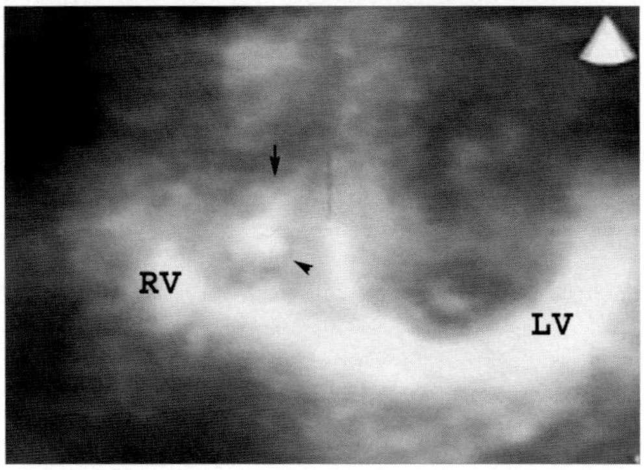

Fig. 5. A real-time 3D full-volume data set is shown with cropping revealing a mass on the pacing wire going through the tricuspid valve. (*From* Pothineni KR, Nanda NC, Patel V, et al. Live/real-time 3D transthoracic echocardiographic detection of vegetation on a pacemaker/defibrillator lead. Am J Geriatr Cardiol 2006; 15(1):62–3; with permission.)

The future

Surprisingly, electrophysiology procedures where catheter guidance perhaps would benefit most from RT3DE have yet to be studied extensively. This may be in part because of the limited ability of currently available transthoracic real-time 3D systems to image the atria where much of the anatomy relevant to treatment of arrhythmias is situated. The value of 3D anatomic information in electrophysiology procedures has been demonstrated by nonreal-time reconstructed 3D intracardiac ultrasound imaging [14–16]. Future developments in intracardiac real-time 3D ultrasound [17–19] and real-time 3D transesophageal echocardiography [20] may address the challenges posed in acquiring high-quality 3D visualization of the atria.

Presenting the information gathered by three-dimensional echocardiography to the physician performing the procedure is an additional area that may benefit from future work. 3D echocardiography data so far have been presented either as a volume-rendered image on a 2D display or by means of a series of 2D slices extracted from the 3D dataset. Although depth cues may be presented in the form of shading and other rendering techniques, they do not mimic the full set of cues that are available when directly viewing an object with one's eyes; thus information on spatial relationships that make 3D imaging powerful may be lost. Handke and colleagues explored the use of stereoscopic glasses to reconstruct some of the binocular cues lost in rendering 3D data onto a 2D display [20]. Wang and colleagues investigated the ability of a true 3D display to improve physician perception of physical relationships within 3D ultrasound data and found that with the use of a true 3D display, the time to perform a task requiring assessing spatial relationships between objects in the ultrasound image was reduced by nearly 50% when compared with volume-rendered images on a 2D display [21].

Summary

RT3DE already has demonstrated its utility in guiding intracardiac procedures. With further enhancements in image quality and display techniques, RT3DE has great potential for serving as an essential tool for visualizing minimally invasive and catheter-based therapies within the heart.

References

[1] Amitai ME, Schnittger I, Popp RL, et al. Comparison of three-dimensional echocardiography to two-dimensional echocardiography and fluoroscopy for monitoring of endomyocardial biopsy. Am J Cardiol 2007;99(6):864–6.

[2] McCreery CJ, McCulloch M, Ahmed M, et al. Real-time 3-dimensional echocardiography imaging for right ventricular endomyocardial biopsy: a comparison with fluoroscopy. J Am Soc Echocardiogr 2001; 14(9):927–33.

[3] Scheurer M, Bandisode V, Ruff P, et al. Early experience with real-time three-dimensional echocardiographic guidance of right ventricular biopsy in children. Echocardiography 2006;23(1):45–9.

[4] Daher IN, Saeed M, Schwarz ER, et al. Live three-dimensional echocardiography in diagnosis of interventricular septal perforation by pacemaker lead. Echocardiography 2006;23(5):428–9.

[5] Pothineni KR, Nanda NC, Patel V, et al. Live/real-time three-dimensional transthoracic echocardiographic detection of vegetation on a pacemaker/defibrillator lead. Am J Geriatr Cardiol 2006;15(1): 62–3.

[6] Downing SW, Herzog WR Jr, McElroy MC, et al. Feasibility of off-pump ASD closure using real-time 3D echocardiography. Heart Surg Forum 2002;5(2):96–9.

[7] Suematsu Y, Takamoto S, Kaneko Y, et al. Beating atrial septal defect closure monitored by epicardial real-time three-dimensional echocardiography without cardiopulmonary bypass. Circulation 2003; 107(5):785–90.

[8] Suematsu Y, Marx GR, Stoll JA, et al. Three-dimensional echocardiography-guided beating-heart surgery without cardiopulmonary bypass: a feasibility study. J Thorac Cardiovasc Surg 2004;128(4): 579–87.

[9] Suematsu Y, Marx GR, Triedman JK, et al. Three-dimensional echocardiography-guided atrial septectomy: an experimental study. J Thorac Cardiovasc Surg 2004;128(1):53–9.

[10] Suematsu Y, Martinez JF, Wolf BK, et al. Three-dimensional echo-guided beating heart surgery without cardiopulmonary bypass: atrial septal defect closure in a swine model. J Thorac Cardiovasc Surg 2005;130(5):1348–57.

[11] Vasilyev NV, Martinez JF, Freudenthal FP, et al. Three-dimensional echo and videocardioscopy-guided atrial septal defect closure. Ann Thorac Surg 2006;82(4):1322–6 [discussion: 1326].

[12] Suematsu Y, Kiaii B, Bainbridge D, et al. Live 3-dimensional echocardiography guidance for the insertion of a retrograde cardioplegic catheter through the coronary sinus. Heart Surg Forum 2007;10(3):E188–90.

[13] Baklanov DV, de Muinek ED, Simons M, et al. Live 3D echo guidance of catheter-based endomyocardial injection. Catheter Cardiovasc Interv 2005;65(3): 340–5.

[14] Knackstedt C, Franke A, Mischke K, et al. Semiautomated 3-dimensional intracardiac echocardiography: development and initial clinical experience of a new system to guide ablation procedures. Heart Rhythm 2006;3(12):1453–9.

[15] Simon RD, Crawford FA III, Spencer WH III, et al. Electroanatomic mapping of the right atrium with a right atrial basket catheter and three-dimensional intracardiac echocardiography. Pacing Clin Electrophysiol 2004;27(3):318–26.

[16] Scaglione M, Caponi D, Di Donna P, et al. Typical atrial flutter ablation outcome: correlation with isthmus anatomy using intracardiac echo 3D reconstruction. Europace 2004;6(5):407–17.

[17] Gentry KL, Smith SW. Integrated catheter for 3D intracardiac echocardiography and ultrasound

ablation. IEEE Trans Ultrason Ferroelectr Freq Control 2004;51(7):800–8.

[18] Light ED, Idriss SF, Wolf PD, et al. Real-time three-dimensional intracardiac echocardiography. Ultrasound Med Biol 2001;27(9):1177–83.

[19] Smith SW, et al. Feasibility study of real-time three-dimensional intracardiac echocardiography for guidance of interventional electrophysiology. Pacing Clin Electrophysiol 2002;25(3):351–7.

[20] Handke M, Heinrichs G, Moser U, et al. Transesophageal real-time three-dimensional echocardiography methods and initial in vitro and human in vivo studies. J Am Coll Cardiol 2006;48(10):2070–6.

[21] Wang AS, et al. An evaluation of using real-time volumetric display of 3D ultrasound data for intracardiac catheter manipulation tasks. In: Volume Graphics 2005, 20–21 June 2005. Stony Brook (NY): IEEE; 2005.

ELSEVIER
SAUNDERS

Cardiol Clin 25 (2007) 341–355

CARDIOLOGY
CLINICS

Three-Dimensional Echocardiography for Studies of the Fetal Heart: Present Status and Future Perspectives

Boris Tutschek, MD, PhD[a,b], David J. Sahn, MD[b,*]

[a]*Prenatal Medicine Munich, Heinrich Heine University, Lachnerstr 6, 80639 München, Düsseldorf, Germany*
[b]*Oregon Health & Science University, Pediatric Cardiology Department, Mailcode L608, Portland, OR 97239, USA*

Structural congenital heart disease (CHD) occurs in about 1% of live births and contributes a large proportion of the perinatal mortality [1–3]. Although it is also among the most frequently missed anomalies in prenatal ultrasound studies, prenatal detection can improve perinatal outcome significantly at least in certain types of CHD [4–7]. Prenatal detection rates depend on different factors like operator training and experience and vary widely [8–10]. Screening for and diagnosis of fetal heart disease are two distinct aspects of prenatal ultrasound, with differences in indications, levels of operator training and experience required, and the complexity of the technology used [11]. Teaching the correct technique for prenatal screening, for example, to include the outflow tracts in addition to the four-chamber view, is the main aspect of all attempts to improve prenatal screening for CHD [12]. Regarding technology, three-dimensional echocardiography has been shown to improve detection rates of cardiac malformations in adults and children [13], and it also promises to improve the prenatal diagnosis of CHD.

This article reviews the current clinical applications of three-dimensional echocardiography in fetal echocardiography. After a brief introduction and historical overview focuses on the application of fetal cardiac 3D imaging from automatically reconstructed mechanical sweeps, providing exemplary references of an already large and rapidly growing body of literature. Finally, the emerging field of fetal cardiac volume and mass quantification and real-time 3D ultrasound systems using 2D matrix arrays is described briefly.

* Corresponding author.
E-mail address: sahnd@ohsu.edu (D.J. Sahn).

Two- and three-dimensional fetal echocardiography

Fetal echocardiography was introduced more than 25 years ago [14,15], and today is an established tool in prenatal diagnosis. Guidelines for 2D fetal echocardiography have been established [16,17]. Most routine studies aiming at the detection of structural heart disease are done at around 20 weeks of gestation, but attempts at even earlier gestational ages such as at 11 to 14 weeks also have been made and evaluated [12,18–22].

Over the last decade, prenatal 3D ultrasound has been used increasingly, both for general imaging and with regard to the fetal heart [23–26]. In addition to the general technical challenges of 3D ultrasound imaging of the human heart, in the human fetus, there are several additional specific obstacles.

At the time of the typical screening examination of the developing fetus in midgestation (at about 20 weeks' gestation), the fetal heart is about the size of a cherry, and the fetal heart rate is high, between 110 and 160 beats per minute, requiring high temporal resolution. Additionally, the fetus moves and assumes random positions, often making it impossible to obtain standard views. Fetal echocardiography in general, and three-dimensional echocardiography in particular, also are limited by the physical properties of the intervening tissue (eg, maternal abdominal wall, placenta,

0733-8651/07/$ - see front matter
doi:10.1016/j.ccl.2007.05.006

or amniotic fluid or lack thereof). Finally, an ECG cannot be recorded routinely (eg, for gating of reconstruction algorithms).

Conventional prenatal ultrasound screening for CHD can be time-consuming and involves a very operator-dependent acquisition and mental reconstruction of a sequence of individual cross-sectional images. Ideally, the instantaneous acquisition of a sequence of full fetal cardiac volumes (ie, 3D for at least one complete cardiac cycle) with the ability to review all possible sections from these volumes at any time during the cardiac cycle might facilitate fetal cardiac screening. Different technical approaches for fetal three- and fourth-dimensional screening have been used.

Reconstructed fetal 3D echocardiography

Reconstructed 3D echocardiography (as opposed to real-time 3D fetal echocardiography) currently is the dominant clinical technology. It makes use of computational power of the diagnostic ultrasound system, which stores large amounts of data, integrates cross-sectional information, and displays the volume data in various views or aspects, either as static or moving displays. Typically, a sequence of sonographic data from a series of cross-sectional images is obtained over time and stored in the computer memory while the sonographer or an automated probe sweeps the ultrasound plane across the fetal heart. Then, off-line reconstruction yields either one cardiac volume acquired over a short period of time (less than 1 second) randomly with respect to cardiac cycle, or one virtual cardiac cycle comprising data from multiple heart beats that have been arranged using some form of spatial and temporal correlation [27].

For reconstruction of data obtained over periods longer than a fraction of a heart cycle duration, a form of assignment of temporal order (so-called gating) has to be applied to arrange the cross-sectional images according to the timing of their acquisition [28]. Another distinction in data recording of reconstructed 3D volumes uses the different technologies that have been employed with regard to acquisition of the sweep, either manual or automatic [13,29,30]. Manual sweeps and ungated 3D acquisition of B-mode sequences and using Power Doppler also have been used to study the normal and abnormal fetal heart and vasculature [31,32].

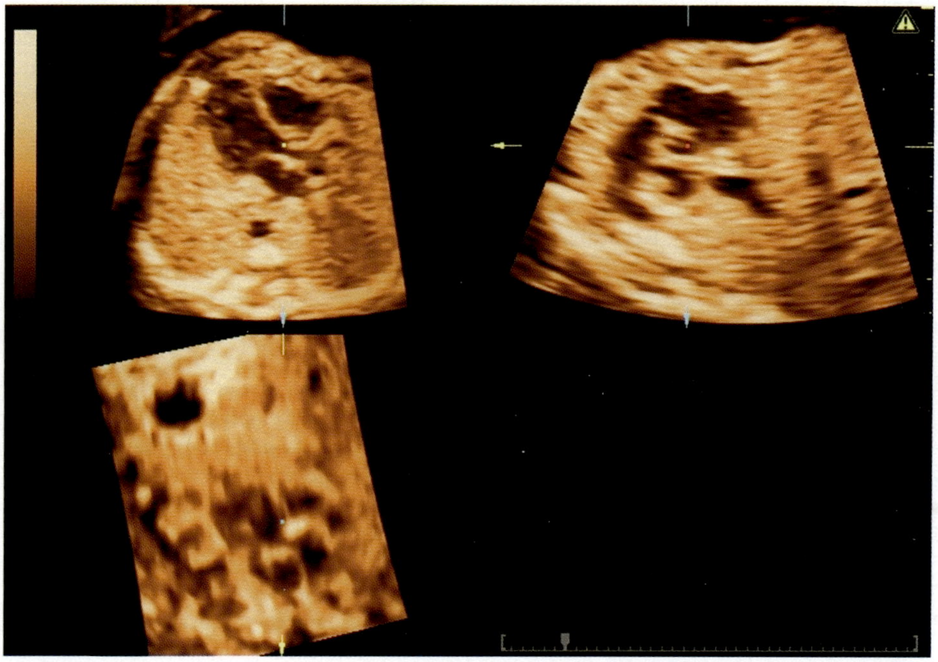

Fig. 1. Multiplanar imaging of a volume containing three orthogonal cross sections of a normal fetal heart (21 weeks' gestation) with the aortic valve in the center of all three planes. Top left: five-chamber view with the aorta arising from the left ventricle. Top right: adjacent aortic and pulmonary artery origin. Bottom left: third orthogonal plane.

Nelson and colleagues [13] were the first to suggest using tissue excursion concurrent with the cardiac contraction or relaxation to extract the temporal information regarding the cardiac cycle. This was used to compute the correct order in which cross-sectional images had to be rearranged to compensate for heart movements during the acquisition time of the volume. 2Another similar technique had been proposed using M-mode [33] and more recently using tissue Doppler data for fetal cardiac gating [34].

There were also successful studies using free-hand acquisition of volumetric data using power Doppler for vascular studies [31,32] or using an external position sensor attached to a conventional high-resolution 2D ultrasound system plus Doppler gating from the umbilical artery sampled immediately before free-hand sweep volume acquisition [35,36] or from concurrent Doppler recording of cardiac motion filtered for gating of a free-hand sweep over the fetal heart [37].

Spatial–temporal image correlation

The technique of computing cardiac gating from tissue excursion first was introduced into a commercially available ultrasound system by Kretz Ultrasound (now GE Kretz Medical Systems, Zipf, Austria) and was termed spatial-temporal image correlation or STIC. STIC now is incorporated in ultrasound systems also from other companies (Philips, Bothell, Washington; Medison, Seoul, Korea).

The most widely used approach is the STIC technique, because it has been integrated successfully in systems ready for clinical use. After its initial description [38–40], STIC has become a most valuable diagnostic tool for fetal echocardiography. Multiplanar imaging, reconstruction of 3D views (so-called rendering), the combination with color Doppler [41] and tomographic and invert mode [42–44], and the ability to quantify fetal

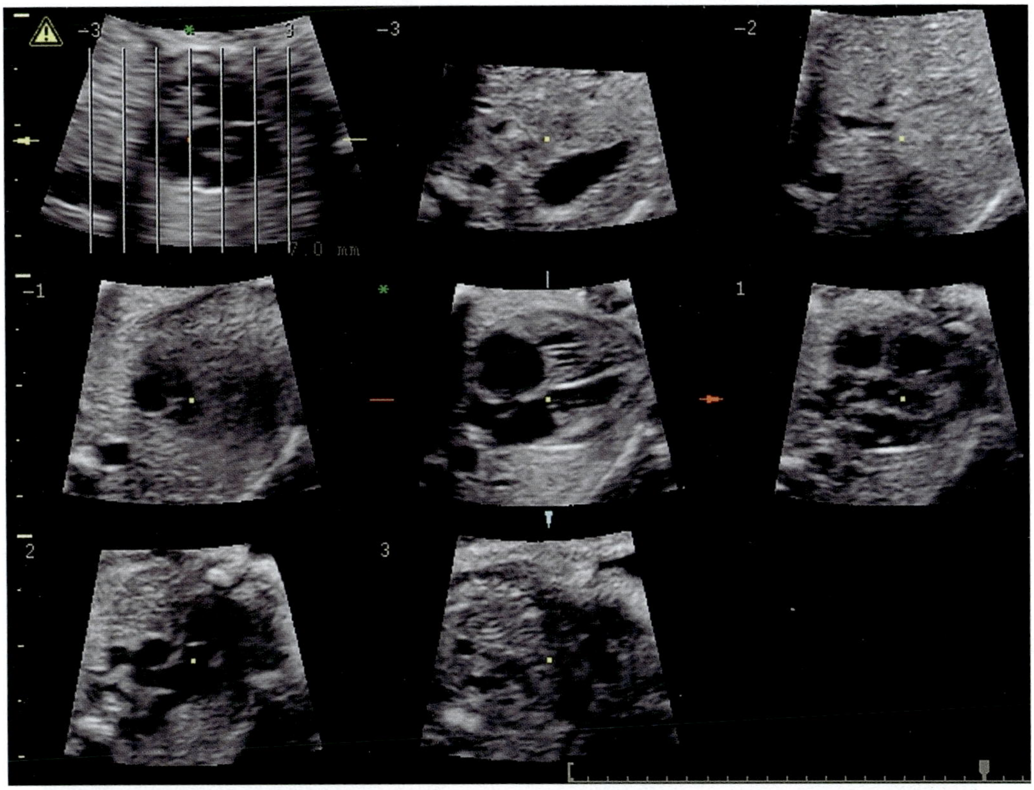

Fig. 2. Tomographic imaging of a volume containing parallel cross sections of the upper fetal abdomen (images 2 and 3 with the fetal stomach) and the thorax (image 1 with aorta and inferior vena cava; *indicating the level of the four-chamber view; images 1 and 2 with longitudinal sections of the ascending aorta and branching pulmonary artery, respectively, and image 3 with the upper mediastinum). The top left image shows a sagittal section orthogonal to the other views, indicating the spatial relationships of the horizontal sections (see also "Video TI abd thor.avi").

cardiac volumes [45–47] have provided exciting new insights into the fetal heart.

Display modalities

3D volumes or volumes sequences of the fetal heart can be displayed in different ways. A cross-sectional plane (or several planes orthogonal to each other) can be placed at any angle through the volume, enabling the examiner to interactively scroll through a volume either in the plane of acquisition (highest spatial resolution) or any other plane that is reconstructed (or calculated)

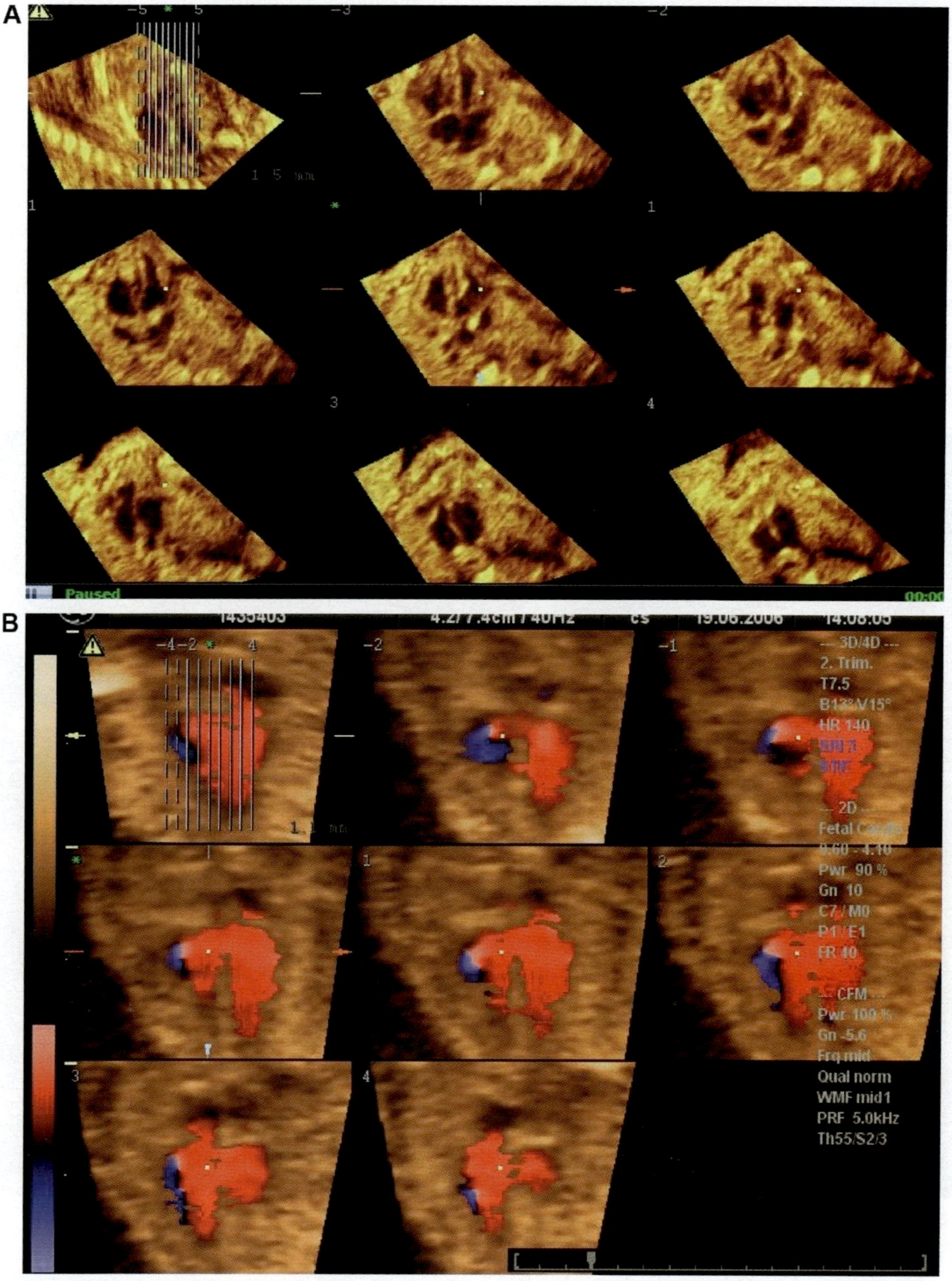

Fig. 3. Tomographic imaging through parallel planes neighboring the four-chamber view of (*A*) a normal fetal heart and (*B*) biventricular inflow with color Doppler.

from the volume. Multiplanar imaging typically describes a display with three orthogonal planes that can be rotated freely in the volume data set (Fig. 1). If a volume sequence has been generated encompassing a whole cardiac cycle, every structure can be inspected at different time points during the cardiac cycle.

Obtaining neighboring cross-sectional planes from a volume scan is particularly useful for the examining the great arteries, one of the key elements to be included in the fetal cardiac screening examination beyond the four-chamber view. In principle, the outflow tracts can be visualized using 2D echocardiography only by moving the transducer beam cephalad to obtain cross sections and by rotation to obtain views along the entire vessel. This may be difficult in many instances, however, because of fetal position, fetal movements, or lack of experience in obtaining these sections [48]. In 3D echocardiography, generating a stored volume (sequence) that can be manipulated off-line, these limitations can be eliminated or at least ameliorated. Because of the fixed relative position of the normal structures toward each other, it should be possible to navigate and display the advanced views like the outflow once the standard four-chamber view has been identified, provided the volume scanned covers all structures of the heart and its vessels, and there is no extensive shadowing from adjacent bones (ribs, spine, or a fetal extremity between the transducer and the heart). Failure to be able to do so may even indicate structural anomalies. In most clinical situations, the acquisition of a fetal cardiac volume will be done from the four-chamber view, and cross or longitudinal sections of these vessels can be extracted from the volume following a simple algorithm (eg, the spin technique) [48].

Traditionally, 2D echocardiography uses imaging planes based on standard sections aligned with one of the ventricular axes. Other digital imaging modalities like MRI and CT typically display and describe the structures in relation to standard anatomical orientations (sagittal, coronal, transverse) as stacks of parallel planes or cross sections. 3D echocardiography can combine the accepted 2D imaging and orientation standards to provide a combination of both approaches. The term tomographic imaging refers to the simultaneous display of several cross-sectional planes through the same volume similar to a typical CT or MRI image sequence (Fig. 2 and accompanying "Video TI abd thor.avi").

Available at: "Video TI abd thor.avi"

The tomographic representation of parallel sections through a volume obtained by ultrasound

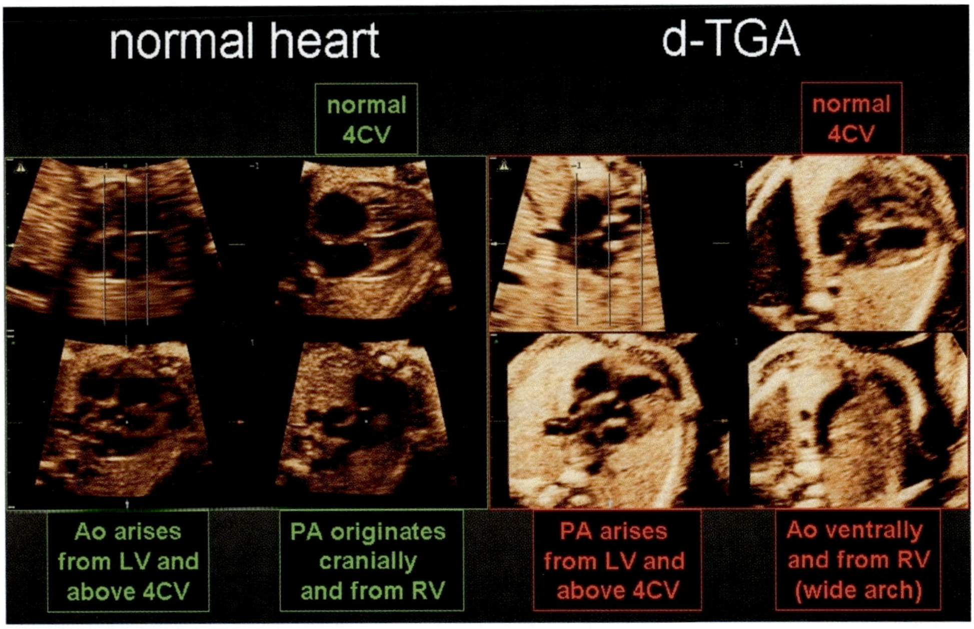

Fig. 4. Tomographic imaging derived from spatial-temporal image correlation sequences showing a normal fetal heart (*left*) and a fetal heart with d-transposition of the great arteries displayed using the same settings for parallel sections at three different levels at and above the four-chamber view (see also "Video TI_nl_TGA.avi").

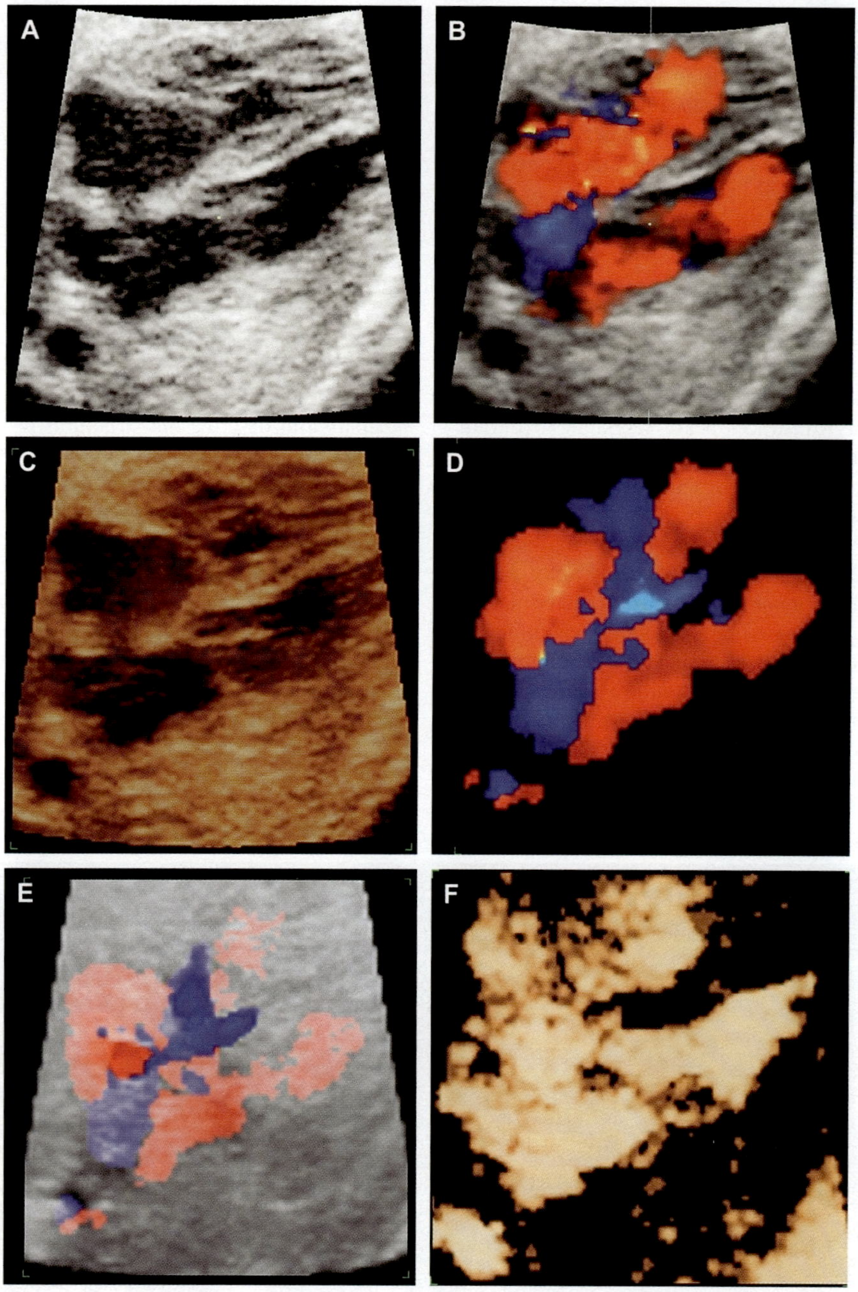

Fig. 5. Examples of cross-sectional and rendered views of a volume acquired from an initial four-chamber view (normal fetal heart at 29 weeks' gestation). All images were generated from the same diastolic frame seen from caudally. *Cross-sectional images:* (*A*) B-mode. (*B*) Color duplex with biventricular inflow (in red). *Rendered images:* (*C*) Surface-rendered view, cropped to display only the cranial half of the heart. (*D*) Color-only rendering of the whole volume with display of hepatic veins and inferior vena cava (*blue*) and ventricular inflow. (*E*) Glass-body region of interest as in (*D*), but with transparent tissue rendering over color Doppler. (*F*) inversion mode (thin volume slice cropped to display only the four-chamber plane).

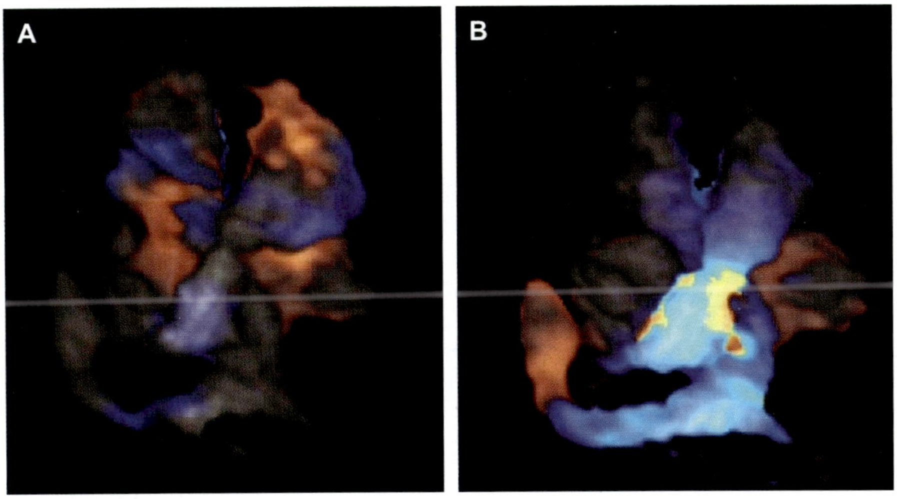

Fig. 6. Color invert mode of a normal fetal heart at 29 weeks' gestation. Full cardiac volume rendering (seen from cranially) in (*A*) diastole and (*B*) systole.

has been given different commercial names ("Multislice," "Tomographic ultrasound imaging/TUI," "iSlice"). Tomographic imaging of three-dimensional volumes of the fetal heart (Fig. 3) can be used to elegantly display different normal or structurally abnormal planes from one insonation angle (Fig. 4 and video "TI_nl_TGA.avi").

Available at: "TI_nl_TGA.avi"

Taking into consideration the anatomy of organ growth, tomographic imaging has been both tailored to the growing heart and applied to CHD successfully [49]. Algorithms (both semiautomatic and automatic) have been described to successfully display the relevant cardiac structures in one or several tomographic and/or multiplanar panels comprising sections generated semiautomatically [50–52]. In the newest release of the Voluson ultrasound system (GE Kretz), such an automated approach (VCAD) is now available in a commercial system [53].

The different rendering (or rendered) modes are an alternative to the simple or complex cross-sectional display modes. Rendering describes the display of either external or internal surfaces of organs with data derived from multiple 2D sections. Using certain values for display thresholds (suppression of weaker signals mainly between the transducer and the object to be displayed), transparency (reduction of tissue signals, giving them a transparent appearance and revealing underlying objects) and shading produce photo-realistic 3D appearances on a two-dimensional display like a computer monitor or in a printed image. Surface rendering originally was developed to display the outer surfaces of

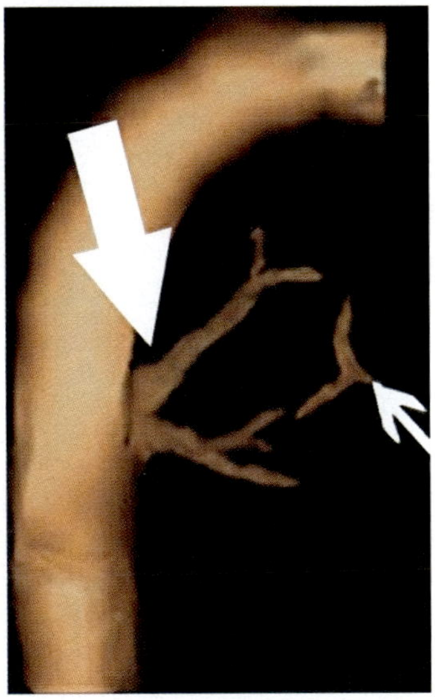

Fig. 7. B-flow 3D rendering from a spatial temporal image correlation volume of a major aortopulmonary collateral artery (*small arrow*) (*large arrow:* pulmonary arteries). (*From* Volpe P, Campobasso G, Stanziano A, et al. Novel application of 4D sonography with B-flow imaging and spatio-temporal image correlation (STIC) in the assessment of the anatomy of pulmonary arteries in fetuses with pulmonary atresia and ventricular septal defect. Ultrasound Obstet Gynecol 2006;28:40–6; with permission.)

solid objects like the fetal face in three dimensions [54]. In a surface rendering mode of the fetal heart, however, cropping into the heart will display its internal surfaces [55,56], for example cutting the heart in halves at the level of the four-chamber view or from an en face view of the valve plane, generating a more plastic impression than the thin slice usually displayed in a conventional B-mode image (Fig. 5). A modification of the surface-rendering mode, the so-called inversion mode (or invert mode), displays only fluid-filled spaces (see Fig. 5F), because it shows negative images of surface rendering. The inversion mode has been shown to produce digital casts of the fetal heart and vasculature both in normal and structurally abnormal cases [43,57–59].

STIC also can be used to include color and power Doppler information, generating detailed structural and functional cardiac information and even angiography-like images including directional information [26,41,60,61]. Power Doppler, with its high sensitivity even for low flow velocities, can display not only ventricular and great artery anatomy, but also extracardiac structures like pulmonary vasculature, teratoma, and chorioangioma [62,63]. The most recent addition to the color Doppler rendering modes from STIC volumes is Color Invert mode (currently available on the HD11 ultrasound system, Philips Medical Systems), combining the anatomic detail of fluid-filled structures in invert mode with the dynamic information of color Doppler (Fig. 6).

Another technically different approach for flow detection, B-flow, extracts Doppler-independent flow information generated from a particular digitally processed B-mode that retains the conventional gray-scale information and spatial resolution (B-flow, GE Medical Systems). B-flow, combined with STIC and these rendering techniques, provides even more detailed visualization of small normal and aberrant vessels [42,64] (Fig. 7).

Another promising new application of volumetric fetal echocardiography (from STIC and from real-time 3D echocardiography) is the functional and quantitative analysis of the dynamics of cardiac ventricular volumes and of chambers

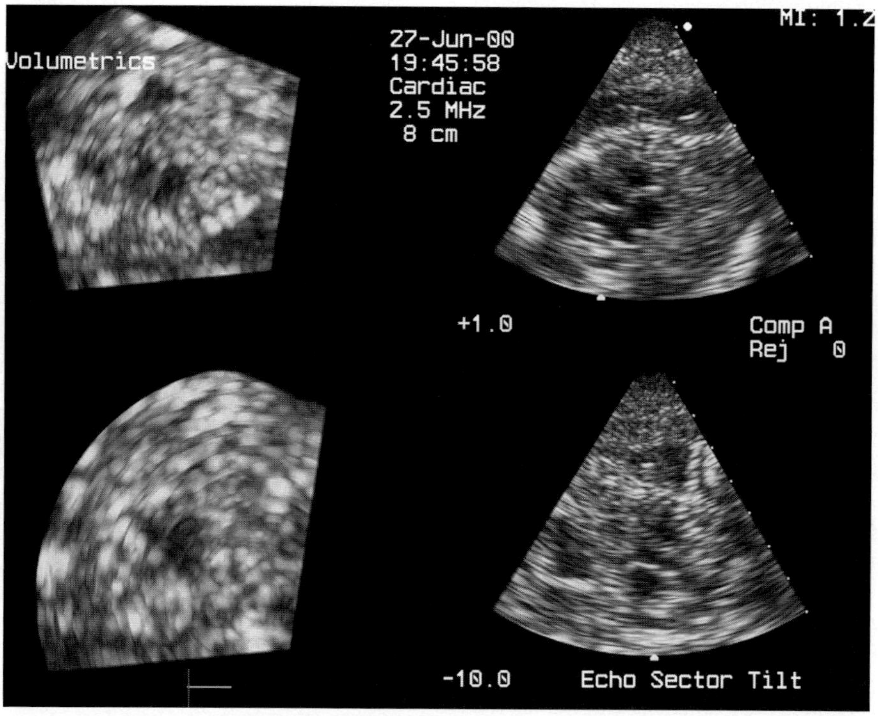

Fig. 8. Real-time fetal 3D echocardiography using the first-generation 2D matrix array (Volumetrics, 2.5 MHz matrix transducer). Fetal echocardiography at 25 weeks' gestation shows the acquisition orientation (four-chamber view on the top right, a section perpendicular to it (through the aortic outflow) in the lower right and two perpendicular images from the elevation plane (cross sections through the two ventricles in short axis) (see also "4CH_25_vlm.avi" and the article by Tutschek et al (2000) [71]).

masses. It can be done using different technical approaches from B-mode or inversion mode and has been shown to be feasible and sufficiently accurate [26,45–47,65].

Finally, volumetric ultrasound, because of its digital nature and off-line analysis feature, naturally lends itself to the application of telemedicine, enabling the separate the acquisition of data (cardiac and other volumes or volume sequences) from manipulation, extraction of relevant views, and interpretation [66–68].

Real-time fetal echocardiography using 2D matrix array transducers

Real-time 3D echocardiography acquires volume sequences of sonographic data instantaneously by using transducers with a 2D array. These 2D arrays insonate volume blocks rather than tissue cross sections. Theoretically, real-time 3D ultrasound with 2D array transducers is the direct and easiest way of acquiring 3D data of the fetal heart, because it obviates the need for fetal gating, a potential source of artifacts [69].

Its wide-spread application, however, so far has been limited by the lower temporal and/or spatial resolution. For high-resolution fetal echocardiography, gated reconstruction to date provides superior spatial and temporal resolutions approaching 2D B-mode quality. Despite advances like STIC, however, the reconstruction required precludes the ease of real-time assessment and makes this method prone to motion

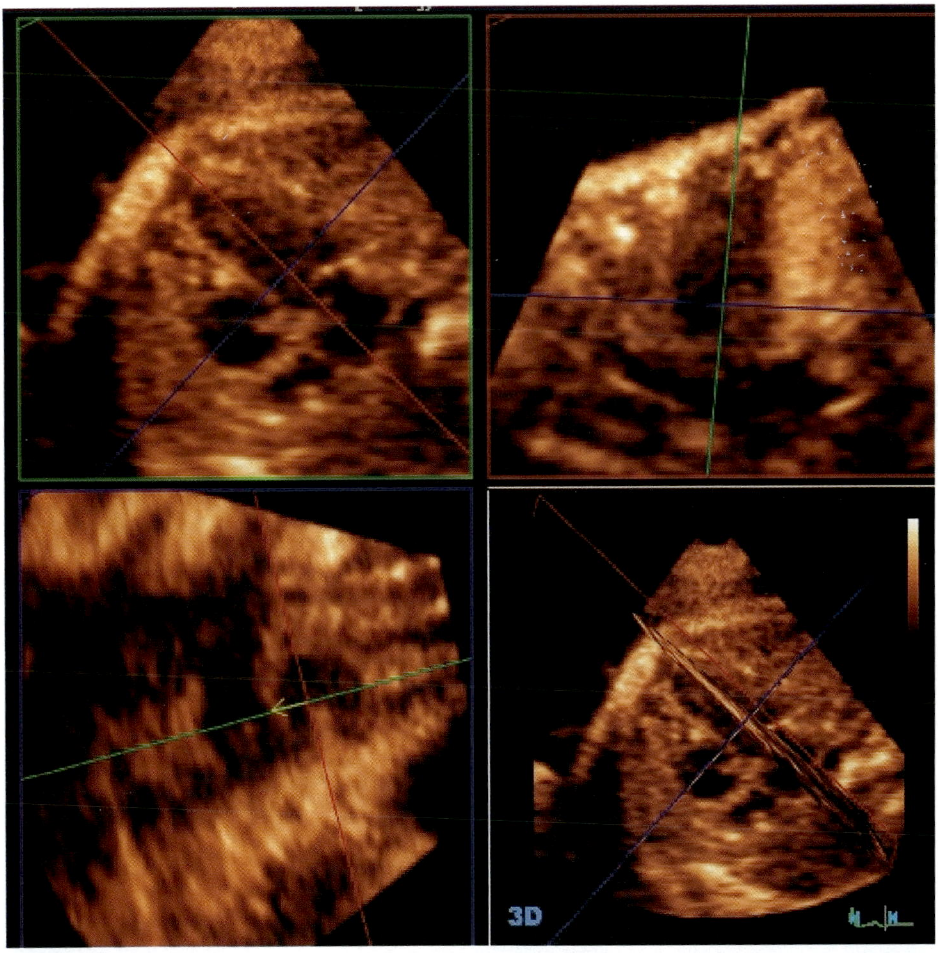

Fig. 9. Real-time fetal 3D echocardiography using a fully electronically steerable two-dimensional matrix array transducer (x3-1, iE33, Philips Medical Systems, Bothell Washington). (*A–C*) Cross-sectional images. (*D*) 3D niche-view of a normal 29-week-old human fetus.

artifacts. In contrast, real-time 3D echocardiography acquires a sequence of pyramidal volumes virtually instantaneously using a 2D matrix phased-array transducer. Although theoretically superior, with regard to fetal echocardiography the main limitation so far has been image resolution. The first prototypes of matrix array transducers had only 256 active elements and limited image quality. It still could be applied to fetal studies acquiring 20 volumes per second in an initial study [70]. Spatial resolution, however, is limited and inferior to comparable 2D systems [71] (Fig. 8 and video "4CH_25_vlm.avi").

Available at: "4CH_25_vlm.avi"

The second generation of matrix array transducers is based on 2D arrays with about 3000 active ultrasound elements. This ultrasound system provides rendered images of the scanning sector in real time with a temporal resolution of 40 to 50 ms, equivalent to a volume rate of 20 to 25 images per second. Sklansky and colleagues [70] were the first to report a initial feasibility fetal echocardiography study. Maulik and colleagues [72] used the same 4 MHz 2D array transducer to study fetal hearts with CHD, suggesting that this technology could be a significant tool for prenatal diagnosis and assessment of congenital heart disease in the human fetus. More recently using a sweep modification. especially for larger fetal hearts that cannot be acquired instantaneously using this transducer, an acceptable diagnostic rate could be shown [73]. Fig. 9 shows an example of a normal fetal heart visualized in real time three dimensionally using such a system. The utility of this transducer designed for adult studies for detailed fetal echocardiography remains limited, however, by its resolution, which is still inferior to the typical high-resolution 2D systems for fetal studies currently in use, and by its relative dependency on cardiac gating. Acar and colleagues [74] performed real-time imaging using such a system. They applied two modalities, the live 3D and the biplane scanning modes, in normal and CHD fetal hearts and could complete successfully the examinations in the majority of fetuses. Also in their study, the main limitations were comparatively low resolution and 3D artifacts.

There are technical advantages to real-time 3D echocardiography and the subsequent data processing, however, that already can be exploited

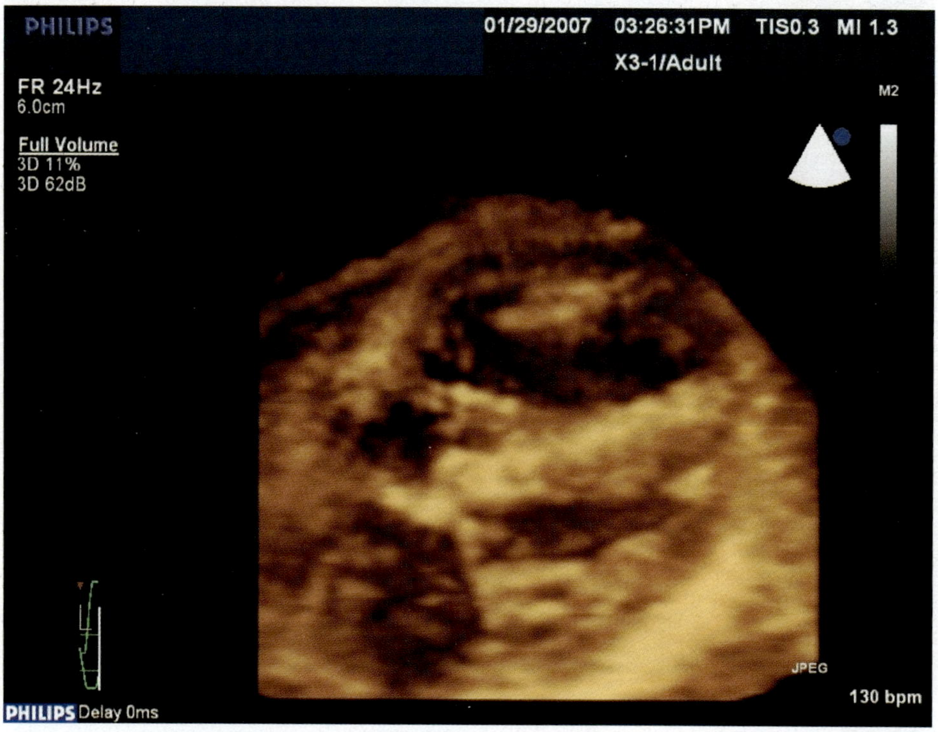

Fig. 10. Fetal echocardiography with a higher resolution program for fetal volumes running on the Philips IU22.

using such a system. Semiautomatic volume quantification of cardiac cavities has been reported [33,75]. Using a 3 MHz 2D matrix array transducer for real-time 3D fetal echocardiography (Figs. 10 and 11) followed by quantitative analysis of the volumetric loops showed that semiautomatic endocardial border detection can generate volume–time curves of fetal ventricular function and that ventricular volumes and ejection fractions can be calculated in human fetuses between 20 weeks and term (Fig. 12) [65]. These data compare favorably with volumetric measurements derived from STIC measurements [65] using a validated technique [45,46].

Real-time 3D echocardiography theoretically obviates the need for cardiac gating (no artifacts from fetal or maternal body movements). With improving transducer technology (mainly higher transducer frequencies), it can be speculated that real-time three-dimensional echocardiography using 2D matrix array transducers will become the dominant technology. As a first step in this direction, a 7 MHz 2D matrix array transducer was introduced recently for a commercially available ultrasound system (iU22/iE33, Philips, Bothell, Washington). Initial studies show an encouraging resolution for fetal studies, but its usefulness for fetal echocardiography remains to be determined.

Summary

The present status of instrumentation for obtaining high-resolution three-dimensional images of the fetal heart is in transition. Expected advances should include large aperture matrix arrays more suitable for obstetric scanning—and with frequency ranges from 4-8 MHZ, flexible volume adjustment acquisition to target the fetal heart area with highest line density and frame rate available, and ultrasonic navigator sampling to clock motion of a region within the fetal heart as a trigger for obtaining full volume coverage when truly live scanning coverage is not capable of encompassing the entire cardiac volume. Continuing advances will change fetal imaging and

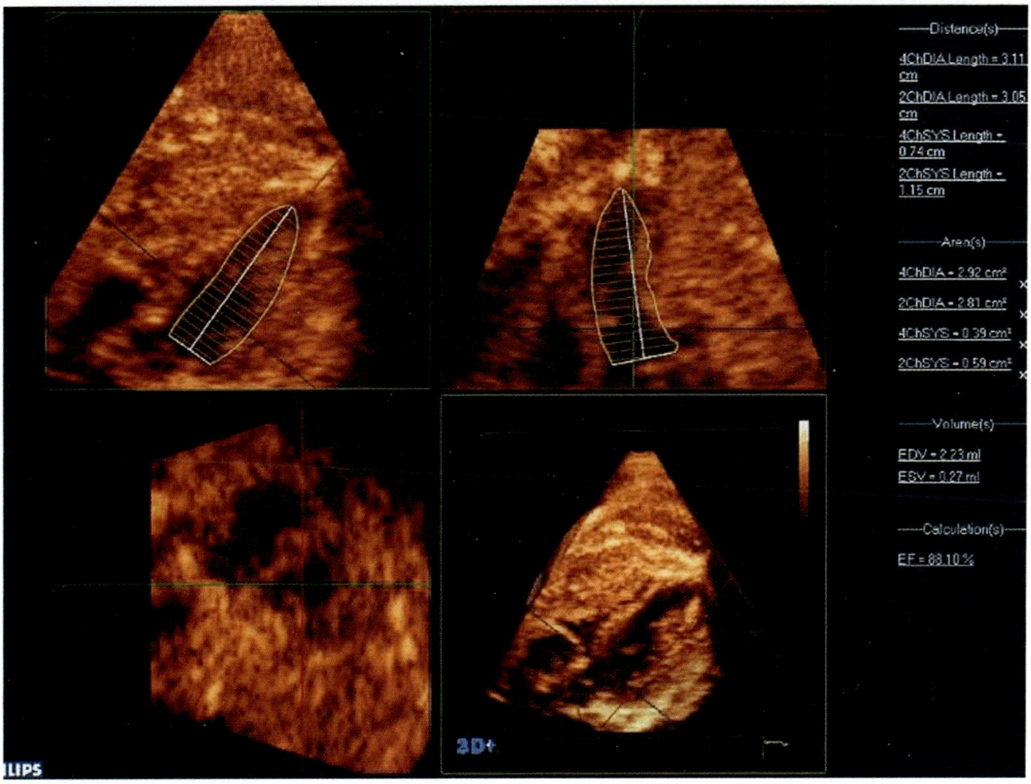

Fig. 11. Fetal left ventricular volume calculation: volumes measured with QLab version 5, no longer requires an apex-up orientation.

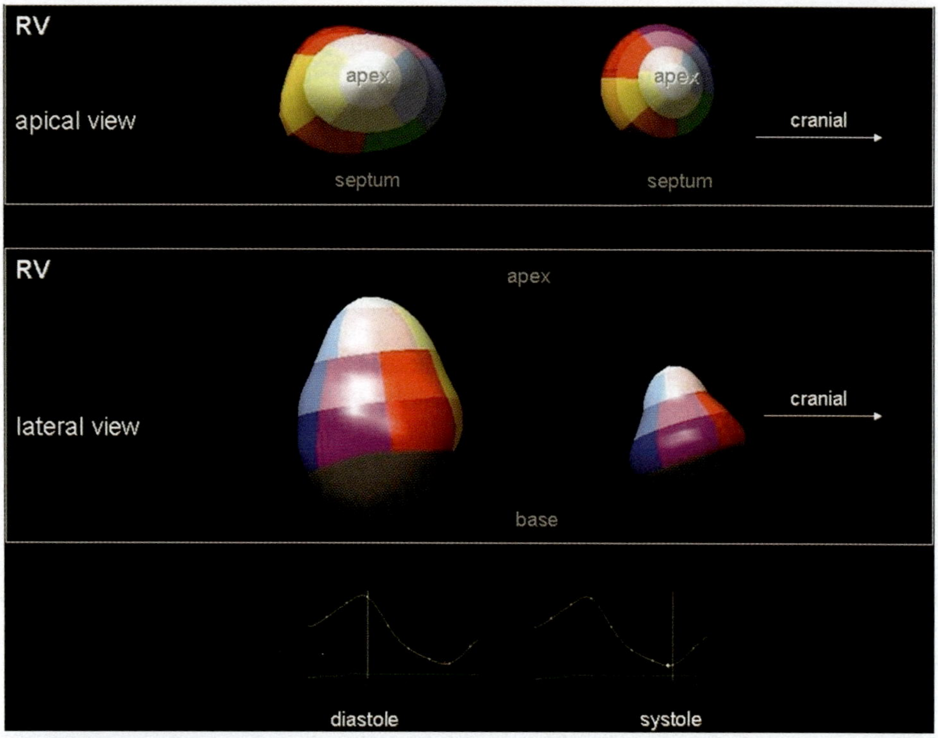

Fig. 12. Virtual endocardial casts of the normal human right cardiac ventricle in a 28-week fetus in diastole and systole and endocardial volume curves, generated using semiautomatic volume calculation software from a volume loop acquired using real-time 3D echocardiography (QLab 3DQAdvanced and x3-1/iE33; Philips Medical Systems).

provide new methods for diagnosing heart disease prenatally and understanding the in-utero natural history of congenital heart diseases by providing improved methods for visualization, and more importantly, for quantitatively evaluating fetal cardiac chamber volumes. New technologies will require new protocols for evaluation and new skills that will need to be learned by sonographers and by obstetricians/perinatologists and pediatric cardiologists.

References

[1] Ferencz C, Rubin JD, McCarter RJ, et al. Congenital heart disease: prevalence at live birth. The Baltimore–Washington infant study. Am J Epidemiol 1985;121:31–6.

[2] Meberg A, Otterstad JE, Froland G, et al. Outcome of congenital heart defects—a population-based study. Acta Paediatr 2000;89:1344–51.

[3] Rosano A, Botto LD, Botting B, et al. Infant mortality and congenital anomalies from 1950 to 1994: an international perspective. J Epidemiol Community Health 2000;54:660–6.

[4] Crane JP, LeFevre ML, Winborn RC, et al. A randomized trial of prenatal ultrasonographic screening: impact on the detection, management, and outcome of anomalous fetuses. The RADIUS study group. Am J Obstet Gynecol 1994;171:392–9.

[5] Bonnet D, Coltri A, Butera G, et al. Detection of transposition of the great arteries in fetuses reduces neonatal morbidity and mortality. Circulation 1999;99:916–8.

[6] Tworetzky W, McElhinney DB, Reddy VM, et al. Improved surgical outcome after fetal diagnosis of hypoplastic left heart syndrome. Circulation 2001;103:1269–73.

[7] Fuchs IB, Muller H, Abdul-Khaliq H, et al. Immediate and long-term outcomes in children with prenatal diagnosis of selected isolated congenital heart defects. Ultrasound Obstet Gynecol 2007;29:38–43.

[8] Tegnander E, Eik-Nes SH. The examiner's ultrasound experience has a significant impact on the detection rate of congenital heart defects at the

second-trimester fetal examination. Ultrasound Obstet Gynecol 2006;28:8–14.
[9] Tegnander E, Williams W, Johansen OJ, et al. Prenatal detection of heart defects in a nonselected population of 30 149 fetuses—detection rates and outcome. Ultrasound Obstet Gynecol 2006;27:252–65.
[10] Simpson LL. Screening for congenital heart disease. Obstet Gynecol Clin North Am 2004;31:51–9.
[11] Ville Y. Fetal imaging: a brief history of the future. Ultrasound Obstet Gynecol 2007;29:1–5.
[12] Allan L. Screening the fetal heart. Ultrasound Obstet Gynecol 2006;28:5–7.
[13] Nelson TR, Pretorius DH, Sklansky M, et al. Three-dimensional echocardiographic evaluation of fetal heart anatomy and function: acquisition, analysis, and display. J Ultrasound Med 1996;15:1–9.
[14] Lange LW, Sahn DJ, Allen HD, et al. Qualitative real-time cross-sectional echocardiographic imaging of the human fetus during the second half of pregnancy. Circulation 1980;62:799–806.
[15] Allan LD, Tynan MJ, Campbell S, et al. Echocardiographic and anatomical correlates in the fetus. Br Heart J 1980;44:444–51.
[16] Lee W. Performance of the basic fetal cardiac ultrasound examination. J Ultrasound Med 1998;17: 601–7.
[17] International Society of Ultrasound in Obstetrics & Gynecology. Cardiac screening examination of the fetus: guidelines for performing the basic and extended basic cardiac scan. Ultrasound Obstet Gynecol 2006;27:107–13.
[18] Carvalho J, Moscoso G, Ville Y. First-trimester transabdominal fetal echocardiography. Lancet 1998;351:1023–7.
[19] Hyett JA, Perdu M, Sharland GK, et al. Using fetal nuchal translucency to screen for major congenital cardiac defects at 10-14 weeks of gestation: population-based cohort study. Br Med J 1999;318:81–5.
[20] Huggon IC, Ghi T, Cook AC, et al. Fetal cardiac abnormalities identified prior to 14 weeks' gestation. Ultrasound Obstet Gynecol 2002;20:22–9.
[21] Makrydimas G, Sotiriadis A, Huggon I, et al. Nuchal translucency and fetal cardiac defects: a pooled analysis of major fetal echocardiography centers. Am J Obstet Gynecol 2005;192:89–95.
[22] Rasiah SV, Publicover M, Ewer AK, et al. A systematic review of the accuracy of first-trimester ultrasound examination for detecting major congenital heart disease. Ultrasound Obstet Gynecol 2006; 28:110–6.
[23] Benacerraf BR, Benson CB, Abuhamad AZ, et al. Three- and 4-dimensional ultrasound in obstetrics and gynecology: proceedings of the American Institute of Ultrasound in Medicine consensus conference. J Ultrasound Med 2005;24:1587–97.
[24] Dyson RL, Pretorius DH, Budorick NE, et al. Three-dimensional ultrasound in the evaluation of fetal anomalies. Ultrasound Obstet Gynecol 2000; 16:321–8.
[25] Goncalves LF, Lee W, Espinoza J, et al. Three- and 4-dimensional ultrasound in obstetric practice: does it help? J Ultrasound Med 2005;24:1599–624.
[26] Yagel S, Cohen SM, Shapiro I, et al. 3D and 4D ultrasound in fetal cardiac scanning: a new look at the fetal heart. Ultrasound Obstet Gynecol 2007; 29:81–95.
[27] Deng J. Terminology of three-dimensional and four-dimensional ultrasound imaging of the fetal heart and other moving body parts. Ultrasound Obstet Gynecol 2003;22:336–44.
[28] Sklansky MS, Nelson TR, Pretorius DH. Three-dimensional fetal echocardiography: gated versus nongated techniques. J Ultrasound Med 1998;17: 451–7.
[29] Meyer-Wittkopf M, Cook A, McLennan A, et al. Evaluation of three-dimensional ultrasonography and magnetic resonance imaging in assessment of congenital heart anomalies in fetal cardiac specimens. Ultrasound Obstet Gynecol 1996;8: 303–8.
[30] Zosmer N, Jurkovic D, Jauniaux E, et al. Selection and identification of standard cardiac views from three-dimensional volume scans of the fetal thorax. J Ultrasound Med 1996;15:25–32.
[31] Chaoui R, Kalache KD, Hartung J. Application of three-dimensional power Doppler ultrasound in prenatal diagnosis. Ultrasound Obstet Gynecol 2001;17:22–9.
[32] Chaoui R, Schneider MB, Kalache KD. Right aortic arch with vascular ring and aberrant left subclavian artery: prenatal diagnosis assisted by three-dimensional power Doppler ultrasound. Ultrasound Obstet Gynecol 2003;22:661–3.
[33] Deng J, Gardener JE, Rodeck CH, et al. Fetal echocardiography in three and four dimensions. Ultrasound Med Biol 1996;22:979–86.
[34] Brekke S, Tegnander E, Torp HG, et al. Tissue Doppler gated (TDOG) dynamic three-dimensional ultrasound imaging of the fetal heart. Ultrasound Obstet Gynecol 2004;24:192–8.
[35] Meyer-Wittkopf M, Rappe N, Sierra F, et al. Three-dimensional (3-D) ultrasonography for obtaining the four- and five-chamber view: comparison with cross-sectional (2-D) fetal sonographic screening. Ultrasound Obstet Gynecol 2000;15:397–402.
[36] Meyer-Wittkopf M, Cooper S, Vaughan J, et al. Three-dimensional (3D) echocardiographic analysis of congenital heart disease in the fetus: comparison with cross-sectional (2D) fetal echocardiography. Ultrasound Obstet Gynecol 2001;17:485–92.
[37] Herberg U, Goldberg H, Breuer J. Three- and four-dimensional freehand fetal echocardiography: a feasibility study using a hand-held Doppler probe for cardiac gating. Ultrasound Obstet Gynecol 2005;25:362–71.

[38] DeVore GR, Falkensammer P, Sklansky MS, et al. Spatiotemporal image correlation (STIC): new technology for evaluation of the fetal heart. Ultrasound Obstet Gynecol 2003;22:380–7.

[39] Vinals F, Poblete P, Giuliano A. Spatiotemporal image correlation (STIC): a new tool for the prenatal screening of congenital heart defects. Ultrasound Obstet Gynecol 2003;22:388–94.

[40] Goncalves LF, Lee W, Chaiworapongsa T, et al. Four-dimensional ultrasonography of the fetal heart with spatiotemporal image correlation. Am J Obstet Gynecol 2003;189:1792–802.

[41] Chaoui R, Hoffmann J, Heling KS. Three-dimensional (3D) and 4D color Doppler fetal echocardiography using spatiotemporal image correlation (STIC). Ultrasound Obstet Gynecol 2004;23: 535–45.

[42] Goncalves LF, Espinoza J, Lee W, et al. A new approach to fetal echocardiography: digital casts of the fetal cardiac chambers and great vessels for detection of congenital heart disease. J Ultrasound Med 2005;24:415–24.

[43] Espinoza J, Goncalves LF, Lee W, et al. A novel method to improve prenatal diagnosis of abnormal systemic venous connections using three- and four-dimensional ultrasonography and inversion mode. Ultrasound Obstet Gynecol 2005;25:428–34.

[44] Goncalves LF, Lee W, Espinoza J, et al. Examination of the fetal heart by four-dimensional (4D) ultrasound with spatiotemporal image correlation (STIC). Ultrasound Obstet Gynecol 2006;27: 336–48.

[45] Bhat AH, Corbett V, Carpenter N, et al. Fetal ventricular mass determination on three-dimensional echocardiography: studies in normal fetuses and validation experiments. Circulation 2004;110: 1054–60.

[46] Bhat AH, Corbett VN, Liu R, et al. Validation of volume and mass assessments for human fetal heart imaging by 4-dimensional spatiotemporal image correlation echocardiography: in vitro balloon model experiments. J Ultrasound Med 2004;23: 1151–9.

[47] Messing B, Valsky DV, Cohen SM, et al. 3D inversion mode combined with STIC: a novel technique for fetal heart ventricle volumetry in congenital heart disease. Ultrasound Obstet Gynecol 2006; 28(Suppl):397.

[48] DeVore GR, Polanco B, Sklansky MS, et al. The spin technique: a new method for examination of the fetal outflow tracts using three-dimensional ultrasound. Ultrasound Obstet Gynecol 2004;24: 72–82.

[49] Paladini D, Vassallo M, Sglavo G, et al. The role of spatiotemporal image correlation (STIC) with tomographic ultrasound imaging (TUI) in the sequential analysis of fetal congenital heart disease. Ultrasound Obstet Gynecol 2006;27:555–61.

[50] Abuhamad A. Automated multiplanar imaging: a novel approach to ultrasonography. J Ultrasound Med 2004;23:573–6.

[51] Abuhamad AZ, Falkensammer P. Automated sonography: defining the spatial relationships of standard diagnostic fetal cardiac planes in the second trimester of pregnancy. Ultrasound Obstet Gynecol 2006;28:359–411.

[52] Espinoza J, Kusanovic JP, Goncalves LF, et al. A novel algorithm for comprehensive fetal echocardiography using 4-dimensional ultrasonography and tomographic imaging. J Ultrasound Med 2006;25: 947–56.

[53] Reichartseder F, Falkensammer P. VCAD—volume aided diagnosis. An automated approach to visualize standard views of the fetal heart. Zipf (Austria): GE Healthcare; 2006.

[54] Sklansky M. Advances in fetal cardiac imaging. Pediatr Cardiol 2004;25:307–21.

[55] Yagel S, Benachi A, Bonnet D, et al. Rendering in fetal cardiac scanning: the intracardiac septa and the coronal atrioventricular valve planes. Ultrasound Obstet Gynecol 2006;28:266–74.

[56] Vinals F, Pacheco V, Giuliano A. Fetal atrioventricular valve junction in normal fetuses and in fetuses with complete atrioventricular septal defect assessed by 4D volume rendering. Ultrasound Obstet Gynecol 2006;28:26–31.

[57] Ghi T, Cera E, Segata M, et al. Inversion mode spatiotemporal image correlation (STIC) echocardiography in three-dimensional rendering of fetal ventricular septal defects. Ultrasound Obstet Gynecol 2005;26:679–86.

[58] Lee W, Goncalves LF, Espinoza J, et al. Inversion mode: a new volume analysis tool for 3-dimensional ultrasonography. J Ultrasound Med 2005;24:201–7.

[59] Goncalves LF, Espinoza J, Lee W, et al. Three- and four-dimensional reconstruction of the aortic and ductal arches using inversion mode: a new rendering algorithm for visualization of fluid-filled anatomical structures. Ultrasound Obstet Gynecol 2004;24: 696–8.

[60] Goncalves LF, Romero R, Espinoza J, et al. Four-dimensional ultrasonography of the fetal heart using color Doppler spatiotemporal image correlation. J Ultrasound Med 2004;23:473–81.

[61] Yagel S, Valsky DV, Messing B. Detailed assessment of fetal ventricular septal defect with 4D color Doppler ultrasound using spatiotemporal image correlation technology. Ultrasound Obstet Gynecol 2005;25(1):97–8.

[62] Ruano R, Benachi A, Aubry MC, et al. Prenatal diagnosis of pulmonary sequestration using three-dimensional power Doppler ultrasound. Ultrasound Obstet Gynecol 2005;25:128–33.

[63] Sciaky-Tamir Y, Cohen SM, Hochner-Celnikier D, et al. Three-dimensional power Doppler (3DPD) ultrasound in the diagnosis and follow-up of fetal

vascular anomalies. Am J Obstet Gynecol 2006;194: 274–81.

[64] Volpe P, Campobasso G, Stanziano A, et al. Novel application of 4D sonography with B-flow imaging and spatiotemporal image correlation (STIC) in the assessment of the anatomy of pulmonary arteries in fetuses with pulmonary atresia and ventricular septal defect. Ultrasound Obstet Gynecol 2006;28: 40–6.

[65] Tutschek B, Hui L, Robertson PA, et al. Fetal cardiac ventricular volumes derived from 3D/4D echo: definitive data from two different types of 3D ultrasound systems. J Am Coll Cardiol 2007; 49(Suppl A):254A.

[66] Michailidis G, Simpson J, Karidas C, et al. Detailed three-dimensional fetal echocardiography facilitated by an internet link. Ultrasound Obstet Gynecol 2001;18:325–8.

[67] Vinals F, Mandujano L, Vargas G, et al. Prenatal diagnosis of congenital heart disease using four-dimensional spatiotemporal image correlation (STIC) telemedicine via an internet link: a pilot study. Ultrasound Obstet Gynecol 2005;25:25–31.

[68] Vinals F, Ascenzo R, Poblete P, et al. Simple approach to prenatal diagnosis of transposition of the great arteries. Ultrasound Obstet Gynecol 2006;28:22–5.

[69] Sklansky MS, DeVore GR, Wong PC. Real-time 3-dimensional fetal echocardiography with an instantaneous volume-rendered display: early description and pictorial essay. J Ultrasound Med 2004;23:283–9.

[70] Sklansky MS, Nelson T, Strachan M, et al. Real-time three-dimensional fetal echocardiography: initial feasibility study. J Ultrasound Med 1999;18: 745–52.

[71] Tutschek B, Buck T, Reihs T, et al. Real-time three-dimensional fetal echocardiography. Ultrasound Obstet Gynecol 2000;16:53–4.

[72] Maulik D, Nanda NC, Singh V, et al. Live three-dimensional echocardiography of the human fetus. Echocardiography 2003;20:715–21.

[73] Sklansky M, Miller D, Devore G, et al. Prenatal screening for congenital heart disease using real-time three-dimensional echocardiography and a novel sweep volume acquisition technique. Ultrasound Obstet Gynecol 2005;25:435–43.

[74] Acar P, Dulac Y, Taktak A, et al. Real-time three-dimensional fetal echocardiography using matrix probe. Prenat Diagn 2005;25:370–5.

[75] Deng J, Ruff CF, Linney AD, et al. Simultaneous use of two ultrasound scanners for motion-gated three-dimensional fetal echocardiography. Ultrasound Med Biol 2000;26:1021–32.

ELSEVIER
SAUNDERS

Cardiol Clin 25 (2007) 357–365

CARDIOLOGY
CLINICS

Three-Dimensional Echocardiography in Congenital Heart Disease

Gerald R. Marx, MD*, Xiaohong Su, MD

Department of Cardiology, Children's Hospital Boston, Farley-2, 300 Longwood Avenue, Boston, MA 02115, USA

Matrix array technology has brought 3D echocardiography into the clinical practice of cardiology [1–3]. Arguably, this advancement [4] is most notable in the field of pediatric cardiology [5,6]. Full-volume acquisitions now can be undertaken in the youngest of infants with excellent image quality. With increasing experience, on-line, live, or simultaneous 3D imaging can be performed, with scanning of the cardiac structures in a true four-dimensional perspective. Moreover, software programs allow for rapid analysis of both global and regional ventricular function. Dedicated software systems provide for summation of disc methodology, which can be applied to measure right and single ventricular size and function. Newer developments in semiautomated border detection have decreased the time for volume measurement determinations, and now allow for complex analysis of regional left and right ventricular function. As familiarity with 3D echocardiography has been gained, a compendium of experienced-based knowledge has been developed to allow recognition and hence rendering of complex congenital heart defects in a 3D imaging domain. Certainly, on-line rendering has aided this process, providing instantaneous image feedback and improved cropping of the desired 3D planes and perspectives of complex congenital heart defects.

A very significant important recent advancement in the application of 3D echocardiography to congenital heart disease has been the development of small dedicated matrix array transducers (Fig. 1). This transducer has a much higher transmit frequency, resulting in increased resolution. Moreover, the frame rate has improved, as well as focusing and imaging in the near field. The much smaller transducer allows for probe placement in either the suprasternal notch or between the rib space for precordial imaging. This article illustrates the clinical application of 3D echocardiography in congenital heart disease.

Atrial septal defects

As has been published in the medical literature, 3D echocardiography can visualize secundum atrial septal defects as they exist in anatomic reality [7]. Rather than assuming the size and shape of the atrial septal defect by visualizing the edges of the defect in multiple 2D imaging cut planes, 3D echocardiography provides a visualization of the entire circumference of the defect (Fig. 2). In particular, secundum atrial septal defects can be rendered from a right or left atrial en face view. An important observation, based on three-dimensional echocardiographic imaging, was that secundum atrial septal defect changes size and shape during the cardiac cycle. Accurate delineation of atrial septal defect size is important in selecting appropriate sized devices for cardiac catheterization device closure. Thus, because of the irregular shape of such defects, and change in size during the cardiac cycle, 3D display of secundum defects would be essential for accurate size measurement. A myriad of 3D echocardiographic rendered planes can detail the anatomic relationship of the defect to other cardiac

* Corresponding author.
E-mail address: gerald.marx@tch.harvard.edu (G.R. Marx).

0733-8651/07/$ - see front matter
doi:10.1016/j.ccl.2007.06.007

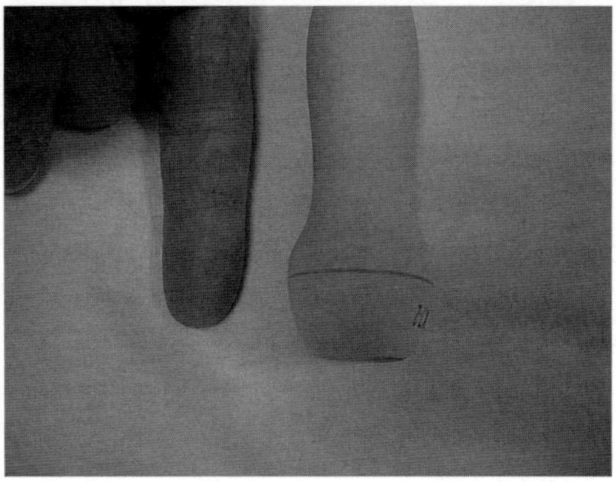

Fig. 1. Example of a small matrix array transducer with imaging frequency of 4 to 6 MHz.

structures, including the superior and inferior vena cava, pulmonary veins, atrioventricular valves, and ascending aorta. Perhaps the most important anatomic relationship to comprehend is the atrial septal defect device to the aortic wall. Although rare, reports have documented aortic wall rupture years after device placement. The amount of retro-aortic rim can be analyzed readily from a succession of serial cut planes from superior to inferior parallel planes. 2D images portray the image in a singular cut plane, which may provide a poor representation of the true extent of the atrial septal defect that is deficient in the retro-aortic region. Not only can 3D echocardiographic imaging be helpful in the preselection of patients for device closure, but it also can analyze the positioning of the device once it has been placed (Fig. 3). Multiple fenestrations in the septum primum of secundum atrial septal defects can be problematic for device closure. Determination of multiple fenestrations may be very difficult to determine either by 2D echocardiographic imaging or angiography. The recent improvements in three-dimensional echocardiographic imaging provide for higher resolution imaging, while reducing imaging artifacts. 3D imaging can provide for very good imaging of the multiple fenestrated secundum atrial septal defect (Fig. 4).

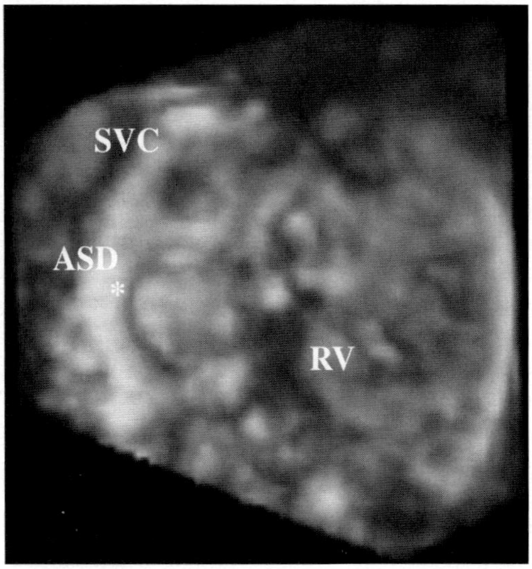

Fig. 2. E -face right atrial view of a secundum atrial septal defect (*). *Abbreviations:* ASD, atrial septal defect; SVC, superior vena cava; RV, right ventricle.

Ventricular septal defects

Irrefutably, for more than 25 years, 2D echocardiography has provided for excellent delineation and diagnostic information as to the relative size, position, and hemodynamics of ventricular septal defects. 3D echocardiography, however, can provide important additional imaging information concerning certain difficult-to-manage muscular ventricular defects [8–10] or a-v septal defects [11,12]. With recent development of catheterization device closure of membranous ventricular septal defects, the extent of rim tissue separating a membranous ventricular septal defect from the aorta can be depicted readily from left ventricular en face views (Fig. 5). Additionally,

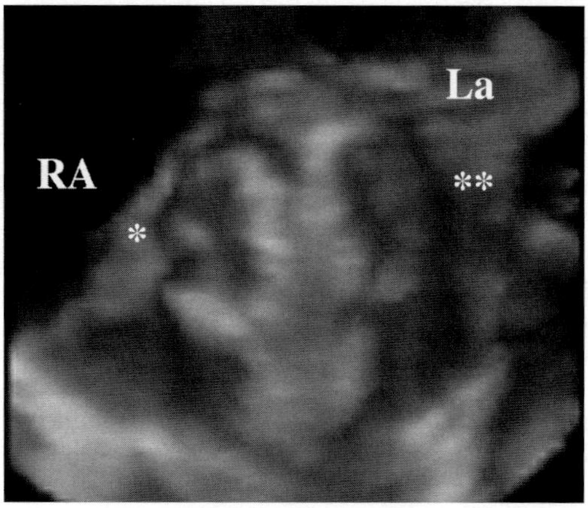

Fig. 3. A 3D echocardiographic image demonstrating the relationship of the right (*) and left (*) atrial discs of an Amplatzer device (AGA Medical, Plymouth, MN) used to close a secundum atrial septal defect. *Abbreviations:* RA, right atrium; LA, left atrium).

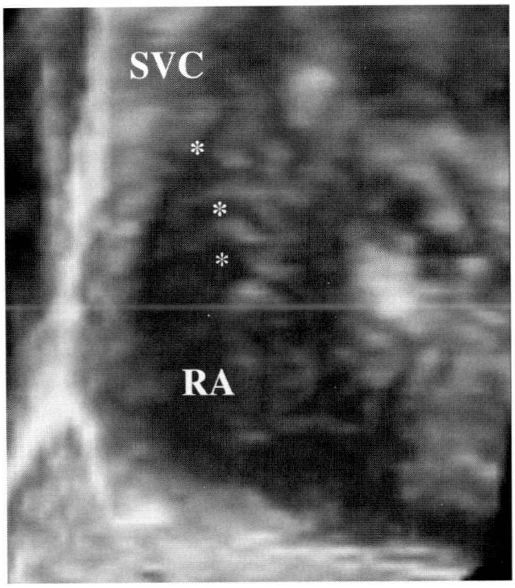

Fig. 4. With improved resolution, multiple fenestrations (*multiple asterisks*) in a secundum atrial septal defect can be seen from this 3D echocardiographic en face view. *Abbreviation:* SVC, superior vena cava.

3D imaging can see the volumetric relationship of the wind socket of tissue covering a membranous defect to the aortic valve. Again, this knowledge would be of paramount importance in considering a patient for device closure.

Certain muscular defects can be very difficult for the surgeon to visualize when operating by means of the right atrium. Such ventricular septal defects include apical and anterior muscular defects. Moreover, important regions of the right ventricular septal surface can be very difficult to see because of large hypertrophied right ventricular muscle bundles, or tricuspid valvar attachments to the septal surface. Previously, the surgeon would perform a left ventriculotomy to gain inspection of the corresponding left ventricular septal surface. This would be advantageous, because there are no trabeculations on the left ventricle, and normally the mitral valve does not have attachments to the left ventricular septal surface. A surgical left ventriculostomy, however, can result in regional wall dysfunction, or create ultimate scar tissue that can become a nidus for future severe dysrhythmias. 3D echocardiography serves as an electronic knife, allowing left ventricular en face views to delineate the size and position of muscular defects. Once the defect (s) can be determined, multiple imaging planes and rotation of the ventricular septum can be undertaken. 3D color-flow imaging can improve the depiction of the number, size, and position of multiple septal defects in relation to the septum and to each other. Several imaging formats of the anatomic gray scale have been developed. One such format shows the heart structures in a transparent format, which heightens color-flow jets and shows the relation to the heart by overlaying the color-flow jets over the transparent shadow of the heart (Fig. 6).

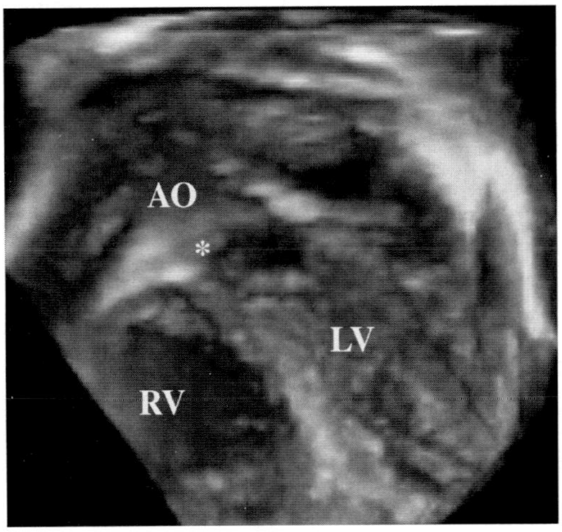

Fig. 5. Left ventricular en face view demonstrating the relationship of a membranous ventricular septal defect (*) to the aortic valve. *Abbreviation:* Ao, aorta.

Complex cono–truncal malformations

The anatomic relationship of the ventricular septal defect is of paramount importance to the surgical undertaking of complex congenital heart defects. The extent and relationship of the ventricular septal defect to the great arteries are of crucial importance for the surgical planning of double outlet right ventricle, or transposition of the great arteries. The prospective pathway from the left ventricular connection to the aorta must be constructed to ensure closure of the ventricular communication, avoidance of subsequent development of subaortic or subpulmonic outlet obstruction, or damage to the atrioventricular valves. Such a pathway may be difficult to conceptualize or even visualize in the flaccid heart at the time of cardio–pulmonary bypass. 3D echocardiographic imaging can provide a more exacting representation of the ventricular septal defect to these anatomic structures (Fig. 7).

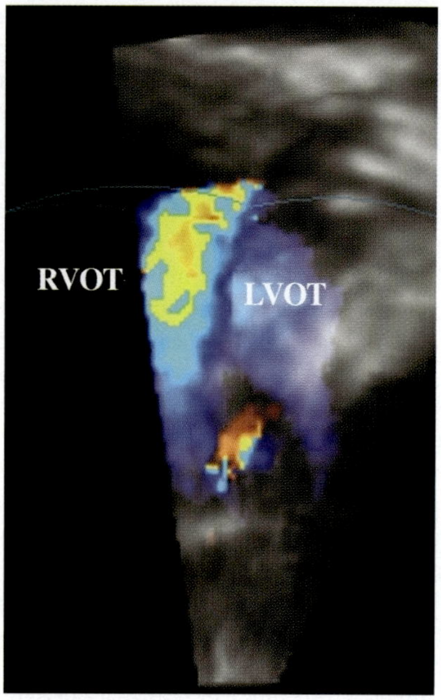

Fig. 6. The heart is displayed in a transparent gray scale format allowing improved imaging of the overlying color flow jets of an anterior muscular ventricular septal defect (*orange jet*) in relationship to the left and right ventricular outflow tracts. *Abbreviations:* LVOT, left ventricular outflow tract; RVOT, right ventricular outflow tract.

Presently, the surgeon and echocardiographers will analyze and render 3D images before surgery to outline the surgical undertaking. At the authors' center, the surgeons have become very knowledgeable of 3D echocardiography and can render the images independently.

Atrioventricular and semilunar valves

Another very important application of three-dimensional echocardiography has been to the understanding of both semilunar [13] and atrial–ventricular valve pathology [14,15]. 2D imaging can depict only the edges of the leaflets in a singular plane. 3D echocardiography demonstrates the surface area of the leaflets, and hence zones of coaptation (Fig. 8). Equally important for atrioventricular valves, 3D echocardiography details the dynamic and coordinated movements of the leaflets and tensor apparatus. Although on cardio–pulmonary bypass, the surgeons can obtain a 3D perspective of the valve leaflets; they cannot obtain an image of the dynamic coaptation of the leaflet structures.

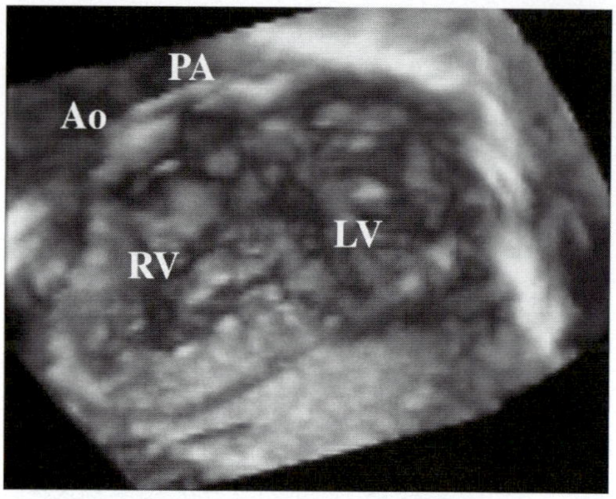

Fig. 7. Double outlet right ventricle demonstrating the relationship of the aorta and pulmonary artery arising from the right ventricle. *Abbreviation:* PA, pulmonary artery.

3D imaging provides direct en face views of the aortic valve from above the surgeon's view, but also from below the aortic valve. With 3D imaging, direct assessment of the most narrowed effective orifice area can be accomplished through multiple parallel cut planes [16]. This can be most important in that, to date, application of the continuity equation to determine the effective orifice area can be very difficult to obtain in young pediatric patients. With 3D echocardiographic imaging, the information is contained within a digital data set. As such, the exact plane from which the cross-sectional views are obtained can be referenced to the corresponding long axis plane. Additionally, because the entire valve surface region can be seen, the extent and locations of valvar deficiency can be seen best. Such examples include 3D echocardiographic visualization of leaflet holes or perforations, or retracted leaflets with

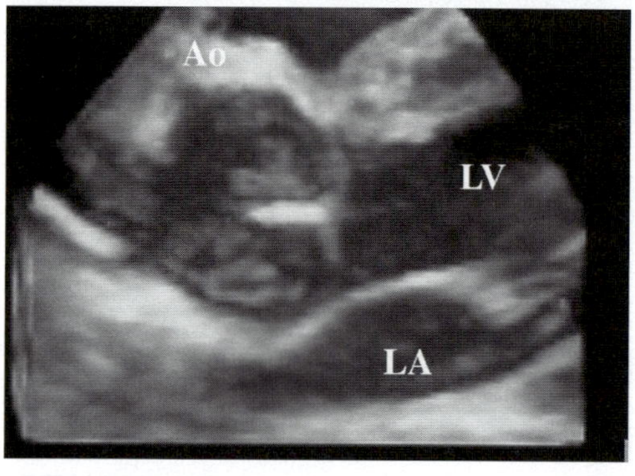

Fig. 8. Long axis view of the aortic valve. In a 3D perspective, the depth of the sinus of Valsalva can be appreciated fully.

diminished surface area, or torn leaflets (Fig. 9). Using superimposed 3D color-flow imaging, the very precise deficient regions can be confirmed. The application of 3D echocardiography is being applied on an everyday clinical practice at the authors' institution for surgical planning for aortic valve repair rather than replacement.

Another aspect of congenital heart disease that has been difficult to precisely diagnose and manage successfully has been left atrioventricular valve abnormalities in a-v septal defects. The incidence for reoperation for left atrioventricular valve stenosis or regurgitation ranges from 15% to 40%. This problem seems related in part to suboptimal imaging and hence diagnosis of the specific pathological problem. 3D imaging can display the a-v valve morphology in improved ways, not available with 2D imaging. The depth and areas of the valve components, and effective dynamic cooptation can be appreciated readily from atrial/and or ventricular en face views. The relative alignment of the common atrioventricular valve to the corresponding left and right ventricle can be discerned with improved clarity. Most importantly, 3D echocardiography can demarcate the full extent of the cleft in the anterior leaflet of the left atrioventricular valve either in patients who have atrioventricular septal defects (Fig. 10), or in the rare case of an isolated cleft. The entire extent or length of the cleft can be seen, and the effective coaptation of the three components of the left a-v valve (ie, the superior anterior, and inferior anterior components of the anterior leaflet) and the mural leaflet. Similar to analysis of aortic valve pathology, 3D echocardiographic color-flow mapping can confirm the anatomic region of ineffective coaptation with the specific 3D color-flow map (Fig. 11).

The pathology of Ebstein's malformation of the tricuspid valve can be extremely difficult to comprehend by 2D imaging. Although the atrialized portion of the right ventricle with septal displacement of the tricuspid valve can be established by 2D imaging, the specific aspects concerning the mechanism of valvar regurgitation can be very difficult to determine. 3D imaging again can display the regions of ineffective leaflet coaptation from direct en face views (Fig. 12) [17]. Fibrous strands, restricting systolic motion and the corresponding regions of lack of coaptation, can be seen. Again, 3D echocardiographic imaging can be used to determine the leaflet surface areas. In particular, the apical view can be used to acquire the tricuspid valve in Ebstein's malformation in almost all patients. Specific serial cut planes can be analyzed in sequence from the apex to base of the right ventricle to best analyze the leaflet abnormalities. In the most severe Ebstein's malformation in newborns and infants, the valve may be displaced into the right ventricular outflow tract and oriented toward the pulmonic valve. A typical 2D apical view will not allow delineation of the valve leaflets. A sub-costal view, however, can delineate the entire atrialized portion of the right ventricle, and the tricuspid valve leaflets. Likewise, the regurgitant jet will not be visualized in a typical 2D echocardiographic apical view, because it will be oriented posterior and inferior toward the diaphragmatic surface. This tricuspid

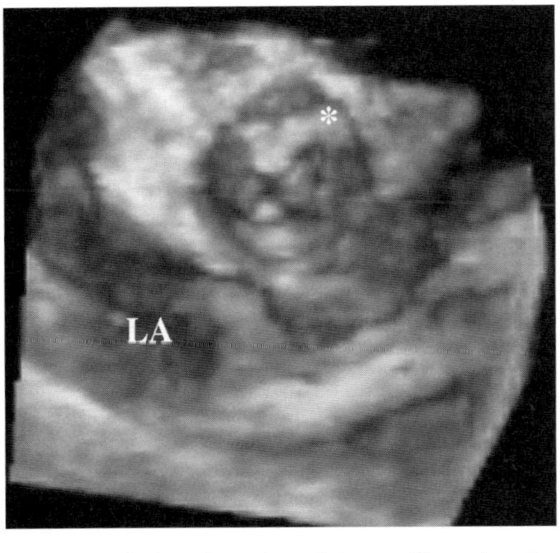

Fig. 9. Surgical en face view of a torn (*) aortic valve leaflet after a balloon dilation valvuloplasty.

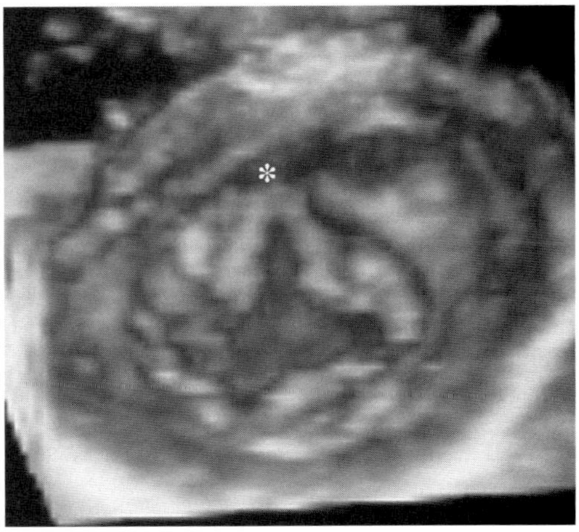

Fig. 10. 3D echocardiographic en face view of the mitral valve from the left ventricular apex to base to demonstrate a cleft (*) in the anterior leaflet.

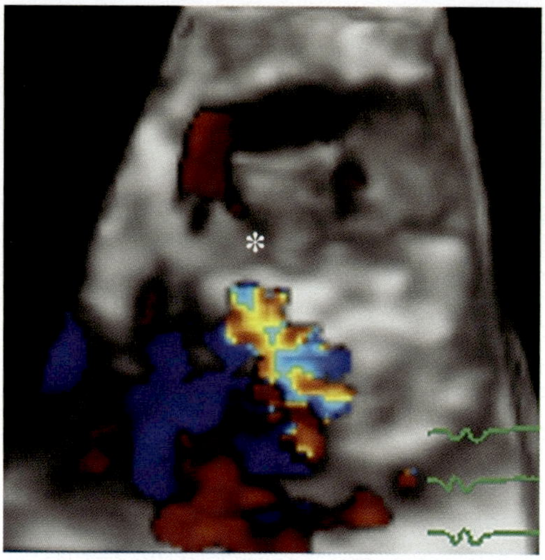

Fig. 11. 3D color flow mapping that confirms origination of the jet (*) through a cleft in the anterior mitral valve leaflet.

regurgitant jet can be appreciated best in a 3D format, especially when acquired from a subcostal plane.

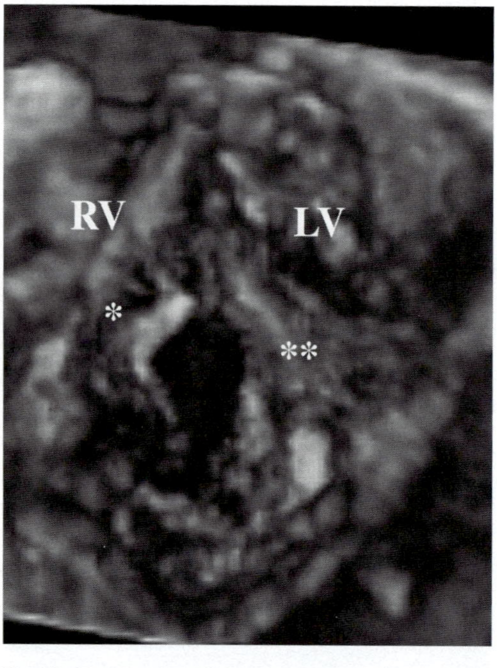

Fig. 12. En face view of the tricuspid valve in an adolescent with severe Ebstein's malformation of the tricuspid valve. Note the large region of noncoaptation of the large anterior (*) and tethered (**) septal leaflet of the tricuspid valve as best seen in this 3D display.

Subaortic stenosis

Subaortic stenosis continues to be a vexing problem, with a high incidence of reoperation. This, in part, is related to the myriad of complex anatomic subtypes. Additionally, complete delineation and understanding of the anatomy have been incomplete with standard 2D imaging. 3D echocardiography can provide an enhanced understanding of this difficult problem. Even for a more routine subaortic membrane, 3D echocardiography allows for visualization of the circumferential narrowing (Fig. 13), whereas 2D imaging depicts only the edges of obstruction. 3D imaging provides a more comprehensive understanding when the mitral valve and/or tensor apparatus is intricately involved in the subaortic obstruction. Often the surgeon will need to know the parts of the mitral valve that can be excised or removed from the subaortic region, without culminating in mitral regurgitation. In the authors' experience, 3D echocardiography has been invaluable to aid in surgical planning for complex left ventricular outflow obstruction.

Three-dimensional imaging of valvar regurgitation

To date, an important application of color flow 2D echocardiography has been the evaluation of the magnitude of valvar regurgitation. To date, the most reliable aspect has been the estimate of the size of the regurgitant vena contracta, which seems to apply best to regurgitant volume. 2D measurements of the vena contracta have relied on diameter measurements, assuming that the regurgitation orifice is circular. Experience with three-dimensional color-flow mapping has shown that the vena contracta can have a myriad of shapes that do not approach that of either a circle or ellipse. Hence, even measurement of the diameter in two orthogonal planes may be inadequate. From the color-flow volumetric digital data set, from the long axis view of the regurgitant jet, a corresponding cut plane can be placed orthogonal at the most narrowed region of the regurgitant. The cut planes then can be visualized in the sequential planes to best depict the true circumference of the vena contracta (Fig. 14).

Right and single ventricular function

Assessment of right ventricular size and function is essential for managing pediatric patients who have congenital heart disease. To date, this

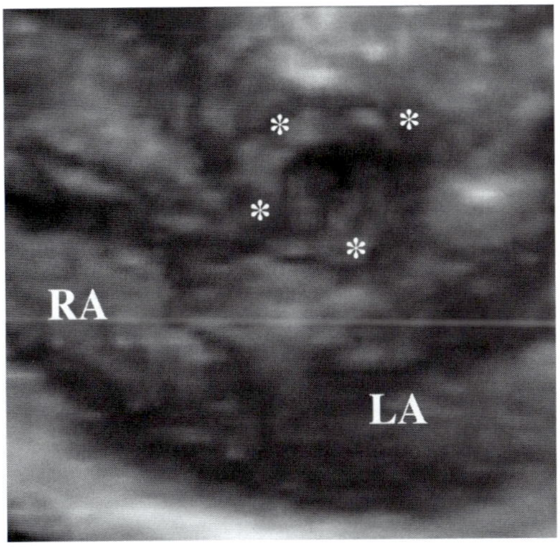

Fig. 13. 3D echocardiogram oriented from the apex of the left ventricle to the aortic outflow tract. The circumferential narrowing from a subaortic membrane (*multiple asterisks*) can be seen in a 3D echocardiographic display.

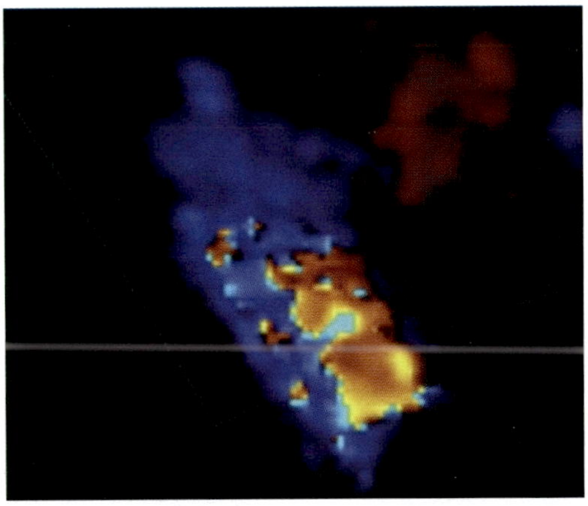

Fig. 14. 3D display of the vena contracta (*orange color*) of severe tricuspid regurgitation. Note that the shape is quite irregular.

has been accomplished by MRI, especially in the adolescent or adult who has postoperative congenital heart surgery. MRI, however, is contraindicated in patients with pacemakers, often occurring in single ventricle patients. Moreover, certain adolescents or adults may suffer from claustrophobia. Young pediatric patients need to anesthetized and ventilated for the best MRI. This can be very difficult for the significantly hemodynamically compromised patient. Moreover, endotracheal intubation and general anesthesia and cannot be applied readily to the serial evaluation of such patients. An important example, to illustrate the importance of single ventricular evaluation, would be in the patients undergoing staged operations for single ventricle with complex systemic outflow tract obstruction. 3D echocardiography would be ideal in the serial evaluation of ventricular function in such patients [18–20].

In the authors' laboratory, the subcostal plane has been used for the three-dimensional echocardiographic analysis of either the single or right ventricular function in young pediatric patients. Analysis of left ventricular size and function has been obtained best from either the subcostal or apical planes. In the authors' experience, the subcostal plane has been the most reliable to acquire the full volume of either the right, left, or single ventricle, especially when dilated or distorted (Fig. 15). Summation of disc methodology allows for analysis of volume, mass, and ejection fraction, again regardless of ventricular size and shape. This methodology, using a matrix array probe for the acquisition and summation of disc for volume determination, has compared well to measurements made by MRI in young pediatric patients in the authors' laboratory. To date, the authors' center has performed two separate studies comparing volumes by three-dimensional echocardiography with those obtained by MRI. The first study was done in infants with single ventricles with a mean age of 7 months. The second study was done to analyze right ventricular volumes in patients with a corresponding normal left ventricle. In the latter study, the mean age was 36 months. In both studies, the echocardiographic and MRI studies were done nearly simultaneously, under similar anesthetic and hemodynamic conditions. Because in both studies the patients were young, they were intubated and anesthetized for the MRI study. For the 3D echocardiographic acquisition, ventilation was suspended during the four-beat acquisition. In the studies comparing 3D echocardiographic right ventricular and single ventricular volumes with MRI, there was good correlation and agreement for end diastolic and end systolic volumes; however, 3D echocardiographic diastolic ventricular volumes were smaller by 7% and 10% respectively. Although these studies were not done under usual clinical conditions, they set the framework for the application of three-dimensional echocardiographic analysis of ventricular size and function in the pediatric age group. In even the youngest of

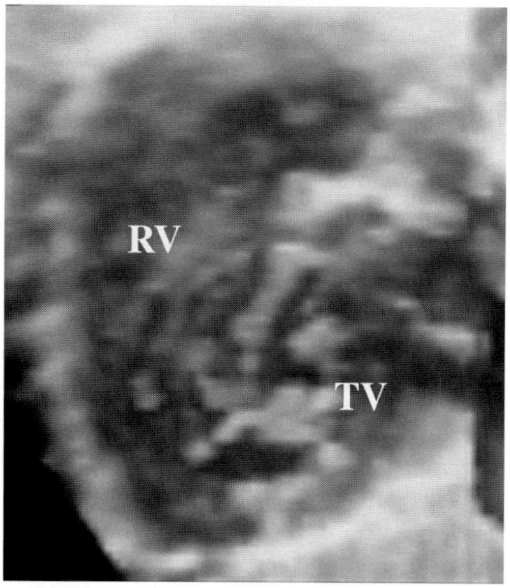

Fig. 15. 3D display of the entire right ventricle in a young pediatric patient with hypoplastic left ventricle. *Abbreviation:* TV, tricuspid valve.

infants, adequate full-volume acquisitions can be obtained with either no or light sedation. These acquisitions have minimal temporal or spatial artifact and can be used for volume determinations.

Matrix array 3D echocardiographic acquisitions and semiautomated border detection allow for rapid analysis of left ventricular volumes in pediatric and adult patients. This technology allows for evaluation of both global and regional ventricular function. Further, it can be used for left ventricular dyssynchrony analysis. Newer software programs also allow for semiautomated border detection of the right ventricle. The right ventricle can be subdivided into inflow, body and outflow sections, thus allowing for detection of regional function.

Summary

Quantum leaps in technological advances have resulted in quantum leaps in the application of 3D echocardiography in congenital heart disease. was Although previously considered to be only in the realm of isolated research, three-dimensional echocardiography is now in the realm of everyday clinical application. With greater learning, continued technological advances, application, and universal acceptance, three-dimensional imaging will become the mainstay of echocardiographic imaging for congenital heart disease.

References

[1] Kisslo J, Firek B, Ota T, et al. Real-time volumetric echocardiography: the technology and the possibilities. Echocardiography 2000;17:773–9.

[2] Sugeng L, Weinert L, Thiele K, et al. Real-time three-dimensional echocardiography using a novel matrix array transducer. Echocardiography 2003; 20:623–35.

[3] Lang RM, Mor-Avi V, Sugeng L, et al. Three-dimensional echocardiography: the benefits of the additional dimension. J Am Coll Cardiol 2006;48: 2053–69.

[4] Marx GR, Sherwood MC. Three-dimensional echocardiography in congenital heart disease. A continuum of unfulfilled promises? No! A current technology with clinical applications and an important future. Yes!. Pediatr Cardiol 2002;23(3):266–85.

[5] Mizelle KM, Rice MJ, Sahn DJ. Clinical use of real-time three-dimensional echocardiography in pediatric cardiology. Echocardiography 2000;17:787–90.

[6] Seliem MA, Fedec A, Cohen MS, et al. Real-time 3-dimensional echocardiographic imaging of congenital heart disease using matrix-array technology: freehand real-time scanning adds instant morphologic details not well-delineated by conventional 2-dimensional imaging. J Am Soc Echocardiogr 2006;19:121–9.

[7] Cheng TO, Xie MX, Wang XF, et al. Real-time 3-dimensional echocardiography in assessing atrial and ventricular septal defects: an echocardiographic–surgical correlative study. Am Heart J 2004;148: 1091–5.

[8] Mercer-Rosa L, Seliem MA, Fedec A, et al. Illustration of the additional value of real-time 3-dimensional echocardiography to conventional transthoracic and transesophageal 2-dimensional echocardiography in imaging muscular ventricular septal defects: does this have any impact on individual patient treatment? J Am Soc Echocardiogr 2006; 19:1511–9.

[9] Chen FL, Hsiung MC, Nanda N, et al. Real-time three-dimensional echocardiography in assessing ventricular septal defects: an echocardiographic–surgical correlative study. Echocardiography 2006; 23:562–8.

[10] Acar P, Abadir S, Aggoun Y. Transcatheter closure of perimembranous ventricular septal defects with Amplatzer occluder assessed by real-time three-dimensional echocardiography. Eur J Echocardiogr 2007;8:110–5.

[11] Singh A, Romp RL, Nanda NC, et al. Usefulness of live/real-time three-dimensional transthoracic echocardiography in the assessment of atrioventricular septal defects. Echocardiography 2006;23:598–608.

[12] Hlavacek AM, Crawford FA Jr, Chessa KS, et al. Real-time three-dimensional echocardiography is useful in the evaluation of patients with atrioventricular septal defects. Echocardiography 2006;23: 225–31.

[13] Sadagopan SN, Veldtman GR, Sivaprakasam MC, et al. Correlations with operative anatomy of real- time three-dimensional echocardiographic imaging of congenital aortic valvar stenosis. Cardiol Young 2006;16:490–4.

[14] Rawlins DB, Austin C, Simpson JM. Live three-dimensional paediatric intraoperative epicardial echocardiography as a guide to surgical repair of atrioventricular valves. Cardiol Young 2006;16: 34–9.

[15] van den Bosch AE, van Dijk VF, McGhie JS, et al. Real-time transthoracic three-dimensional echocardiography provides additional information of left-sided AV valve morphology after AVSD repair. Int J Cardiol 2006;106:360–4.

[16] Xie MX, Wang XF, Cheng TO, et al. Comparison of accuracy of mitral valve area in mitral stenosis by real-time, three-dimensional echocardiography versus two-dimensional echocardiography versus Doppler pressure half-time. Am J Cardiol 2005;95: 1496–9.

[17] Acar P, Abadir S, Roux D, et al. Ebstein's anomaly assessed by real-time 3-D echocardiography. Ann Thorac Surg 2006;82:731–3.

[18] Sugeng L, Mor-Avi V, Weinert L, et al. Quantitative assessment of left ventricular size and function: side-by-side comparison of real-time three-dimensional echocardiography and computed tomography with magnetic resonance reference. Circulation 2006; 114:654–61.

[19] van den Bosch AE, Robbers-Visser D, Krenning BJ, et al. Real-time transthoracic three-dimensional echocardiographic assessment of left ventricular volume and ejection fraction in congenital heart disease. J Am Soc Echocardiogr 2006;19:1–6.

[20] Chen G, Sun K, Huang G. In vitro validation of right ventricular volume and mass measurement by real-time three-dimensional echocardiography. Echocardiography 2006;23:395–9.

ELSEVIER
SAUNDERS

Cardiol Clin 25 (2007) 367–370

CARDIOLOGY
CLINICS

Index

Note: Page numbers of article titles are in **boldface** type.

A

B

C

D

E

F

H

I

doi:10.1016/S0733-8651(07)00070-7

J

L

M

P

R

V